# Engineering Applications of Ultrasonic Time-of-Flight Diffraction

*Second Edition*

**ULTRASONIC INSPECTION IN ENGINEERING SERIES**

*Series Editor:* **Doctor M. J. Whittle**

2. Engineering Applications of Ultrasonic Time-of-Flight Diffraction
 *Second Edition*
 **J. P. Charlesworth** *and* **J. A. G. Temple**

# Engineering Applications of Ultrasonic Time-of-Flight Diffraction

*Second Edition*

**J. P. Charlesworth**
*formerly with AEA Technology plc*
*and*
**J. A. G. Temple**
*AEA Technology plc*

**RESEARCH STUDIES PRESS LTD.**
Baldock, Hertfordshire, England

**RESEARCH STUDIES PRESS LTD.**
**16 Coach House Cloisters, 10 Hitchin Street, Baldock, Hertfordshire, England, SG7 6AE**
and
**325 Chestnut Street, Philadelphia, PA 19106, USA**



## Marketing:

Research Studies Press Ltd.
16 Coach House Cloisters, 10 Hitchin Street, Baldock, Hertfordshire, England, SG7 6AE

## Distribution:

*NORTH AMERICA*
Taylor & Francis Inc.
International Thompson Publishing, Discovery Distribution Center, Receiving Dept.,
2360 Progress Drive Hebron, Ky. 41048

*ASIA-PACIFIC*
Hemisphere Publication Services
Golden Wheel Building # 04-03, 41 Kallang Pudding Road, Singapore 349316

*UK & EUROPE*
ATP Ltd.
27/29 Knowl Piece, Wilbury Way, Hitchin, Hertfordshire, England, SG4 0SX

**Library of Congress Cataloguing-in-Publication Data**

Charlesworth, J. P., 1936-
Engineering applications of ultrasonic time-of-flight diffraction / J.P. Charlesworth and J.A.G. Temple.--2nd ed.
p. cm. -- (Ultrasonic inspection in engineering series ; 2)
Includes bibliographical references and index.
ISBN 0-86380-239-7
1. Ultrasonic testing. I. Temple, J. A. G. II. Title. III. Series.

TA417.4.C47 2001
620.1'1274--dc21) 2001019084

**British Library Cataloguing in Publication Data**
A catalogue record for this book is available from the British Library.

ISBN 0 86380 239 7

Printed in Great Britain by SRP Ltd., Exeter

# Editorial Preface to the Second Edition

Over a decade has elapsed since I wrote the preface to the first edition of this book. Over that period the Time-of-Flight Diffraction (TOFD) Method of ultrasonic inspection has continued to find wider and wider applications as its benefits have been recognised. These include the ability to scan a component, detect and recognise defects extremely quickly compared to more conventional methods. Accurate measurement of defect size is another strength. Of course, correct choice of method is essential for each different set of circumstances and there will be occasions when TOFD is not first choice. However, a very wide range of situations has now been recognised where TOFD is the method of choice. It is, therefore, timely to re-issue this book taking account of the experience which has now been gained in the application of TOFD.

Perhaps the sign that any new innovation has reached maturity is when it becomes the subject of standards which define how it should be applied. This process has started for TOFD with the issue of a British Standard and the launch of a draft European Standard as described in Chapter 10 of the book. The difficulties in gaining acceptance of the latter indicate that this process has still some way to go. Another related area is that of schemes which verify and certificate the competence of those who apply the method and, here again, there is considerable scope for further innovation.

Fortunately, the difficulty of issuing standards no longer provides an insuperable obstacle to the use of new methods such as TOFD. This is due to the widespread adoption of qualification of entire inspections as an alternative way to demonstrate that an inspection is capable of meeting the requirements placed on it. This process, also referred to as performance demonstration, means that inspections do not have to be specified in detail by those requiring it (though they must still be defined in inspection procedures by those implementing the chosen inspection to ensure they are applied in a uniform way). Instead, their performance is assessed by an independent body through the use of theoretical arguments and practical application to test pieces. Inspections are acceptable so long as they meet the stipulated requirements for defect detection, location and size measurement. TOFD has been subjected to qualification of this type on a number of occasions now and has proved equal to the challenge.

This second edition of 'Engineering Applications of Ultrasonic Time-of-Flight Diffraction' therefore provides a welcome update of the subject and again sets out the principles of the method together with a range of recent applications. It continues to be an essential reference for those with a responsibility for the well-being of engineering plant and for those who wish to apply the method.

M. J. Whittle
July 2001

# Editorial Preface to the First Edition

Ultrasonic inspection is now established as a routine method for detecting defects in engineering structures. Unlike most non-destructive test methods, it can detect defects when they are embedded within the material as well as at the surface. Furthermore, it does not require the safety restrictions which attend the use of radiography, which is the alternative method for finding buried defects. Most significantly and uniquely, it can detect cracks and other planar flaws, the defects of most structural concern, and then provide the size information required to assess their significance through the use of fracture mechanics. For these reasons the use of ultrasonics has grown to the point where it is the preferred method of inspection for a wide range of plant and particularly that whose reliability is of special significance.

A consequence of the growing industrial significance of ultrasonics has been the large body of research and development devoted to it. Work has been carried out to establish the performance of ultrasonics, determine the factors which influence performance and so improve reliability. Other activities have sought to mechanise the inspection and improve reliability by increasing automation to avoid the 'human factor'. A further incentive here has been the desire to apply the method to inaccessible or hostile situations such as the internals of nuclear reactors or the submerged parts of offshore oil platforms. All these aspects will be covered by books in the present series. The pace of development has been so intense that there has been little opportunity to take stock and present an account of the state of the art. The essential information is presented in a range of research papers and conference reports. It is now timely to pull this knowledge and experience together and present it in an easily accessible form. That is the incentive behind the Ultrasonics in Engineering series.

The present book on 'Engineering Applications of Ultrasonic Time-of-Flight Diffraction' is the first of the series. The work it describes is one of the most notable pieces of development and application in recent times. Driven by apparent shortcomings in the conventional approach to ultrasonic inspection, workers at Harwell took an interesting but untried idea of Maurice Silk and turned it into an impressive and reliable alternative method for both detection and size measurement of defects. It has now been applied to a wide range of components in a wide variety of shapes and sizes with considerable success. Fortunately for engineering, conventional ultrasonics, if applied properly using well designed procedures, is now accepted as having sufficient reliability in many applications. However, there are others where the Time-of-Flight method has the edge, not least in its simplicity of application. There are other crucial components where the availability of diverse methods of inspection provides confidence that the necessary reliability of defect rejection can be achieved. This book by Philip Charlesworth and Andrew Temple is a timely and expert drawing together of a wide body of work and experience. All those with an interest in or responsibility for the well-being of engineering plant will find it invaluable.

M. J. Whittle
March 1989

# Acknowledgements

Without the pioneering work of Dr Maurice Silk, there would have been no occasion for either edition of this book. We have been greatly encouraged in writing the second edition by the staff at Research Studies Press who have seen the project through from inception to completion: Mrs Veronica Wallace, Guy Robinson and Giorgio Martinelli. We also thank Professor John Whittle for his careful reading of the manuscript.

We have benefited from discussions with three colleagues: Dr Tony Harker, now at University College, London; Dr Steve Burch of AEA Technology plc; and Brian Hawker, now with British Energy whose enthusiasm and practical understanding of the applications of TOFD has been especially helpful.

Our greatest debt of gratitude must go to our families who have encouraged us to complete the second edition and tolerated the anti-social habits that such a project entails.

We are grateful to Derek Yeomans of AEA Technology plc for permission to use the illustration on the front cover. We repeat our acknowledgements of the first edition to: The Welding Institute (as it formerly was) for permission to quote from Report No 3527/11/81; to The British Institute of Non-Destructive Testing (NDT) for permission to quote from an article by Watkins et al; to Harwell Laboratory and to Dr Silk to quote from AERE-12158; and to The Engineering Materials Advisory Services and Dr Duncumb and Mr Mudge for permission to quote from the proceedings of the 20th Annual British Conference on NDT.

All of the figures are original although several from the first edition were based on figures in Authority reports for which UKAEA holds the copyright. We continue to be grateful to the UKAEA for their original permission to publish these. In addition, we are grateful to Elsevier Science for permission to reprint Figure 3.6.

The TSSD typesetting system we used for the first edition has unfortunately disappeared without trace. However, we have found a more than adequate substitute in LaTeX, using LyX as a more user-friendly front end. The main text is in Times Roman with compatible mathematical symbols provided by the `mathptmx` package. Most of the figures have been scanned from the original prints but some have been redrawn and some new ones added using METAPOST, a variant of Donald Knuth's METAFONT. All the programs have been run on a PC under Gnu/Linux with the final output generated by pdfLaTeX. We are grateful to the many people who have contributed to all of these projects.

# Preface to the Second Edition

Ultrasonic Time-of-Flight Diffraction was invented in the early 1970s and initially developed as a research tool. Its rate of development was dramatically changed by the decision at the beginning of the 1980s to plan for a Pressurised Water Reactor (PWR) in the United Kingdom. Although such reactors were common in other countries, a considerable body of opinion in the UK was sceptical of the safety of PWRs. A thorough safety case was therefore required to present to the public enquiry which was almost inevitable once a site for the power station had been named.

Nuclear reactors of the PWR type have thick steel walls withstanding considerable internal pressure. It is therefore necessary to establish with a very high level of confidence that there are no cracks bigger than the critical size, in the parent metal, or in the welds. At about the time that the decision to build one of these reactors in the UK was taken, results were published which suggested that conventional ultrasonic inspection techniques could not size planar cracks bigger than the critical size as accurately as would be necessary to achieve the confidence level required.

This led the nuclear industry in both the United Kingdom and Europe, to invest heavily in a research and development programmes aimed at improving ultrasonic inspection of thick-section steel. The programme in the UK covered conventional ultrasonic inspection techniques but also devoted considerable effort to ultrasonic Time-of-Flight Diffraction because it had already shown great promise as a tool capable of accurately sizing planar, through-wall cracks — exactly what was required.

The first edition of our book, published in 1989, came at a time when much of the development work had been completed and several test-block trials had also been undertaken. The technique had proved itself and was being adopted as one of the essential tools, alongside enhanced pulse-echo inspection, for nuclear reactor inspection. Our hope then was that the technique would spread into other industrial sectors. In the intervening years, this has taken place and the technique is now a mature one.

As we enter a new millennium, it seems the right time to bring our exposition of the technique up-to-date. To do this we have kept much the same form as the previous edition, starting with the theoretical background. One of the strengths of ultrasonic Time-of-Flight Diffraction is that theoretical understanding was developed at an early stage and this has been used consistently to develop the inspection techniques used in real applications. The technique, if used correctly, is capable of yielding very accurate measurements of crack size but, to achieve this, it is necessary to have a good understanding of potential sources of error. We have therefore considerably extended the section on errors and how to minimise them.

Since the technique now has more data to back it up, both from more complex test-block trials and more realistic field applications, we have extended the sections covering both these aspects. As a mature technique it has begun to be specified in codes and standards and we have described the current status in this area.

No other industry has been pressing for such a thorough understanding as the safety case for a PWR required, so only a small amount of additional development work has been done since the first edition of the book. Somewhat surprisingly, some of the signal processing techniques that were covered in the first edition are still not regularly applied, despite computer processing power having increased a thousand-fold since then. There is room for further work in this area to demonstrate what could be achieved with modern technology.

This book aims to provide a thorough background to the theory and practice of the technique and we hope that it will encourage an even wider range of applications and further advances in capability.

J. P. Charlesworth, Dartmouth, Devon
J. A. G. Temple, Upton, Oxfordshire
September 26, 2001

# Preface to the First Edition

Modern engineering has made possible longer bridges, vessels to withstand greater pressures, and components generally which are expected to work under high stresses. Developments in materials technology have contributed to this, and, in particular, many of these items rely on welded metal construction for their strength and integrity. The economics of designing components with huge safety margins, often by vastly increasing the thickness of material used, has given way to designs based on an understanding of the critical defect size and fracture properties of materials, allowing lighter, safer, structures.

Failure is often caused by cracks which enhance the local stress so failure occurs at a load which would be acceptable in the absence of cracks. Fracture mechanics has given us an understanding of the critical cracks which need to be detected and removed if a given component is to survive given applied loads. The sizing of defects is therefore crucial to an economic ideal of minimum lifetime cost, that is the minimum sum of the cost of manufacture, of maintenance and of disposal at the end of life. A crucial part of the approach to this is in-service inspection, in which any cracks likely to pose a threat to the integrity of the component are detected and sized accurately so that their significance can be determined. Accurate sizing is important to avoid the economic penalty of scrapping safe components and to minimize the risk of failure of apparently sound ones, with the consequent threat to safety of individuals or the public at large. Although several non-destructive testing techniques can be used to detect and size cracks, only ultrasound is currently capable of the sizing accuracy required in fracture mechanics assessments of many components, such as those made of thick steel sections. One ultrasonic technique, that of Time-of-Flight Diffraction, has proved to be a very accurate way of measuring the through-wall extent of cracks in such components. Since the through-wall extent of a crack is always one of the parameters determining the severity of the defect, and is often the most important, the ultrasonic Time-of-Flight technique is clearly of interest to anyone concerned with structural integrity or fitness-for-purpose of components.

This book considers the need for accurate size measurement and the underlying basis of the Time-of-Flight Diffraction method in sufficient technical detail to enable it to be implemented by people otherwise unfamiliar with it. Mathematical detail has been largely restricted to the appendices, so that the body of the text can also be read by non-experts. The capability of the technique is illustrated by discussions of the various experimental tests which have been undertaken internationally. Examples of its current use in the field and potential for further exploitation are given. There is also an extensive bibliography in which detailed discussion of issues raised can be followed up in greater depth.

J. P. Charlesworth
J. A. G. Temple
Harwell Laboratory, 7th March 1989

# Contents

# List of Tables

# List of Figures

# Chapter 1

# Introduction

Whenever we turn on a domestic appliance, fill the petrol tank of a car, travel by road, rail, sea or air, we rely directly or indirectly on some equipment or structure working reliably under stress. For example: most electricity generation involves high pressure steam boilers heated either by the burning of fossil fuel or by a nuclear reaction; gas is transported from the North Sea to the users by high pressure pipelines; hydrocarbon fuels are produced in refineries containing much high pressure plant; most modern forms of transport rely on the integrity of components subjected to large and rapidly varying stresses.

Components are designed with more than adequate strength to resist the stresses arising in normal service and even to tolerate certain levels of abnormal conditions. When failure occurs, it is often because the component contained a defect, normally of a crack-like nature, sufficiently large to cause a major reduction of strength. Such defects may arise from faulty manufacture or the effects of service in a corrosive environment and may be enlarged by fatigue. To ensure their absence after manufacture or to detect them in service, a variety of non-destructive testing (NDT) techniques may be used. Of these, ultrasonic testing is the most widely applicable, being capable of detecting and sizing cracks in a wide variety of locations and orientations, in many materials used in engineering and even for considerable thickness of material (greater than 300 mm in steel, for example). A particular type of ultrasonic testing technique is the subject of this book.

Ultrasonic testing makes use of high frequency, but very low amplitude, sound waves to detect, characterise and size defects in components. The sources and receivers of these ultrasonic waves are transducers, usually, but not always, made from a piezoelectric material which deforms under the application of a voltage. Applying a voltage generates a mechanical distortion which propagates into and travels through the component as a wave. When such a wave arrives at the receiver, the piezoelectric material converts this into a voltage which depends on the orientation and magnitude of the distortion.

Other methods of creating and detecting ultrasonic waves are possible, such as electromagnetic acoustic transducers (EMATs) which essentially use (electro)magnetostriction as the method of translating a distortion into a voltage and vice versa, or the use of lasers to ablate part of the surface to generate an ultrasonic pulse coupled with an interferometer to read the surface ripples on the component when signals arrive back. While most of what we discuss in this book is independent of the mode of generation or reception of the ultrasonic waves, we usually have in mind ceramic piezoelectric transducers.

The physical method of sending and receiving signals may be unimportant but the characteristics of the signals generated and received can be important. As we shall see later, the pulse length, the angular spread of the ultrasonic beam, the polarisation of the waves in the signal and their phase are all important.

Pulse-echo ultrasonic inspection techniques rely on the amplitude and range of a signal returned from the defect to the interrogating equipment in order for the defect to be detected, sized and, possibly, characterised. The process governing the amplitude is usually specular reflection, in which any crack acts like a mirror for the ultrasound. For a given arrangement of ultrasonic transducers on the component undergoing inspection, this process of specular reflection can only occur for a limited range of orientations of the defect. In the absence of a specular reflection, the signals returned will be those arising from diffuse scattering from the surfaces of the crack and by diffraction from the edges of the crack. These diffracted signals are of particular interest, since, being associated with the extremities of the defect, they may be used to determine the size of the defect accurately and thus assess the integrity of the component. The ultrasonic Time-of-Flight Diffraction technique is based on the exploitation of these signals diffracted from the defect edges.

## 1.1 The need for accurate measurement of defect size

Engineering structures can fail catastrophically by rapid brittle fracture if they contain defects above a certain critical size for the load applied. The theoretical maximum strength of a solid, based on the chemical bond strength of the elements, is never achieved in bulk solids but only in very thin fibres or whiskers [Gordon, 1976]. In practice, the resistance to brittle fracture is determined by critical cracks either on the surface or in the bulk of the material. When a material is strained, energy is stored in the elastic displacement. If the material contains a crack which increases in size, for a given applied load, then the crack will open slightly and the two faces become more separated. The material behind the crack faces is therefore relaxed and the strain energy stored there is released. However, the process creates new crack surface — a process which requires a certain amount of energy. By balancing these two energies, a relationship can be found for the theoretical critical crack size $a_c$ as [Gordon, 1976]:

$$a_c = \frac{2WE}{\pi\sigma^2} \tag{1.1}$$

where $a_c$ is in metres, $W$ is the work of fracture of the solid in $\mathrm{J/m^2}$, $E$ is an elastic modulus dependent on the mode of stressing, and $\sigma$ is the applied stress (in $\mathrm{N/m^2}$).

A typical value of $W$ would be $6\,\mathrm{J/m^2}$ for glass, a brittle material with a very small critical crack size, and a value of $W$ for a ductile material such as steel or aluminium might be in the range $10^4$ to $10^6\,\mathrm{J/m^2}$. The corresponding critical crack sizes, at realistic loads of 100 MPa, but for plates infinitely wide and thick, would be about 27 μm for glass and 1.3 m for steel. For realistic sized structures these critical sizes are further reduced. The critical defect is a crack orientated perpendicular to the principal applied stresses and the critical defect parameter is usually the through-wall extent of these crack-like defects. Accurate measurement of this parameter of defects is therefore of great importance in ensuring the structural integrity of many components.

The ultrasonic Time-of-Flight Diffraction technique described in this monograph is one method of carrying out the measurement of the through-wall extent of defects accurately. In the early use of pulse-echo ultrasonics, defects could be located but there was often little precision in defect sizing. To overcome this limitation the inspection procedures were used principally in a test of *good workmanship* by requiring components, and welded components in particular, to have fewer than a specified number of defects of a given estimated size per unit volume (or weld length). While this is a reasonable way of ensuring the quality of the manufacture, it can lead to unnecessary repair or replacement of components under stress in service. The move, by various industry sectors, such as aerospace and the nuclear industry in particular, towards an approach to non-destructive evaluation based on fitness-for-purpose considerations, prompted considerable development of improved NDT techniques, particularly in the field of ultrasonics. Techniques now available, of which Time-of-Flight Diffraction (TOFD) is one, have great accuracy for measuring the all-important through-wall size of crack-like defects. This accuracy is, in many cases better than $\pm 1$ mm, and can be obtained in the wide range of material thickness from which pressurised components are constructed.

## 1.2 History of Time-of-Flight Diffraction

The development of the Time-of-Flight Diffraction technique grew out of an appreciation of the difficulties of achieving accurate defect sizing with conventional pulse-echo ultrasonic techniques; a brief discussion of such techniques is therefore presented first. This is followed by an elementary description of the basis of the Time-of-Flight Diffraction technique and a brief history of its invention and development. More detailed descriptions of all aspects of the technique appear in later chapters of the book. A review of earlier crack depth measurement by ultrasonics can be found in Doyle and Scala [1978], following early work by Cook [1972]. Details of the development of Time-of-Flight Diffraction can be traced through a series of published papers by Silk [1979a,e, 1982a,b,c, 1984]; Silk and Lidington [1974b, 1975] and Silk, Lidington and Hammond [1980].

### 1.2.1 Conventional ultrasonic testing

Conventional ultrasonic testing uses the pulse-echo technique. A piezoelectric transducer, which often has a rectangular piezoelectric active element, fires a short-duration pulse of ultrasound in a narrow beam into the metal and any echoes coming back are received with the same transducer. The finite-width beam is a result of a finite-sized piezoelectric crystal element. The ultrasonic echoes are normally displayed on a modified oscilloscope, called a flaw detector, which displays the rectified waveform using a time-base which starts at the firing pulse and is calibrated horizontally (from a knowledge of the ultrasonic velocity) in terms of distance within the metal.

The system is calibrated vertically by adjusting the amplifier gain so that the signal from a standard feature in a calibration block appears at a standard height on the screen. The amplitude of other signals can be obtained by adjusting the calibrated gain or attenuation controls to give the same screen height. This establishes a reporting level, signals larger than the level being assessed as flaws and those below it being ignored. The size of flaws is assessed either simply from amplitude relative to signals from a calibration reflector, in terms of (say) flat-bottomed hole or side-drilled hole sizes for very small flaws, or, in the case of larger flaws, either from the amount of probe movement required to cause a standard fall in signal strength, or from observation of features in the echodynamic signal as the probe is scanned. This is a very simplified description of the basis of the method which, in an important safety-related inspection, can involve a great deal of manual skill or sophisticated computer controlled scanning, signal acquisition and processing.

### 1.2.2 The problems with pulse-echo techniques

The problem with pulse-echo techniques is simply put. These techniques are based on the assumption that echoes come from planar features which are suitably angled to give a specular reflection back to the transducer. Clearly it must be quite rare for defects to be exactly normal to the beam as would be required for a perfectly smooth large specular reflector. The failure of various national standard inspection codes to give the necessary confidence in detecting misoriented defects was highlighted by Haines, Langston, Green and Wilson [1982]. Fortunately, in practical cases there is some relaxation of this strict requirement, since diffraction causes reflection energy to be spread over a wider angle and for rough defects surface roughness will also produce an angular spread. Thus there is rather more likelihood of a randomly oriented defect being detected than one might think and a range of beam angles is used to ensure that this happens. However, methods of sizing by probe movement require judgment of when the beam has reached the edge of the defect. The net result is that thorough inspection by the pulse-echo technique requires the use of probes sending beams in at a range of angles depending on the orientation of the defects being sought and requires a very careful examination of echoes down to an amplitude level well below that expected from a favourably oriented defect. The lack of capability of conventional ultrasonic inspections to detect significant defects when the sensitivity is too low and the range of angles is too limited was highlighted by the round-robin

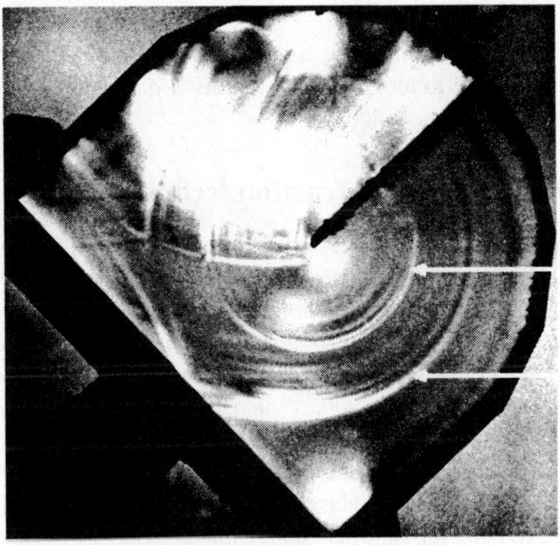


**Fig. 1.1** Stroboscopic visualisation of ultrasonic diffraction at the tip of a slot in a glass block. The ultrasonic transducer is at top centre, with its beam aimed at the tip of the slot.

exercise organised by the Programme for Inspection of Steel Components (PISC I) [PISC, 1979].

### 1.2.3 The diffraction process

The reason that defect sizing can be done at all on defects which are not favourably aligned is that there are other signals in addition to the specular reflection. When an obstacle is placed in the path of a beam of light, some of the light is bent into the shadow zone by diffraction. The effects of diffraction of light only become noticeable, for example, for slits or stops of a few wavelengths across. The same effect can be seen with ripples on water. If waves are propagating across a water surface, say because a stone has been dropped into otherwise calm water, and these ripples encounter an object, they reflect from the side of the object and diffract round the ends of the object. In this case the effects are easy to see because of the longer wavelength of the water ripples compared to that of visible light. The same phenomenon occurs with elastic waves, where the wavelength (in the case of ultrasound) is typically of the order of a few millimetres, the effects are easily observed. The picture of sound travelling in a glass block, Figure 1.1, taken by K. G. Hall at British Rail Engineering, Derby, shows some of the many interactions between an incident compression wave and a defect and shows particularly clearly the diffracted waves which appear to radiate from the edge of the defect. Similar results can be predicted from theoretical modelling work using finite difference solutions to the elastic wave equations

[Harker, 1984].

Experienced pulse-echo practitioners make use of these edge waves to obtain accurate defect sizes, but they have to look for them against a background of larger and probably variable specular reflection signals.

### 1.2.4 The basic Time-of-Flight Diffraction technique

The thought process which led to the Time-of-Flight Diffraction technique may have been something like this: *if pulse-echo inspection, while usually based on a search for specular reflections, is actually relying in some cases on diffracted waves for accurate sizing, would it not be advantageous to design a technique which is aimed directly at those diffracted waves and which deliberately avoids the specular reflections which may mask them? In addition, timing measurements may be made to high accuracy and if this can be used to size defects, the defect size would be measured accurately.* This is the basis of the Time-of-Flight Diffraction (TOFD) technique invented at the National NDT Centre, Harwell, by Dr Maurice Silk. Although Miller [1970] appears to have been the first person to publish evidence of detecting diffracted signals from crack tips, he did not recognise that this was the source of his signals and so missed the opportunity of inventing the TOFD technique. Time-of-Flight Diffraction was developed, mainly by Silk and his co-workers at the Harwell Laboratory, over a period of about 10 years starting in the early 1970s, from a laboratory curiosity into a sophisticated full-scale inspection method capable of detecting and sizing defects in components from 1 mm thick sheets or tubes up to the massive 250 mm thick shell of the pressurised water reactor (PWR) pressure vessel.

In order to optimise the strength of the diffraction signal and to avoid specular reflection signals, the probes are deployed as shown in the upper part of Figure 2.1. A typical signal consists of a first pulse from a wave travelling by the most direct route, called the *lateral wave*, followed by zero or more diffracted wave pulses from defects and finally a specular reflection from the back wall of the component (assumed to be a plate here). The lateral wave and the *back-wall echo* act as natural reference signals, delimiting the time zone within which defect signals can be expected. Note that the upper and lower edges of the defect give signals of fairly similar amplitude but, theoretically, at least, of opposite phase, so that for any individual signal, one should be able to tell from the phase whether it originated from a defect top or a bottom.

The timing of the diffracted signals, relative to the lateral wave and back-wall echo can be used to calculate the depth of the defect edges as shown in the upper part of Figure 2.1. This assumes that the defect is symmetrically placed between the probes, a position which can be found by moving the probes (while maintaining constant separation) along the line joining them until the delay of the diffracted signals becomes a minimum. The depth resolution deteriorates as the inspection surface is approached but, if necessary, depth resolution can be maintained near the surface by moving the probes closer together. This is discussed in Section 2.3.2. Experience and theory agree in predicting an angular zone for accurate and reliable inspection, stretching from about 45° to 80° to the normal to the plate surface, so this, together with the accuracy which must be achieved, determines whether the depth zone of interest can be covered by one probe separation. This is discussed in Section 3.1.1.

Note that, provided adequate sound amplitude reaches the defect and is subsequently received at the receiver probe, the nominal beam angles of the probes do not matter, nor has the amplitude of the signal any relevance provided the signal can be recognised within the background noise. The only significant information is in the signal timing and this is why it has been called the Time-of-Flight Diffraction technique.

Although the technique can be, and has been, used with shear waves, it is normally used with compression waves. Whenever ultrasound strikes a surface or defect at other than normal incidence, some of the energy will be converted to other wave modes; e.g. if the incident wave mode is compression then some shear mode energy will be present in the reflected and diffracted waves. Because the wave velocity of shear waves is only about half that of compression waves, it is necessary to know the mode of the signals to calculate the defect depth. The TOFD technique is normally used with compression wave probes so that the primary diffracted signals are compression waves and arrive well ahead of any signals which have travelled over all or part of the path as shear waves. There is, however, no fundamental reason for avoiding shear waves.

## 1.3 Development of experimental techniques for Time-of-Flight Diffraction

The technique developed in the early 1970s as a laboratory, hand-held tool with one transmitter transducer and one receiver transducer [Silk, Lidington, Montgomery and Hammond, 1976]. This was supplemented with a variety of crawler devices for the inspection of ferritic pipes and other geometries [Silk, 1976]. In the early days of the development of Time-of-Flight Diffraction, it was regarded as a potentially very accurate sizing method for cracks which were either readily visible or had been found by conventional ultrasonic techniques. This placed the emphasis on accurate measurements of the timing of the crack-tip diffraction signals; consequently ultrasonic flaw detectors, which commonly rectify and smooth the signal before displaying it, were considered less suitable as a measurement tool than were conventional oscilloscopes on which the unrectified signal could be displayed and timed to a fraction of a cycle.

There has been discussion from time to time of whether single probe techniques, in which the signal is both transmitted and received by a single transducer can be included under the title Time-of-Flight Diffraction. Provided a single probe technique makes a timing measurement and relies primarily on diffracted wave energy, rather than specular reflection, the authors see no reason why it should not be included. However, we are mainly concerned in this book with techniques using two or more probes, and refer briefly to single probe techniques only when they have some particular feature of interest.

### 1.3.1 The first digital gauge

The technique was initially applied to cracks growing from the inspection surface and for this purpose the total length of the diffracted pulse is not of much significance as long as the time of arrival of the leading edge can be accurately assessed. It was recognised at an early stage that compression waves should be used so that the diffracted compression wave pulses would arrive at the receiver before any mode converted pulse. By this means ambiguities of mode identification were avoided. Commercial angled compression wave probes were not available, so simple narrow band probes were constructed by clamping discs of PZT (lead zirconate titanate) to polystyrene shoes of the appropriate angle. Two such probes were mounted, with their beams pointing towards each other, in a holder which maintained a constant probe separation and orientation while allowing the assembly to be manually or mechanically scanned along the defective sample. Provided that the diffracted signal could be recognised in the oscilloscope trace, very accurate measurements could be made of crack depth.

Because the transit time in the probe shoe is significant, it must be accurately known if the transit time of the diffracted wave within the workpiece is to be measured. In principle, this calibration process is best done by timing a signal along a known path, close to that of the diffracted signal of interest. Hence, blocks containing calibration slots were sometimes used. However it was found that a sufficiently accurate calibration on parallel sided plates could be obtained by timing either the direct subsurface signal, later always referred to as the *lateral wave*, or the reflection from the back surface of the sample, usually called the *back-wall echo*.

This method of operation led to the development of a digital gauge which could be used to measure the time of arrival of the diffracted signal, relative to that of a direct subsurface signal in an uncracked part of the sample. However, it proved difficult to ensure that the gauge always triggered on the correct signal. Later developments, to be described, moved away from this kind of system. Other work on corrections to ultrasonic time-delay measurements of crack depth [Silk and Lidington, 1974a], and crack depth measurement using a single surface wave probe [Lidington and Silk, 1975], consolidated the foundations laid for this technique of accurate sizing for the through-wall dimension of cracks.

### 1.3.2 The B-scan display

The accurate results which had been obtained in the early stages led to inclusion of the Time-of-Flight Diffraction technique in a study organised by the Welding Institute on sizing of internal defects in butt welds. In this case the location of the defects was not known and, although they could have been first located by pulse-echo ultrasound, that was found to be unnecessary. For a given, fixed, position of the transmitter and receiver relative to a defect, the unrectified signal amplitude as a function of time observed at the receiver is called an *A-scan* (see, for example the lower part of Figure 2.1). As the transmitter and receiver moved relative to the defect, the peaks and troughs in the A-scan will come at different times. By capturing A-scans from a number of consecutive probe positions, and displaying them in a stacked formation side by side, a display called a *B-scan* is produced (see Section 5.2 for a description of B- and D-scans and Figure 2.2 for an example of a B-scan).

Initially, a simple B-scan display was implemented by producing a slowed down representation of the signal by means of a boxcar integrator and displaying the output as a quantified grey-level line on a facsimile recorder. As the probe assembly was scanned along the workpiece, the successive traces on the facsimile recorder built up a picture of the pattern of signals, from which identification and measurement of the diffracted signals, relative to a suitable timing reference, could be carried out directly.

Because the signal for the facsimile recorder was produced by sweeping a gate through the ultrasonic signal by means of an analogue sweep generator, there was no fixed relationship between the time scale of the original signal and that on the B-scan. It was necessary therefore to calibrate the B-scan picture and the most convenient method proved to be to use the positions (along the time axis) of the lateral wave and back-wall echo signals visible on the B-scan, together with the probe separation, probe shoe delay, plate thickness and ultrasonic velocity. If all these items of information are known, it is an over-determined system and so can be checked for consistency. If up to two pieces of information are unknown they can be determined from the others. In practice, the probe delay and the velocity were usually treated as unknown and the depth calibration worked out in terms of the other known parameters, without explicit calculation of probe delay and velocity.

This method proved very successful for defect detection because the characteristic pattern and phase coherence of the unrectified signals were easy to recognise even when the signals were little above the noise level. This use of visual assessment of phase coherence to estimate the significance of a signal has been a feature of the Time-of-Flight Diffraction technique since that time but there is no reason why it should not be applied to pulse-echo signals, provided they are displayed before rectification. Problems were, however, encountered with obtaining accurate through thickness sizes for internal defects because, with narrow band probes, the long duration of the signal diffracted from the top edge of a defect would often cause it to overlap the start of the diffracted signal from the bottom edge. To combat this problem, heavily damped probes, producing pulses of about 1.5 cycles, were introduced. This greatly improved the resolution of signals in the time domain and also first drew attention to the fact that signals from the top and bottom edges of a defect are in antiphase. The signals from these probes had lower amplitude, however, than the narrow band ones used earlier and this led to a search for ways of further improving the signal-to-noise ratio, above what could be achieved with the boxcar system.

### 1.3.3 Digital signal processing

At about the time that short pulse probes were introduced, small minicomputers had become inexpensive enough to be used as an NDT research tool and the possibilities of digital signal processing had become apparent. A start was made by using a

Tektronix Digital Processing Oscilloscope to digitise the signals from the boxcar integrator, since the digitisation rate was still too low to be used directly. The data was displayed either as a stack of A-scans, or as a B-scan on a Tektronix storage type graphics terminal. This enabled rapid plotting of B-scan pictures with two intensity levels or, by the use of shading patterns, much slower plotting of four level pictures, each level representing a range of signal voltage. Hard copies of these pictures could be produced directly from the terminal on a Versatec electrostatic printer/plotter and software was subsequently developed to plot B-scans with about ten distinguishable grey levels directly on the Versatec, from the stored data. These techniques were used throughout the later stages of the Welding Institute study (see Section 8.3). The results of that study suggested that the Time-of-Flight Diffraction technique had performed significantly better in through thickness sizing than any other technique.

### 1.3.4 First application to thick-section steel

The technique had been confined to the inspection of small components and seemed, therefore, to be mainly of academic interest up to that time. However, with the decision of the Central Electricity Generating Board (CEGB) to build a pressurised water reactor at Sizewell, coupled with the public concern which had been expressed about the integrity of the pressure vessel, it became urgent to demonstrate that there were NDT techniques available which could ensure that the vessel was free from significant defects. The results of the Welding Institute study encouraged the view that the Time-of-Flight Diffraction technique had reached a stage of development at which it could take part in a large scale comparative trial on samples which realistically simulated critical regions of the pressure vessel. The Defect Detection Trials (DDT) were organised by the United Kingdom Atomic Energy Authority (UKAEA) for this purpose (see Section 8.4).

The DDT samples posed a number of new problems for the technique which had not been addressed before. The samples were about 250 mm thick, being representative of the actual thickness of a pressure vessel, whereas the thickest samples previously studied were only 90 mm thick. The plates were covered on one face by a double layer of austenitic strip cladding which shows marked anisotropy in its ultrasonic properties. One of the plates had small defects extending only a few millimetres into the ferritic base material from the interface between plate and cladding. Finally one of the samples was a full size simulation of the nozzle crotch corner region of the vessel, presenting by its complex geometry, problems both of interpretation of the signals and of accurate location of the defects relative to surfaces of compound curvature.

Because of the scale of the exercise, it was clear that a great increase in sophistication was needed quickly at that time. Fortunately, much better digitisers and displays became available, together with more powerful computers. Scanning had, in the past, been done very simply by mounting the relatively small samples on the bed of a modified milling machine so that they could be moved under the probe assembly. The new test-blocks were too large for this technique so a 2 m square X-Y scanning frame was procured. The frame was driven by stepping motors under computer control. The test plates were set up level in a water tank which was straddled by the frame. In order to shorten the inspection process, rather than carrying out several scans with different probe separations successively, an array of probes was constructed enabling many combinations of transmitter and receiver at different separations and lateral displacements to be used within the same traverse of the plate (see Chapter 4).

To avoid the problems with multiplexing, 8 separate transmitter units drove the 8 transmitter probes and could be independently triggered from the computer. The eight receiver probes were connected to eight 20 MHz CAMAC-compatible digitisers each triggered from a delay generator.

While even more complex systems have been used for the inspection of large components of complex geometry, the application of Time-of-Flight Diffraction to more routine tasks was also eased by the appearance on the commercial market of integrated digital ultrasonic test sets. One such early piece of equipment, called Zipscan, grew directly out of the Harwell work described above and was manufactured under licence by Sonomatic Ltd. It provided all the hardware and software for application of the Time-of-Flight Diffraction technique in a single portable package. Sonomatic still make equipment which is based on the principles described in this book, although modern electronics has allowed a considerable reduction in the overall size of the equipment. A fairly typical modern instrument is described briefly in Section 4.5. Instruments of similar type are now a part of standard ultrasonic inspection equipment and available from various sources.

## 1.4 Outline of the remainder of the book

One of the strengths of the Time-of-Flight Diffraction technique is that many aspects of the underlying theory were used in the development of the technique. This book follows the same course; giving the underlying theoretical background, including a theoretical treatment of measurement errors, before giving details of practical applications. In the next chapter, basic theoretical aspects of Time-of-Flight Diffraction are reviewed together with a discussion of errors in its use for measurement of defects sizes. Understanding sources of error is the basis of successful implementation of the technique. Even if you are impatient to read about practical applications of the technique, Chapter 2 should not be skipped. The chapter ends with a brief discussion of some single probe techniques which complement the more generally accepted use of two or more probes.

In Chapter 3 we consider theoretical prediction of the amplitude of the diffracted signal. This chapter could be skipped at a first reading but is placed here in its logical relationship to the other material. In this chapter we also compare Time-of-Flight Diffraction with other methods. As an example, an early criticism of the Time-of-Flight Diffraction technique was that the signal amplitudes are small compared with those from conventional techniques. While this is true if specular signals are compared with diffracted signals, in many conventional inspections for defects of arbitrary orientation, signals of comparable magnitude to diffracted signals may have to be used. This aspect of Time-of-Flight Diffraction is discussed in Chapter 3 together with a discussion of the angular range over which the diffracted signals can be received and the choice of optimum beam angles. The relative insensitivity of Time-of-Flight Diffraction to the tilt or skew of defects is contrasted with the narrow range of defect orientations that can be successfully detected and sized with techniques based on specular reflection when only one transducer is used.

With these essential underlying theoretical aspects covered, Chapter 4 deals with the design of Time-of-Flight Diffraction equipment for situations where the inspection geometry is of simple flat-plate form. Choice of frequency is governed by a compromise between resolution and signal attenuation. The arrangement of the probes and scanning patterns for various defect orientations, such as defects nearly parallel or nearly perpendicular to the weld direction, are discussed. Near surface defects require a slightly different treatment.

This chapter also describes the characteristics of an instrumentation system suitable for use with the TOFD technique.

Chapter 5 deals with the display and analysis of Time-of-Flight Diffraction signals. Part of the success of the technique is the B-scan display in which the human eye has proved adept at detecting the characteristic arcs arising from defect signals as the probe scans over the inspection surface. Although the technique does not rely on signal amplitude, it is often necessary to increase the signal-to-noise ratio. This can be readily carried out by signal averaging. Fitting of shaped cursors to the characteristic arcs is one way of discriminating between valid defect signals and other unwanted information in the image. The measurement of defect through-wall extent and length together with characterisation of defects are all covered.

While the Time-of-Flight Diffraction technique gives an accurate measurement of defect through-wall size, the measurement of defect length is carried out in a similar way to that used in conventional techniques. Various methods of improving the accuracy of length measurement exist and some of these, particularly synthetic aperture processing, are discussed in Section 5.8.1.

Application of the technique to complex geometries is another complication which we treat in Chapter 6. Inspection of nozzles and associated welds is at least as important an engineering problem as the inspection of flat plates. Experience has been gained on specimens representing nozzles of nuclear reactor pressure circuits and the nodes of offshore structures.

Additional complexities may interfere with either defect detection or interpretation of signals so that defects become more difficult to size correctly. Some of these complexities are discussed in Chapter 7. In particular, we consider the effects of a cladding layer which is isotropic only in one plane, or of a bulk material which may be wholly anisotropic. The effects of compressive stress on cracks and how this affects the signals and the effects of component curvature are all discussed.

The results of the experimental tests of capability of the technique over the last 25 years or so are covered in Chapter 8. Some caveats concerning the validity of test-block trials are noted before we examine the detailed results of several sets of trials, including a collaborative project with the Welding Institute, the Defect Detection Trials organised by the United Kingdom Atomic Energy Authority, and the international PISC I, II and III series of trials. The trials are discussed in historical order since test-block trials themselves evolved through increasing attempts at realism. Such attempts were not always wholly successful since it is actually relatively difficult to make artificial defects closely resemble those that occur naturally. The chapter brings out these difficulties. Some smaller trials involving comparison of TOFD with other NDT techniques are also described. We end the chapter with a brief discussion of the implications of the results of test-block trials for the structural integrity of pressurised components.

In Chapter 9, we look at the wide range of engineering applications of the technique which have been reported in the literature. While little fundamental development of the technique took place through the 1990s, much was done in establishing the technique in various industry sectors. Part of the maturing process for new non-destructive testing techniques is the assimilation of the technique into codes and standards. We present a relatively brief review of this aspect of Time-of-Flight Diffraction in Chapter 10.

An extensive Appendix contains the more mathematical theory relevant to some of the chapters and the book is completed by a bibliography and an index.

# Chapter 2

# Theoretical Basis of Time-of-Flight Diffraction

In this chapter we consider the technique from a theoretical point of view. We do not present detailed theory but we illustrate conclusions drawn from modelling work and discuss the way in which these conclusions affect the design of TOFD inspection. We give the types of waves which can propagate and examples of their wavespeeds. We explain elementary diffraction with emphasis on the radiation of the diffracted energy into a wide range of angles. This gives the technique one of its advantages over conventional methods of defect detection and sizing — its relative insensitivity to defect orientation. We explain how the TOFD technique is used to measure defect sizes and we discuss the accuracy of such measurements in considerable detail. We also describe some important features of the signals observed when a TOFD probe assembly is scanned across the location of a defect. Finally, we very briefly describe ways of using diffracted signals with only a single transducer.

## 2.1 Waves in homogeneous and isotropic media

The term ultrasound is used to describe sound waves with frequencies above the audible range. While sound is commonly understood as a wave motion in gases such as air, the term is also used for elastic waves in solids. The possible wave motions in solids are, however, more complex than those arising in gases. A gas cannot support shear stress and so the particle displacement is always parallel to the direction of propagation of the waves. These waves consist of alternate regions of compression and rarefaction in a periodic pattern. A solid body can support shear stress, so the displacement $\vec{u}$, now a vector, need not be parallel to the direction of propagation of the wave.

At this stage we need only consider isotropic and homogeneous media. Two distinct cases emerge: first the displacement is parallel to the direction of propagation and this wave is called a *compression wave*; second, the displacement is perpendicular to the direction of propagation and the wave is a *shear wave*. In a shear wave, the displacement can be in any direction perpendicular to the direction of propagation but for convenience is usually resolved into two perpendicular directions. These two directions define the polarisation of the shear wave. In an isotropic medium, remote from boundaries, all shear wave polarisations are equivalent but, at boundaries between media, the behaviour of the wave depends on the direction of polarisation. It is usual, therefore, to resolve a shear wave of arbitrary polarisation into components with mutually perpendicular polarisation directions defined with respect to the plane of the boundary.

The common terminology for the different types of wave is taken from seismology. The surface of the component on which the transducers are placed is taken to define the directions along which the polarisation of the shear waves is resolved; in seismology this surface is, of course, the surface of the Earth. Shear waves propagating at some angle to the normal to this surface are said to be *SV waves* if the particle displacement lies in the plane, perpendicular to the surface, containing the direction of propagation, and *SH waves* if the particle displacement is parallel to the surface. The terms SV and SH stand for *shear-vertical* and *shear-horizontal* with obvious interpretation for the seismologist but less clear descriptive properties for the NDT practitioner; nevertheless the terms are commonly used. The compression wave is often also called a *P wave*, which stands for primary wave, as it is the first signal to arrive at the receiver. Most Time-of-Flight Diffraction studies carried out to date have used compression waves rather than shear waves for this very reason.

### 2.1.1 Wavespeeds in terms of elastic constants

We shall use the symbols $C_p$ and $C_s$ for the speeds of compression waves and of shear waves respectively. In an isotropic material there can be only two distinct elastic constants. These quantities are usually denoted $\lambda$, $\mu$ and are called Lamé constants. The wavespeeds are related to these elastic constants of anisotropic material through the relations:

$$C_p = \sqrt{\frac{\lambda + 2\mu}{\rho}} \tag{2.1}$$

$$C_s = \sqrt{\frac{\mu}{\rho}} \tag{2.2}$$

where $\lambda$, $\mu$ are the Lamé constants and $\rho$ is the density. Other elastic constants are Young's modulus $E$, Poisson's ratio $\nu$ and the bulk modulus $K$ and these are related to the Lamé constants through the relationships:

$$E = \frac{\mu(3\lambda + 2\mu)}{\lambda + \mu} \tag{2.3}$$

**Table 2.1** Wavespeeds and densities for some common materials

| Material | Compression wavespeed (mm/μs) | Shear wavespeed (mm/μs) | Relative density |
|---|---|---|---|
| Aluminium | 6·42 | 3·04 | 2·7 |
| Brass | 4·7 | 2·1 | 8·6 |
| Nickel | 5·89 | 3·22 | 8·97 |
| Sodium | 3·08 | 1·43 | 0·9 |
| Steel | 5·9 | 3·2 | 7·9 |
| Titanium | 6·07 | 3·13 | 4·5 |
| Zinc | 4·2 | 2·4 | 7·1 |
| Alumina | 13·2 | 6·4 | 4·0 |
| Haematite | 6·85 | 3·91 | 4·93 |
| Manganese sulphide | 7·4 | 4·3 | 4·0 |
| Martensite | 7·5 | 3·1 | 7·8 |
| Silica | 6·0 | 3·77 | 2·66 |
| Perspex | 2·68 | 1·10 | 1·18 |
| Polyethylene | 1·95 | 0·54 | 0·9 |
| Polystyrene | 2·35 | 1·12 | 1·06 |
| Glycerine | 1·92 | | 1·26 |
| Ice | 3·59 | 1·81 | 0·9 |
| Water | 1·498 | | 1·0 |

$$\nu = \frac{\lambda}{2(\lambda+\mu)} \tag{2.4}$$

$$K = \lambda + \frac{2\mu}{3} \tag{2.5}$$

but we shall use only the wavespeeds $C_p$, $C_s$ and the density $\rho$ to characterise isotropic media. Typical wavespeeds encountered in engineering materials are given in Table 2.1. We use natural (metric) units throughout this text. In ultrasonic testing, we are usually dealing with frequencies of a few Megahertz, wavelengths and component dimensions in millimetres, and times of a few microseconds. Therefore, we quote frequencies in the formulae in Megahertz, linear dimensions in millimetres, the times in microseconds and hence wavespeeds in millimetres per microsecond.

It is worth observing that, in non-destructive testing applications, the amplitude of the waves is very small and so the materials behave in a linear elastic way. In other applications, where amplitudes may be large enough for non-linear behaviour to occur, wave propagation can be more complicated than described here.

### 2.1.2 Other wave motions in isotropic media

So far we have only mentioned the waves which exist in infinite unbounded media, although we have pointed out that the different polarisations of shear wave are only defined when there is a reference surface. Once such a surface exists, as it always will in practice, various complications arise. The first complication is that, at such a free surface, which is taken to be stress free, incident waves which are purely compression or purely shear (SV) give rise, in general, to reflected waves containing both compression and shear (SV) components. This is known as *mode conversion*.

Bulk waves can travel parallel to flat interfaces. A compression wave travelling parallel to a flat surface does not satisfy the stress-free boundary conditions by itself and a shear wave is also generated travelling away from the surface at the critical angle. The compression wave travelling parallel to the flat surface we call a *lateral wave* and is sometimes referred to by other authors as a creeping wave. The shear wave which is generated by the compression wave travelling parallel to the flat surface is called a *head wave*. We reserve the term *creeping wave* for those waves which follow curved surfaces by continually interacting with the surface curvature and these are discussed in Section 7.3.

The second complication comes from the fact that other wave motions become possible at boundaries. The most important wave which occurs at stress-free boundaries is called a *Rayleigh wave* after Lord Rayleigh who first studied it. A Rayleigh wave is confined to the surface with an amplitude which decays exponentially with distance from the surface. The Rayleigh wave propagates along the surface at a speed which is distinct from the speed of the waves in the body of the material. This speed, denoted by $C_r$, is given by the solution of Equation A.6 in Section A.2 of the Appendix, and has a value of $C_r \sim 0.92C_s$ in steel. Because the Rayleigh wave expands in only two dimensions, conservation of energy requires that the amplitude of the wave falls off only as $1/\sqrt{r}$, whereas the body waves transmitted into the medium from a point source expand in three dimensions and so have an amplitude which falls off as $1/r$, where $r$ is the distance from the source. In seismology it is the Rayleigh wave which causes most destruction because it carries energy further from the epicentre; in ultrasonic non-destructive testing large signals arising from Rayleigh waves generated either at inspection surfaces or crack faces can be confused with bulk wave signals in certain cases.

## 2.2 Diffraction of waves

When waves of any sort: electromagnetic waves such as light or radio waves; sound waves in air; waves on the surface of water, or elastic waves in solids; impinge on discontinuities of material properties they are scattered by the discontinuity. At the edges of the discontinuity, the waves will be diffracted. Diffraction is a result of blocking or attenuation of part of the original wavefront by the discontinuity and is not a property of the edges as such. However, it is convenient to visualise the process as one of scattering at the edges, as this correctly gives the shape of the ensuing wavefront. In this way, energy which originally may have been propagating in one direction can be radiated into a wide range of angles. Familiar examples of this are: the way in which waves fill a harbour no matter which way the incident predominant sea swell approaches the harbour mouth; and the production of intensity fringes of light passing through small apertures. Diffraction thus results in energy being redistributed into a greater range of angles, with a consequent reduction in the energy travelling in the original direction of propagation. A familiar example of edge diffraction is that of light waves at a straight edge, producing a pattern of fringes in the shadow zone. This illustrates that the dependence of the energy on the propagation angle from the edge can be complicated. The diffraction of plane SH-waves at a semi-infinite plane crack edge is analogous to the optical case, while further complications arise for compression and SV-waves. Thus while the simple picture of diffracted energy radiating from the edge is a useful one, it is necessary to consider in more detail the distribution of energy with angle to see where detectable signals will occur.

### 2.2.1 Diffraction of plane elastic waves by infinite straight crack edges

The results of the mathematical analysis of diffraction of elastic waves are important for the successful implementation of Time-of-Flight Diffraction studies and are, therefore, noted in the next chapter and reproduced in more detail in Section A.4 of the Appendix. It turns out that the angular distribution of diffracted energy from a smooth crack edge, like reflection from a smooth surface, does not depend on the frequency of the wave. This means that there is no natural length scale in the diffraction problem, so the angular distribution of energy can be found by solving a kind of universal problem called a *canonical problem*. For a crack in a plane perpendicular to the line joining the transmitter and receiver index points, with the defect straddled by the two transducers, as is common in TOFD inspections, the canonical problem is that of an infinitely long crack, infinitely thin but with no contact between the crack faces. Although it may seem strange that such an apparently unrealistic model can give correct results, experiments have shown that this model is a good one in many real cases, as we show in Section 3.1.2. The results were first produced by Maue [1953] and were developed by Coffey and Chapman [1983] as the basis of a model of pulse-echo and tandem inspection of misoriented smooth flat cracks. The theoretical approaches of Maue and Coffey and Chapman were compared by Ogilvy and Temple [1983], who also derived results appropriate to the development of Time-of-Flight Diffraction technique. A complete theoretical description of the diffraction from cracks at arbitrary angles, including both tilt and skew, has been given by Achenbach, Gautesen and McMaken [1982].

## 2.3 Time-of-Flight Diffraction in Isotropic Media

As we have already pointed out, the Time-of-Flight Diffraction technique is based on timing measurements made on the signals diffracted by the crack. The general situation is depicted in Figure 2.1. Let us consider a buried crack in a plate of some isotropic and homogeneous material. The transmitting transducer $T_x$ emits a short burst of ultrasound into the component. This energy spreads out as it propagates into a beam with a definite angular variation, as described in Section A.3.2 of the Appendix. Some of the energy is incident on the crack and is scattered by it. If the crack face is smooth, there will be a mirror-like reflection of the wave incident on the face. This, just like an optical reflection, occurs at an angle of reflection equal to the angle of incidence, both angles measured from the normal to the crack face.

In many real situations the crack, which tends to grow in a plane perpendicular to the direction of maximum stress, will be oriented much as shown in Figure 2.1 and the reflected energy will be directed away from both transmitter and receiver transducers. For a rough crack some energy is scattered in all directions. For any crack, whether smooth or rough-faced, scattering from the edges of the crack, properly called diffraction, causes some fraction of the incident energy to travel towards the receiving transducer $R_x$. If the crack is big enough, the signals from the two extremities of the crack will be sufficiently separated in time to be recognised as coming from separate sources. As well as these two signals, there will be some energy which arrives at the receiver directly from the transducer by the shortest possible path, the lateral wave — just below the surface of the component — and there may be an echo from the back wall. Such a set of actual signals is displayed in the lower part of Figure 2.1. This type of time trace is known as an *A-scan*.

A typical experimental result showing these signals is presented in Figure 2.2, although the defect in this case is a hole, not a crack. This type of presentation is known as a *B-scan* and is created by stacking together A-scans recorded at successive positions of the transducer pair. The voltage fluctuations in the A-scan are represented by intensity variation in the B-scan. In the example shown, the transducers were moved, at constant separation, in the vertical plane containing their index points, over a cylindrical hole drilled perpendicular to that plane. The signals appearing are, from the top of the figure to the bottom, the lateral wave, signals from the top and bottom of the hole, mode converted signals from the top of the hole, and finally the back-wall echo. The significance of the mode converted signals will be described in the next section.

From the time differences indicated in Figure 2.2, the through-wall extent of the crack or other defect and its depth from the inspection surface can be obtained, provided the speed of the waves in the component is known. This is where the assumption that the material is isotropic and homogeneous is important. In such material the speeds of propagation of different types of elastic wave are constant and independent of direction. This is not true of materials which are anisotropic or inhomogeneous, and we return to this point in Section 7.1.

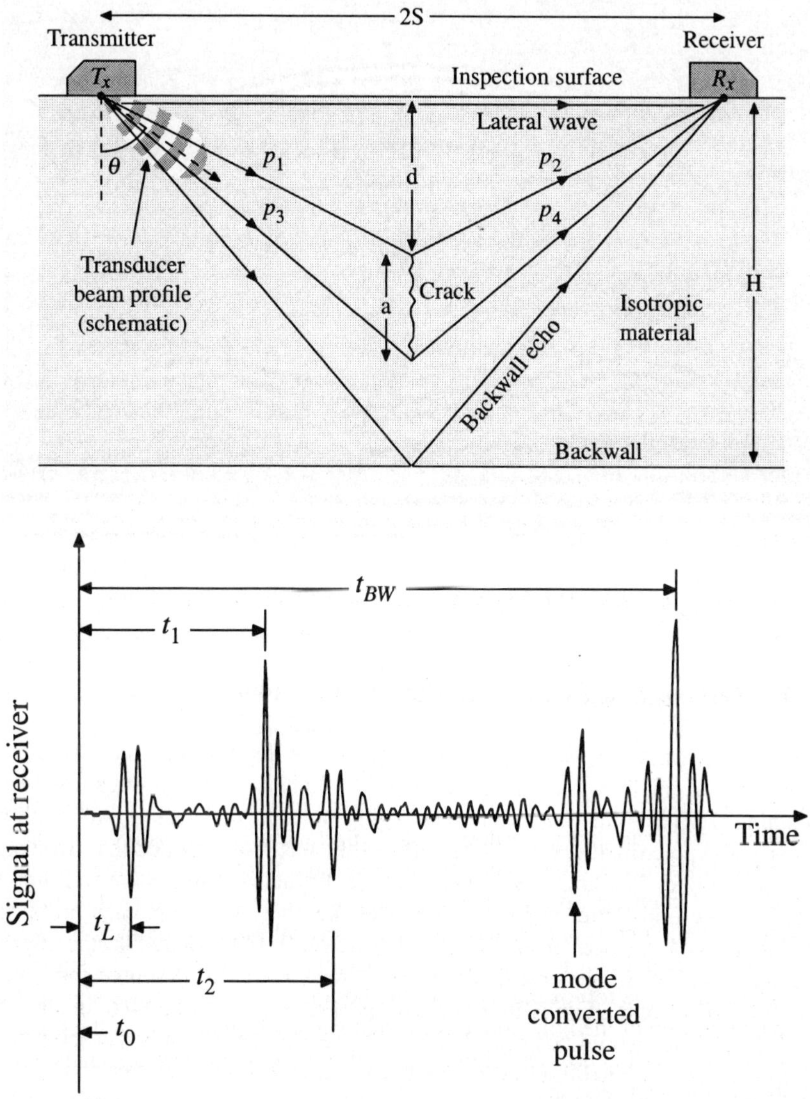


**Fig. 2.1** The two probe basis of the Time-of-Flight Diffraction technique. The locations of the tips of the crack are determined from the time differences between the lateral wave and the pulses which follow paths $p_1 + p_2$ or $p_3 + p_4$. These paths correspond to $t_1$ and $t_2$ respectively in the lower figure.

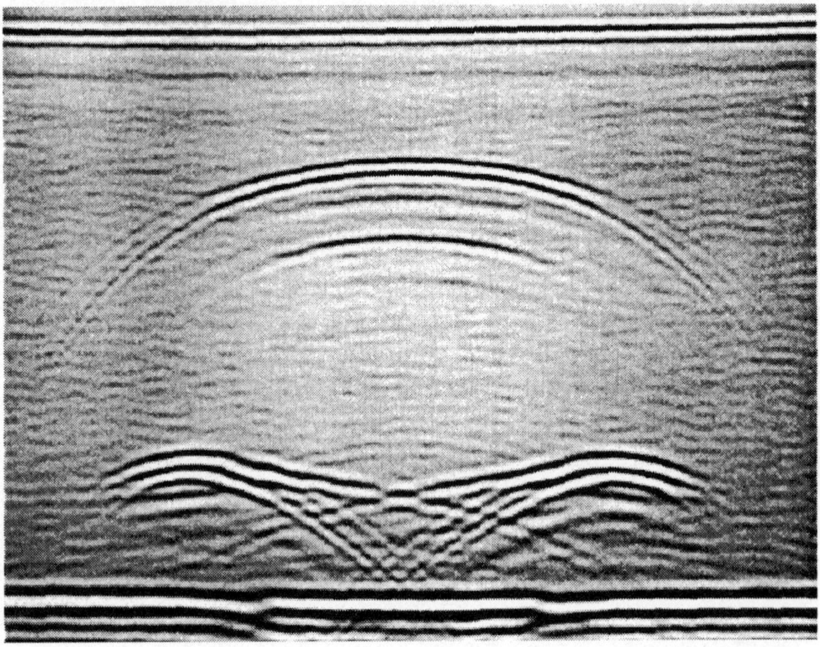

**Fig. 2.2** Experimental diffraction signals from a buried hole.

### 2.3.1 Through-wall size and depth of cracks

In order to simplify the discussion of calculating the depth from which the diffraction signals originate, we shall assume that the ultrasonic wavefront can be treated as coming from a point source and converging on a point detector. Although this is clearly an approximation, it will be sufficiently accurate provided that two conditions are fulfilled. The first condition is that the diffraction sources are well into the *far field* of the transmitter and receiver probes, i.e. the range from each probe substantially exceeds the *near-field distance*, defined as $D^2/4\lambda$, where $D$ is the effective diameter of the vibrating element of the probe, treated as a piston source and $\lambda$ is the ultrasonic wavelength. For 10 mm diameter probes vibrating at 5 MHz in steel, the near-field distance would be about 21 mm. The second condition is that the diffraction source lies reasonably close to the beam axes of the transmitter and receiver probes. The central lobe of the beam extends to an angle of approximately $\lambda/D$ radians from the beam axis and for the probe quoted above would be little more than $8°$. If these conditions are fulfilled, we should be able to measure the time interval between signals following different paths to a small fraction of a period. In practice these condition are often not completely fulfilled but it is convenient to postpone discussion of the consequences until later in the chapter. The effects of working in the near field on the pattern of signals observed will be discussed in Section 2.3.4. The effect of finite probe size and the consequent limited beam width on the accuracy with which signals can be timed will be discussed in Section 2.3.2.7. For the initial discussion, we shall also ignore the transit time of the ultrasound in the probe assemblies, probe shoes, coupling media etc., and assume that we can measure the travel times in the workpiece accurately, relative to the transmitter firing pulse. We shall return to a discussion of probe, shoe and coupling effects in Section 2.3.2.

To calculate the crack through-wall size and depth from the inspection surface requires nothing more than Pythagoras's theorem. Suppose, at present, that the crack is oriented in a plane perpendicular to both the inspection surface and the line joining transmitter and receiver along the inspection surface. Suppose also that the crack is midway between the transmitter and receiver (i.e. the probe pair has been moved until the time-of-flight of the defect signal is at the minimum), with the extremity nearest the inspection surface at a depth $d$ below it, and that the crack itself has through-wall extent $a$. Referring to Figure 2.1, if the separation between the centres of the transmitter $T_x$ and receiver $R_x$ is taken to be $2S$, and the speed of propagation of elastic waves is taken to be $C$, then the arrival times of the various signals are

$$t_L = \frac{2S}{C} \tag{2.6}$$

$$t_1 = \frac{2\sqrt{S^2+d^2}}{C} \tag{2.7}$$

$$t_2 = \frac{2\sqrt{S^2+(d+a)^2}}{C} \tag{2.8}$$

$$t_{bw} = \frac{2\sqrt{S^2+H^2}}{C} \tag{2.9}$$

where $t_L$, $t_1$, $t_2$ and $t_{bw}$ are as marked on Figure 2.1 and $H$ is the plate thickness. The times $t_1$ and $t_2$ are the arrival times of the signals diffracted by the extremities of the crack. The first signal to arrive, $t_L$, is due to the lateral wave and that marked $t_{bw}$ is the time of arrival of a back-wall echo. $C$ is taken to be either $C_p$ or $C_s$, the speed of propagation of bulk compression or shear waves respectively.

Rearranging the above equations, we find the depth of the top of the crack from the inspection surface is $d$ with

$$d = \frac{1}{2}\sqrt{C^2t_1^2 - 4S^2} \tag{2.10}$$

and the through-wall extent $a$ is given by

$$a = \frac{1}{2}\sqrt{C^2t_2^2 - 4S^2} - d \tag{2.11}$$

and the value of the separation of the probes need not be known, since we can substitute

$$2S = C_L t_L \tag{2.12}$$

for this, where $C_L$ is the speed of the lateral wave. On a flat plate this speed is identical to the bulk wave velocity $C_p$ or $C_s$ of compression or shear waves respectively. This brings out an interesting question: which wave mode would be most advantageous to use? The shear wave has a wavelength roughly half that of compression waves and therefore offers an enhanced resolution but has the disadvantage that the speed of propagation is only half that of the compression waves. This slower speed means that in many cases the signals of interest from the defect will arrive in amongst other, possibly spurious, signals generated by mode converted compression waves which have travelled further, or by Rayleigh waves. Hence, in many cases, the shear wave signals will be more difficult to interpret than those from compression waves. For this reason the normal choice is to use compression wave signals. Although compression waves are usually preferable, because of their earlier arrival time than shear waves, there may be other considerations, such as the anisotropy of the material to be inspected, which might make the use of shear waves preferable in certain cases, and this will be discussed in Section 7.1.

If compression wave signals are to be used, we can choose the probe separation so that any signals which travel over their complete path as shear waves arrive after the compression wave back-wall echo. Referring to Figure 2.1, this will be the case if

$$t_L(\text{shear}) > t_{bw}(\text{compression}) \tag{2.13}$$

or

$$\frac{2S}{C_s} > \frac{2\sqrt{S^2 + H^2}}{C_p} \tag{2.14}$$

Since $C_p \simeq 2C_s$, the condition reduces to $S > H/\sqrt{3}$. We cannot, however, exclude the possibility of signals which travel part of their path as compression waves and part as shear waves, undergoing a mode conversion at a defect. Some such signals appear in the lower part of Figure 2.2. Their main intensity arises where the shear wave beam from one transducer intersects the compression wave beam from the other. Since there are two such positions, a single defect gives rise to two sets of signals, compression wave converting to shear waves and vice versa.

Effects of this kind can be confusing in isolation, but a consideration of all the signals arriving and their relation to each other will normally make clear the origins of each; where any ambiguity remains, an additional scan with a different transducer separation will resolve it. In some circumstances these mode converted signals can be used to advantage. This is further discussed in Section 5.5.1.

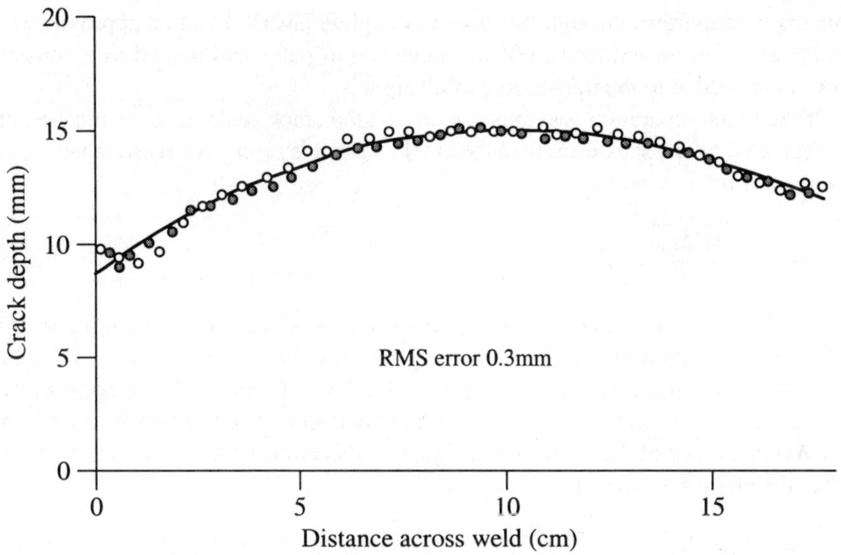


**Fig. 2.3** Sizing a fatigue crack with Time-of-Flight Diffraction. The filled and open circles are TOFD measurements at beam angles of 10° and 20° to the normal, from the surface from which the crack grew. The solid line gives the actual crack profile determined destructively.

## 2.3.2 Accuracy of through-wall size measurements

An example of the accuracy achievable over a limited range of defect depth, between about 8 and 15 mm, is presented in Figure 2.3 where the measured defect depths are plotted against the actual defect depths for a defect with an irregular profile.

The defect in this case is a fatigue crack. On the figure, the actual profile is given by the solid line, while the experimental values are given by the circles and are taken from Silk [1979a]. The root-mean-square (RMS) error is found to be 0.3 mm.

The accuracy of depth measurements by the Time-of-Flight Diffraction technique was discussed in detail by Lidington, Silk, Montgomery and Hammond [1976]. The importance of the subject is such, however, that it is worth presenting it again here from a somewhat different viewpoint.

### 2.3.2.1 Probe shoe effects

The idealised discussion of the previous section has ignored some important features of actual measurements. In order to propagate the ultrasound into the workpiece at an appropriate angle and to receive the diffracted signals, the probes, if of the contact type, will have to have wedge-shaped shoes, or, if coupled by immersion, have their axes tilted, in order to achieve the appropriate angle of incidence on the inspection surface. The primary effect of this is to increase the transit time of all signals by the time required to travel through the shoes or coupling layers. To a first approximation the increase can be assumed to be the same for all paths and treated as a constant *probe delay* added to the transit time of all signals.

If the probe separation is symmetric around the crack, and the beam entry points are separated by a distance $2S$, then the crack depth $d$ is given, to a reasonable degree of accuracy by

$$d = \sqrt{\frac{(C\Delta t)^2}{4} - S^2} \tag{2.15}$$

where $\Delta t$ is the transit time in the component. However, from our measuring instruments, we can only measure the interval $\Delta t_0$ between the transmitter firing pulse and the arrival of the diffracted signal; to arrive at the transit time in the component, we need to subtract the probe delay. The probe delay is most easily determined from the time of occurrence of the lateral wave signal. If it occurs at a time $t_{L0}$ after the firing pulse, the probe $p$ is given by

$$p = t_{L0} - t_L = t_{L0} - 2S/C \tag{2.16}$$

An equivalent approach is to measure the difference between transit time of the lateral wave and that of the defect signal. Then the defect depth can be obtained from

$$C\Delta t = 2\sqrt{S^2 + d^2} - 2S \tag{2.17}$$

$$d = \sqrt{\left(\frac{C\Delta t}{2} + S\right)^2 - S^2} \tag{2.18}$$

The assumption of a fixed probe delay amounts to ignoring the fact that the path length in the probe shoes or coupling layer will vary with angle. The degree to which this is justified needs to be examined in more detail. Because of refraction at the component surface, the exact relationship is the solution of three simultaneous equations [Lidington et al., 1976]

$$\Delta t = 2\left(\frac{h}{C_1 \cos\psi} + \frac{d}{C_2 \cos\theta}\right) \tag{2.19}$$

$$S = h\tan\theta + d\tan\theta \tag{2.20}$$

$$C_1 \sin\theta = C_2 \sin\psi \tag{2.21}$$

where $h$ is the vertical thickness of the probe shoe at the centre of the probe face, $d$ is the through-wall depth of the diffracting crack edge, $\psi$ is the beam angle in the probe shoe, $\theta$ is the refracted beam angle in the component, $C_1$ is the elastic wave speed in the probe shoe, $C_2$ is the elastic wave speed in the component and $2S$ is the

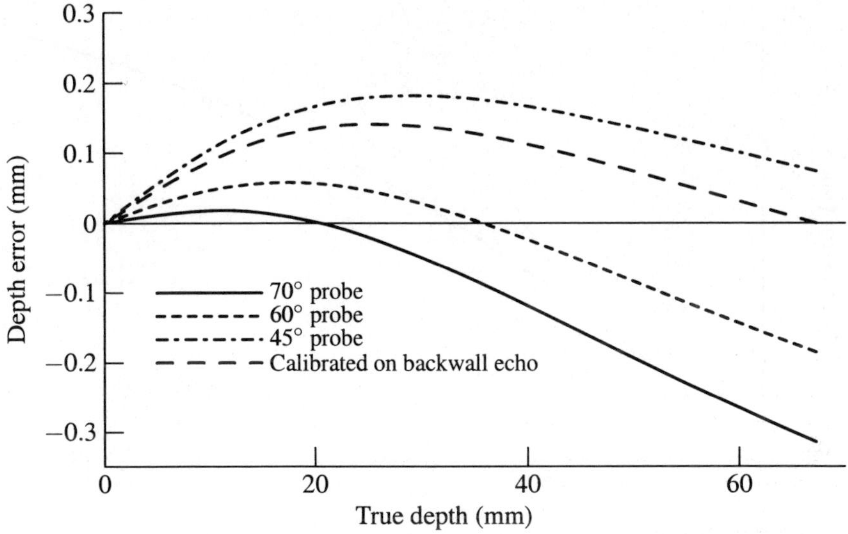


**Fig. 2.4** The effect of probe shoes on the accuracy of depth estimation. The separation of the centres of the probe elements is 80 mm, the shoe thickness at that point is 5 mm and the various curves show the effect of different ways of estimating the effective probe separation (see text for details).

separation of the centres of ultrasonic vibrating elements. $\Delta t$ is the total transit time, including that within the probe shoes

Although an expression for the depth can be obtained from these equations, it is complicated and does not readily bring out the size of the effects. An example is more illuminating. Figure 2.4 shows the difference in the calculated depth derived from Equations 2.19 – 2.21, compared with that derived from Equation 2.17, for probes on 5 mm thick shoes and a nominal separation of 80 mm. Note that the shape of the variation with depth depends on what is assumed for the effective probe separation. The usual practice is to derive the probe index points (and hence the effective probe separation) by projecting the beam axes from the probe crystals, through the shoes, to meet the inspection surface. Figure 2.4 shows the effect of making this assumption for 45°, 60° and 70° probes. It is clear that this procedure is satisfactory, in that the maximum depth errors for defects near the beam axis will be very small. However, the procedure is not necessarily optimum. An alternative is to use a figure for the effective probe separation which will reduce the depth error to zero at some particular depth. This can most easily be achieved by calibrating on a signal at known depth. A common practice is to use the reflection from the back wall of the workpiece as a calibration point. This has often been applied as a means of checking the ultrasonic velocity, as discussed below, but, in this case, it would be used to derive a figure for the effective probe separation, using a velocity figure obtained some other way. The additional curve in Figure 2.4 shows the result of this

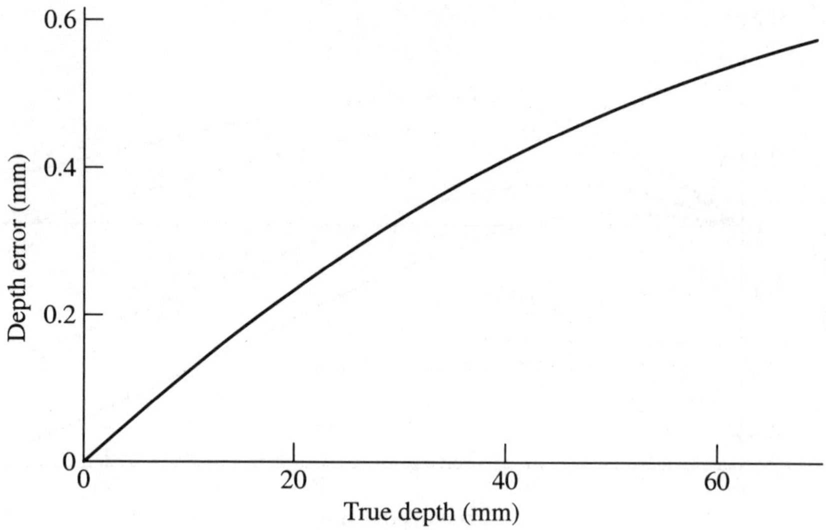


**Fig. 2.5** Depth error as a function of depth, for a 1 mm error in $S$ when S = 40 mm.

approach. It ensures accurate results near the two surfaces and the calculated depth at intermediate depths will be a slight overestimate.

It should be noted that, unless very thick shoes, or coupling layers, are used, the shoe or coupling layer corrections to the calculated depth are small enough to be ignored in all but the most accurate work.

### 2.3.2.2 Probe separation errors

One of the features which comes out of the above discussion is that the figure used for the probe separation has a noticeable influence on the accuracy of depth measurement. To explore this further, let us discard the added complication of the shoes and go back to simple point probes on the inspection surface. We shall again measure the transit time $\Delta t$ of a diffracted signal relative to that of the lateral wave. We can simplify Equation 2.17 thus

$$(C\Delta t)^2 + 4C\Delta t\, S = 4d^2 \tag{2.22}$$

Here $\Delta t$ is what we have measured and we want to look at the effect of the value we use for $S$ on the derived value of $d$. Treating $d$ as a function of $S$ and differentiating, we obtain

$$\frac{\partial d}{\partial S} = \frac{C\Delta t}{2d} \tag{2.23}$$

Thus, for small changes in $S$, the depth error is proportional to the error in $S$. As an example, for probes with $S$= 40 mm, (i.e. separated by 80 mm), for a defect on the centreline of a 60° beam, every 1 mm error in $S$ gives an error of 0.27 mm in $d$. To calculate the depth dependence, it is necessary to substitute for $C\Delta t$ in terms of $S$ and $d$ from Equation 2.17, obtaining

$$\frac{\partial d}{\partial S} = \frac{\sqrt{S^2+d^2}-S}{d} \tag{2.24}$$

Figure 2.5 shows how the depth error varies with true depth for a 1 mm error in S, when S = 40 mm.

#### 2.3.2.3 Coupling film thickness

In order for contact probes to act as efficient transmitters and receivers of ultrasound on a workpiece of typical surface finish, there must be a thin film of some coupling medium, usually a fluid or gel, between the probe face and the workpiece. Normally this coupling film is so thin that its influence on the timing of the ultrasonic signals is negligible. However, there may be circumstances where a thicker film is necessary. In the case of immersion probes, the coupling layer takes the place of the shoe on a contact probe but its thickness may vary during probe traversal, for instance because the workpiece surface is not flat. The effects of coupling layers, or other layers such as wear protection coatings, can be taken into account by adding to the model represented by Equations 2.16 – 2.18, one or more extra layers of uniform thickness, between the shoe and the workpiece. The effect is again best illustrated by an example. Using the same arrangement as for the data in Figure 2.4 but adding a coupling layer 0.5 mm thick, having the same ultrasonic properties as water, the results shown in Figure 2.6 are obtained.

The effect of the coupling layer is very small compared with the effect of the shoe. For contact probes, variations in coupling layer thickness of 0.5 mm, or greater, would be unusual, so the effect can normally be neglected, in comparison with other sources of error. Similarly, for immersion probes, maintaining the standoff of the probe faces from the inspection surface to this degree of constancy would ensure that the errors from variations in standoff were negligible. However, careful design of probe mountings may be necessary to ensure that much larger variations do not occur in automatic immersion scanning of large components.

In the above discussion of errors, we have assumed that the defect signals were timed relative to the lateral wave signal. To illustrate how critical this procedure is to the achievement of accurate measurement, we show, in Figure 2.7, the depth errors that would result if we increased the coupling layer thickness by 0.5 mm but ignored the resultant change in the lateral wave time.

Such larger errors would, of course, be intolerable. In inspections where the lateral wave cannot be monitored, it is highly desirable, if not always absolutely essential, to find some other signal which can be relied upon as a depth calibration. In a plate workpiece, the obvious candidate is the back-wall reflection; in more complex workpieces, there may be other signals which can be used. This issue will be revisited in Chapter 6, where complex geometries are discussed.

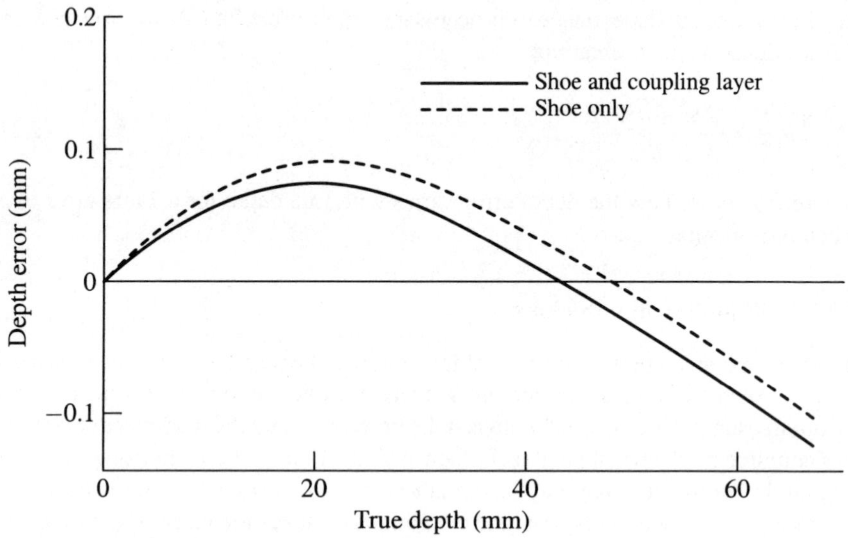


**Fig. 2.6** Effect on depth error of adding a 0.5 mm layer of coupling medium between the shoes and the workpiece. The coupling layer has the same ultrasonic properties as water. An effective value of 38 mm has been assumed for $S$.

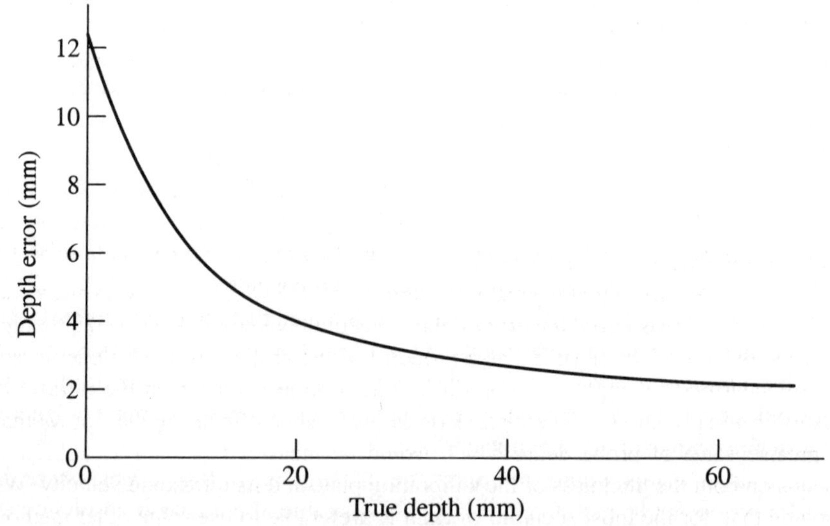


**Fig. 2.7** Effect of the same added coupling layer as in Figure 2.6 but ignoring the change in lateral wave timing caused by the coupling layer.

#### 2.3.2.4 Variations in velocity

Thus far we have assumed that the velocity of the appropriate mode of ultrasonic wave in the workpiece is known accurately. For a plate workpiece of uniform, homogeneous, isotropic material, this requirement is easily met by timing the interval between back-wall reflections for a beam normal to the surface. In more complex geometries or with materials with less ideal properties, the inaccuracy of velocity estimates, or variations in velocity with position or direction may become a significant source of error. To see how a change in velocity would effect the depth measurements, we start, again, with Equation 2.22, treating it as expressing $d$ as a function of $C$ for constant $\Delta t$ and $S$. Differentiating with respect to $C$ and $d$, we obtain

$$\frac{\partial d}{\partial C} = \frac{C\Delta t(C\Delta t - S)}{4Cd} \tag{2.25}$$

Expressing $C\Delta t$ in terms of $S$ and $d$ from Equation 2.17, we get

$$\frac{\partial d}{\partial C} = \frac{\sqrt{S^2+d^2}\left(\sqrt{S^2+d^2} - S\right)}{Cd} \tag{2.26}$$

For $d$ very much smaller than $S$, this simplifies to

$$\frac{\partial d}{\partial C} = \frac{d}{2C} \tag{2.27}$$

from which we deduce that a 1% error in $C$ gives a 0.5% error in $d$, for $d \ll S$. $\partial d/\partial C$ increases with $d$ but not very rapidly, so that for $S = 40$ mm, the depth error has increased to 0.67% for a depth of 60 mm (Figure 2.8).

These results show that it is well worth obtaining an accurate value for the velocity and that where velocity variations occur, significant depth errors can arise. This issue will be revisited in Chapter 7, when anisotropic materials are discussed.

One way of maintaining a check on the velocity is to monitor the timing of the back-wall echo. From Equations 2.6 and 2.9, we can show that

$$C = \frac{2H}{\sqrt{t_{bw}^2 - t_L^2}} \tag{2.28}$$

Here, it should be noted that $t_{bw}$ and $t_L$ are the travel times within the workpiece and they can only be measured if the probe delay is accurately known. However, although the probe delay may be regarded as a property of the probe assembly alone, it can only be measured by applying the probes to a workpiece for which the ultrasonic velocity is already known. The discussion of probe shoe effects, above, shows that the precise value of probe delay which would be measured in such a calibration depends on both the thickness of the calibration plate and its ultrasonic velocity. We conclude that, for the most accurate work, it is preferable to use some other method of measuring the ultrasonic velocity in the workpiece and to use the back-wall echo as a means of estimating an effective probe separation which will minimise the probe shoe effects. In a workpiece in which the velocity may vary, the back-wall echo may provide a useful means of monitoring those variations.

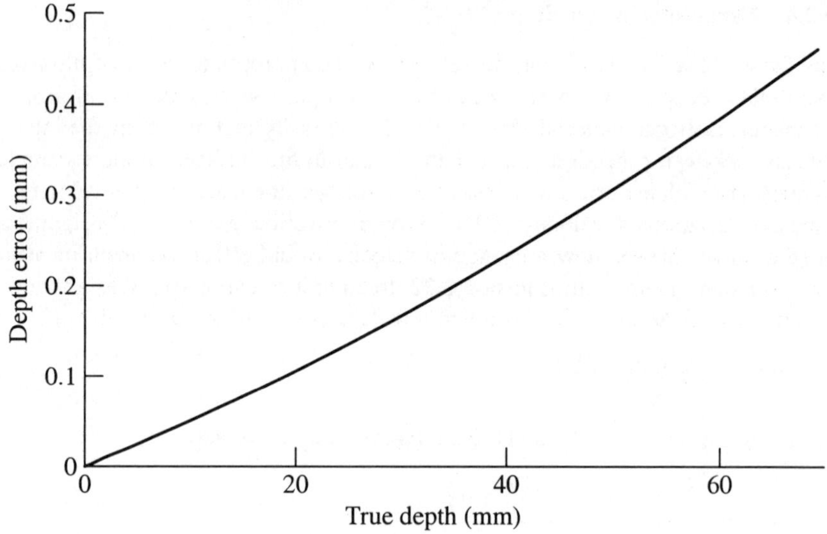


**Fig. 2.8** Effect of a 1% velocity error on the accuracy of depth estimation for $C = 5.9\,\mathrm{mm}/\mu\mathrm{s}$ and $S = 40\,\mathrm{mm}$.

#### 2.3.2.5 Inspection surface characteristics

The discussion of accuracy has been based on the assumption that the inspection surface is a smooth flat plane. Minor departures from flatness will obviously degrade the accuracy somewhat because the probes will be displaced up or down from the assumed position. The depth errors will be of the same order as, or less than, the displacements of the probes. Major departures from flatness introduce geometric considerations and will be considered in more detail in the chapter on complex geometries. If the surface is rough, on a scale comparable with the ultrasonic wavelength, the accuracy may be degraded by variations in the thickness of the coupling layer, as discussed above, or by changes in the shape of the ultrasonic pulse resulting from a variation of coupling efficiency with frequency.

#### 2.3.2.6 Effect of time resolution on depth resolution

Returning to the equations for the depth and through-wall extent of the crack detected and sized by the Time-of-Flight Diffraction technique, we see that the resolution of the through-wall position and extent is determined by the resolution of a timing measurement. The depth resolution $\partial d$ can be derived in terms of the resolution in the time measurement $\partial(\Delta t)$, by differentiation of Equation 2.15 as [Silk, 1978],

$$\partial d = \frac{C\partial(\Delta t)}{2\cos\theta} \tag{2.29}$$

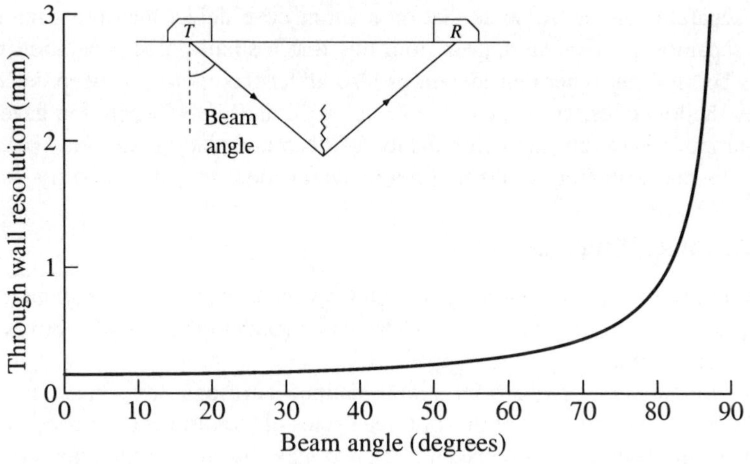


**Fig. 2.9** Depth resolution of Time-of-Flight Diffraction in the through wall direction for buried or surface breaking defects in steel. A time resolution of 50 ns is assumed.

where $\theta$ is the angle, measured from the normal to the inspection surface, of the ray joining the tip of the defect to the transmitter centre, as shown in Figure 2.1. A plot of this function for $\partial(\Delta t) = 50\,\text{ns}$ is shown in Figure 2.9, and is discussed in Section 3.1.1.

The resolution of time measurement, $\partial(\Delta t)$, is related to both the signal frequency and the digital sampling rate. Sampling rates of 20 MHz are common and rates up to 200 MHz are readily available. A resolution of 1 sampling interval (50 ns at 20 MHz) is easily obtainable and higher resolution can be obtained, in favourable circumstances, by interpolation [Charlesworth and Lidington, 1985]. A sampling interval of 50 ns gives satisfactory resolution for thick material where an accuracy of 1 mm is sufficient but for inspecting thin-walled tubes of wall thickness less than 1 mm it would be necessary to use higher frequencies and a higher digitisation rate. The higher sampling rates are only advantageous if the signal has frequency components which require the higher rates (i.e. approach half the sampling frequency) and if the time stability of the electronic system is sufficiently good. The frequency content of the signal is partly determined by the design of the ultrasonic transducers and partly by the propagation characteristics of the material being inspected. We shall not discuss transducer design in this book, but some discussion of the effect of material properties on propagation will be introduced in Section 7.1 with reference to anisotropic media.

The other important feature of Equation 2.29 is the $\cos\theta$ term in the denominator. This encapsulates the decline in resolution for near surface defects. It should be clear that, since $\cos\theta$ is simply $d/\sqrt{S^2+d^2}$, the definition of *near-surface* scales with $S$. Thus the resolution available on a 10 mm deep defect measured with 80 mm probe separation is the same as that on a 2 mm deep defect measure with 16 mm probe separation. It might appear from this that a small probe separation should always be used but other considerations also affect the choice. If deep defects, as well as shallow ones, are sought, the beam angle and probe separation have to be a compromise between the requirements for deep and shallow defects. In critical cases, separate scans for defects in different depth zones may be necessary.

#### 2.3.2.7 Effect of timing accuracy

In addition to the considerations set out above which refer to how small an interval of time can be accurately measured, we have to consider other possible errors in the time measurement.

The typical signal pulse from a well-damped ultrasonic transducer, at a point near the beam axis, consists of two or three cycles of the resonant frequency with an approximately Gaussian envelope. It is easy to make accurate timing measurements on a signal of that type and common practice is to base such measurements on the first really well defined zero crossing of the signal. Although such a measurement may be accurate, in its own terms, to a small faction of a period of the dominant frequency, it does not necessarily follow that defect depths or sizes calculated from it will be correspondingly accurate. For that to be the case, the form of the signal pulse would need to be the same for all the signals involved, a condition which is rarely completely fulfilled in practice.

Two disturbing factors need to be considered: first, measurements often involve pulses which travel by routes far enough from the axis of one or both transducers for distortion of the pulse shape to arise; secondly the phase of pulses can vary, depending on what processes of diffraction, or reflection they undergo en route. We shall consider these two factors separately.

The theory of the variation in pulse form with angle from the beam axis is set out in Section A.5 of the Appendix. Here, we merely draw on two important features of that theory:

- For a beam travelling at an angle from the beam axis greater than the nominal beam width, the pulse is split into leading and trailing components which appear to have originated from the nearest and furthest points of the transducer face. By the nominal beam width we mean $\sin^{-1}(\lambda/D)$ where $D$ is the transducer diameter and $\lambda$ is the wavelength at the centre frequency of the on-axis pulse.

- Because the beam width is frequency dependent, low frequency components become relatively more dominant as the angle from the beam axis increases and can strongly affect the pulse shape, especially at angles very much greater than the nominal beam width. The extent to which this effect is observed depends on the low-frequency response of the receiver amplifier.

The effect of these off-axis effects on defect signals is illustrated in the upper part of Figure 2.14 and discussed in more detail in Section 2.3.4. It is demonstrated in the lower part of Figure 2.14 that the effects can be very much reduced by reducing the effective probe diameter. Here we concentrate on the most important situation where defect signals originate from close to the beam axis of both probes but the lateral wave is used as a timing reference.

It is shown in Section A.5 that, provided the low frequency components are attenuated by the receiver amplifier, the characteristic shape of the lateral wave pulse is that of a central pulse with leading and trailing satellites of about half the amplitude. In practice, the satellites seem to be smaller than that and sometimes hard to detect on a grey-scale B-scan. There is some evidence in Figure 2.2 of a trailing lateral-wave satellite and the leading one may have been present prior to the start of the recording gate. On the whole it seems unlikely that the satellites will be large enough to be a confusing factor.

The central pulse has fewer cycles than the on-axis pulse and a slightly lower frequency. In shape, it matches the central part of the on-axis pulse well and, in particular, its central zero crossing aligns with the central zero of the on-axis pulse. It is clear that this is the measurement point to use and any other will incur some error. If the receiver amplifier has a flat response down to very low frequencies, the central pulse of the lateral wave can be 'blurred-out' as far as the satellite pulses into something like a single cycle. In this case the central zero crossing is still an accurate timing reference.

It is difficult to be precise about the magnitude of errors which might arise from a faulty choice of measurement points, because it is very dependent on the pulse shape. However, it is clear that errors of at least one cycle at the nominal frequency could occur, leading to errors in depth measurement of several mm at 5 MHz for our typical 80 mm probe separation. This is larger than any of the errors previously discussed, except perhaps for uncorrected variations in coupling layer thickness.

We now come to the question of signal phase. In the discussion of pulse shape we have implicitly ignored the effect of the diffraction process on the phase. The theory is described in detail in Section A.4 but the essence of it is that, for the probe angles in common use, 45° – 70°, the phase of the signal from the bottom of a crack should lag that of the lateral wave by $\pi/4$, while that from the top of the crack leads by $3\pi/4$. Ravenscroft, Newton and Scruby [1991] obtained good agreement with theory for an open fatigue crack but found rather variable results for other defects. The conventional approach to signal phase has been to assume that the signal from the bottom of the defect has the same phase as the lateral wave and that from the top of the defect has opposite phase (*vice-versa* relative to the back-wall echo). Measurements based on these assumptions are likely to be, on average, in error by about one eighth of a period at the centre frequency of the pulse, although errors perhaps twice as large could occur, depending on the nature of the defect. This error is typically less than one digital sampling interval, so is not a major source of error although it might be significant in the most accurate work. Burch and Ramsey [1986] demonstrated how signal phase can be accurately measured digitally (see Section 5.8.2) and, by implication, how accurate signal timing can be obtained irrespective of phase. For very accurate work, depth errors arising from phase differences could be eliminated

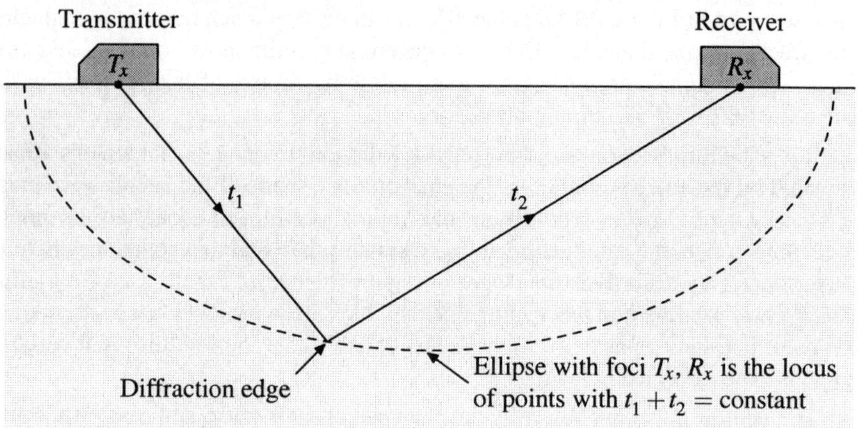


**Fig. 2.10** Elliptical locus of points with constant travel time from transmitter $T_x$ to receiver $R_x$.

by using this method.

From this discussion, we can derive some useful guideline for applying TOFD to obtain accurate measurements.

- Use the smallest probes consistent with adequate signal strength because they will have a larger beam width and so off-axis signals, such as the lateral wave, will be less distorted than with large probes.

- If the lateral wave is to be used for timing, examine its shape, relative to that of a signal from near the beam centreline and choose the precise measurement procedure with care, bearing in mind that the true correspondence is between the centre of the lateral wave signal and the centre of the defect signal. If the first well-defined zero crossing of a defect signal is used for measurement, a correcting offset may need to be added to the lateral wave time.

- For probe angles of much less than 60°, it may be preferable to use the back-wall echo as a reference. Alternatively, on a flat workpiece of constant thickness, it may be better to measure the probe separation and probe delay accurately by calibration on a test block of the same material as the inspection workpiece and use these figures, rather than a lateral wave or back-wall echo time to calculate the defect depths.

- Examine the phases of the defect signals carefully and choose the measurement point correspondingly, otherwise there could be as much as a half period error in the measured time of a defect top relative to a defect bottom.

In a material with high attenuation, significant changes in pulse shape with depth may occur. This arises because the attenuation almost always increases with fre-

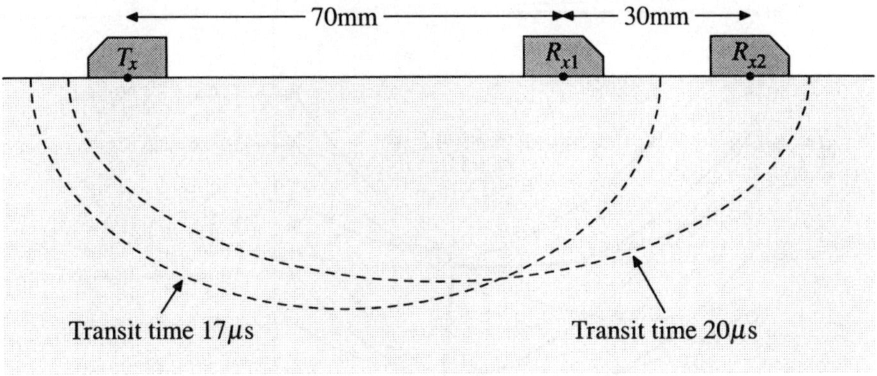


**Fig. 2.11** The elliptical loci of a crack tip determined by time differences. A transmitter and two receivers are shown; two transmitters and one receiver would produce an equivalent diagram. The defect tip is at the intersection of the two ellipses.

quency, so that signals travelling by a longer path have their high frequency components relatively more attenuated than their low frequency components. In this case, a measurement of the interval between equivalent features of the waveform may be difficult to carry out, or may be subject to systematic error, so the accuracy of the technique may be degraded in this type of material.

### 2.3.3 Locus of estimated crack through-wall size or depth

So far, we have considered the simplified case, where the crack is symmetrically placed between transmitter and receiver, but this is not the most general relative position of the probes and defect. In general the crack will lie somewhere between the two probes shown in Figure 2.1, but not necessarily midway between them. The possible locations of the crack tips lie on loci of constant travel time, which are arcs of ellipses with the centres of the two probes as foci. This is shown in Figure 2.10.

From this figure, it is clear that some ambiguity exists in the actual depth from the surface and the through-wall extent of a crack sized with just two probes, although this error will be relatively small if the defect is close to the midway position assumed in deriving Equations 2.10 and 2.11. If we add another transmitter, or another receiver, as shown in Figure 2.11, then the ambiguity is removed — at least for infinitely long defects.

For truly three-dimensional defects, at least four probes, or the equivalent achieved by multiple scans at different separations, are required for unambiguous location and sizing. Often further redundancy, involving more probe pairs, is an important part of ensuring reliable detection and accurate sizing of cracks in thick walled material, such as the pressure vessel of a pressurised water reactor. The rationale for deployment of multiple probes is discussed in more detail in Section 4.1.2 and experience

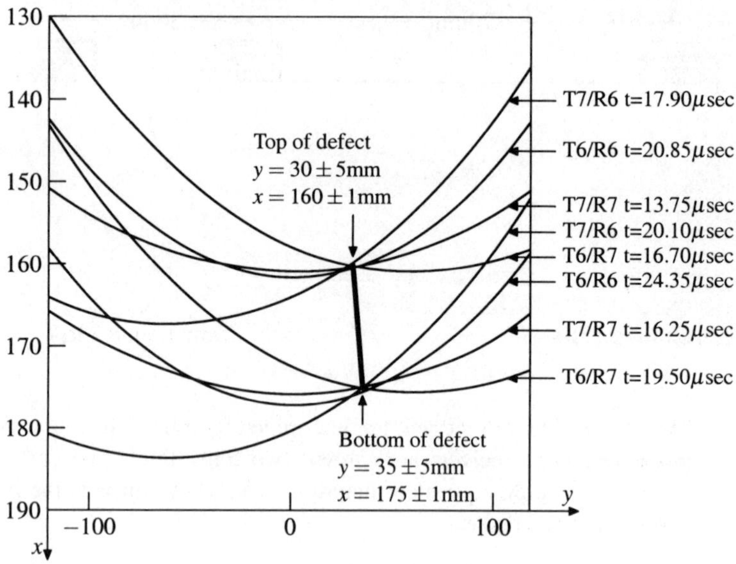


**Fig. 2.12** Loci indicating possible sites of diffraction edges from individual observations collectively locate the top and bottom in both $x$ and $y$. The $z$-coordinates are determined directly from the graphical presentation [from Hawker, 1983].

with deployment of complex probe arrays in the Defect Detection Trials is discussed in Section 8.4. An example of loci from several pairs of transmitters and receivers obtained in scans over a defective region of one of the plates in the Defect Detection Trials is given in Figure 2.12 [from Hawker, 1983] with the $z$ (through-wall) coordinates determined directly from the graphical presentation.

## 2.3.4 Diffraction arcs

Although developed initially as a tool for sizing cracks whose location was already known, the Time-of-Flight Diffraction technique has usually been applied in practice to detect the defects as well. This is made possible by use of the B-scan presentation aided by the excellent sensitivity of the human eye and brain for spatial coherence. The spatial coherence in the B-scan image takes the form of signal arcs generated as the transducers approach and recede from the defect. It is clear that, with the defect symmetrically between transmitter and receiver, crossing the plane passing through both transmitter and receiver and normal to the inspection surface, the transit time of the pulse is at a minimum. As the transducers move away from this position, along a scan line perpendicular to the plane of the defect, the transit time will increase. Hence, if the transducers are scanned from one side of the symmetrical position to the other, the transit time of the diffracted signal will reduce to a minimum and then increase again, forming an arc on the B-scan presentation. Such an arc is clearly visible in Figure 2.2 for a scan over a buried side-drilled hole.

In order to illustrate some of the properties of these arcs we consider a simplified situation in which the transmitting and receiving transducers located on a flat plate surface and we calculate the time-of-flight for a pulse scattered by a small spherical pore at a depth $d$. This defect is essentially a point scatterer. To calculate the effect of scanning the transducers, it is easier to fix the transmitter and receiver and let the defect move along some line parallel to the plate surface. The time-of-flight can then be obtained as a function of the distance of the defect along its scan direction from some arbitrary origin. The origin of coordinates is taken to lie in the surface and we fix the transmitter at $(-S,0,0)$ and the receiver at $(S,0,0)$. Let the defect position be $(x, y, -d)$, then the time-of-flight $t$ is given by

$$t = \frac{1}{C}\left[\sqrt{\left((x+s)^2+y^2+d^2\right)}+\sqrt{\left((x-s)^2+y^2+d^2\right)}\right] \quad (2.30)$$

where $C$ is the appropriate signal velocity. This equation is for a fixed position of the small pore. If we simulate a transducer scan by allowing the defect to move along a path parallel to the surface given by a straight line such as

$$y = mx + \text{constant}$$

then we get an equation which is not of any well known form. There is, however, one special case, when the transducers scan parallel to the $y$-axis with the defect symmetrically placed between them (a D-scan). In this case, $x = 0$ and

$$\frac{C^2t^2}{4k^2} - \frac{y^2}{k^2} = 1 \quad (2.31)$$

where $y$ gives the scan position and $k^2 \equiv S^2 + d^2$ is a constant. Equation 2.31 is recognised as the equation of a hyperbola. This has two branches; in the one of physical interest, $t$ is at a minimum at the point where the scattering point lies in the plane defined by the two beam axes and it increases as the point moves away from that plane. From physical arguments it is clear that signal loci, although hyperbolic only in the special case referred to above, will be of the same general shape for all scan paths in this simple geometry. In particular, the signal loci for a scan parallel to the plane defined by the beam axes (a B-scan) will look very like hyperbolae for deep defects but will appear increasingly flattened near the minimum as the surface is approached (see Figure 5.5).

When the defect is well away from the beam axes of the transducers even simple defects can yield complex patterns of arcs. These arise because signals generated at the separate transducer edges can travel to the defect and back to the receiver as distinct wavepackets without interference, making it appear as though for each pair of probes there were in fact two transmitters and two receivers giving four possible arcs for each defect extremity. These effects are only striking in the near field of the transducers. Figure 2.13 shows schematically the geometry used in the following

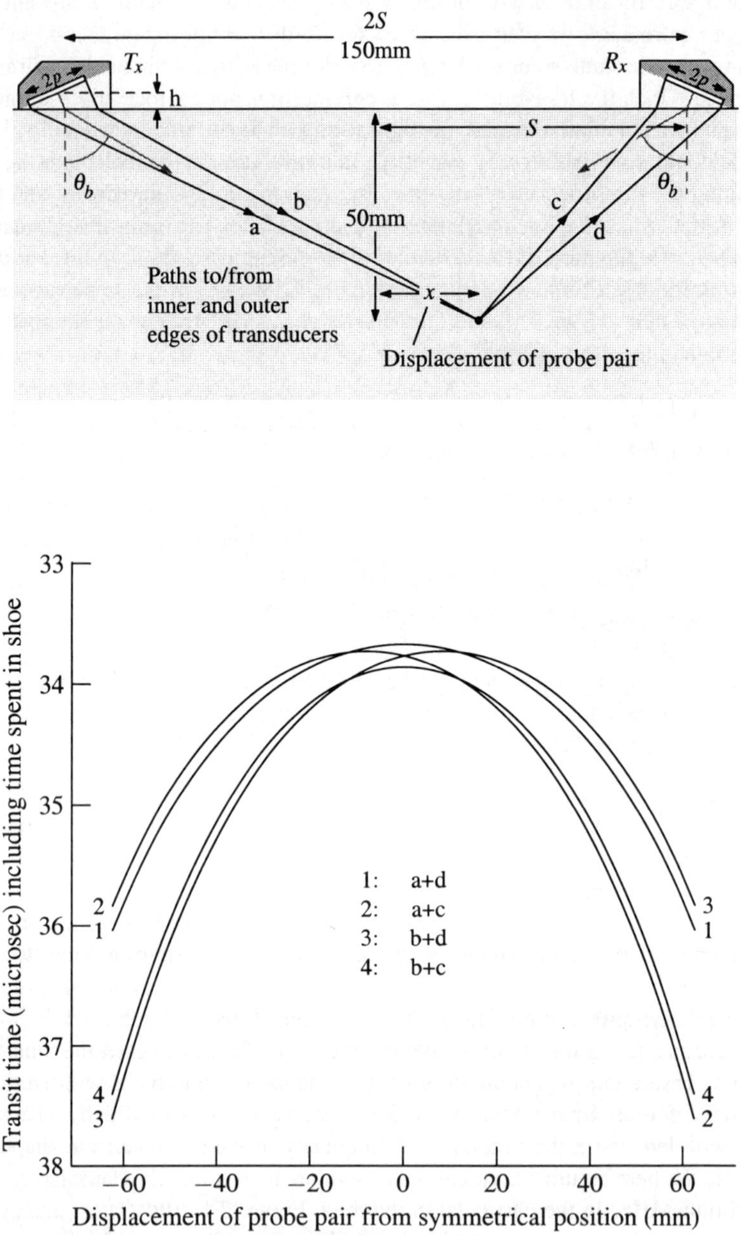


**Fig. 2.13** Multiple arcs produced by the inside and outside edges of the transmitter and receiver probes. The probes are 15 mm in diameter, have a beam angle of 60° and are separated by 150 mm; the defect tip is located 50 mm below the surface.

discussion of the origin of these multiple arcs and shows predictions of their shape for probes of diameter 15 mm, separated by 150 mm, scanning over a point defect 50 mm below the surface. For a crack, there would be a similar pattern of arcs for both the top and bottom crack edges, provided the defect through-wall dimension was greater than the pulse length, or bigger than about $2\lambda$.

In the geometry shown in Figure 2.13 the probes are separated by $2S$ as usual, each probe is of diameter $2p$, the defect is at depth $z$, and $x$ denotes the horizontal distance of the defect from the plane midway between transmitter and receiver, i.e. the offset of the probes from the position of minimum signal travel time. If the full geometry of the probe shoes and the Snell's Law refraction at the workpiece surface is included in the analysis, a solution can only be obtained numerically and that is the way the curves in Figure 2.13 have been calculated. However, an approximate solution can be obtained by using a construction due to Coffey and Chapman [1983], in which the probes and shoe assemblies are replaced by virtual probes of radius $p = a(\cos\theta/\cos\psi)$, where $a$ is the true probe radius and $\theta$ and $\psi$ are the beam angle and shoe angle respectively. The virtual probes are centred at the index points on the workpiece surface, and aligned normal to the beam axes. Paths from these probes to points in the interior of the workpiece are treated as lying entirely within the workpiece material; i.e. the surface is deemed to have been removed.

We define $u = p\sin\theta$ and $v = p\cos\theta$. Then, with these changes, the travel times become $t_i$, with $i = 1,2,3,4$, given by

$$t_i = \frac{1}{C}\sqrt{(S+\alpha_i v+x)^2+(z-\alpha_i u)^2}+\frac{1}{C}\sqrt{(S+\beta_i v-x)^2+(z-\beta_i u)^2} \quad (2.32)$$

where the paths are labelled: $i = 1$ for rays $a+d$, on Figure 2.13, with $\alpha_i = \beta_i = +1$; $i = 2$ for rays $a+c$ with $\alpha_i = +1$, $\beta_i = -1$; $i = 3$ for rays $b+d$ with $\alpha_i = -1$, $\beta_i = +1$; and $i = 4$ for rays $b+d$ with $\alpha_i = \beta_i = -1$. $\theta_b$ is the beam angle. Arcs calculated from these formulae agree very closely in shape with the ones shown in Figure 2.13, but, because the time spent by the ultrasound in the probe shoes has been ignored, they are displaced on the time axis by a constant amount to earlier time.

The arcs themselves show the differences in travel time along the different paths but when considering the effect on the observed signals, the effect of the pulse shape has to be considered. In general, pulses travelling by different paths will overlap and interfere with each other so that the received pulse shape is modified. The precise effects will depend on the fundamental frequency of the pulse and the shape of its envelope. We here assume a typical pulse with an approximately Gaussian envelope centred on 5 MHz. In the particular case which Figure 2.13 illustrates, pairs of arcs are almost coincident over much of their length, so the effect is to split the signal into two arcs each with a pulse shape which differs from the basic pulse shape only in having frequency components which are well above the centre frequency somewhat attenuated. However, where all four arcs cross in the centre, the effects are more severe. Here, destructive interference occurs at the fundamental frequency, leaving a severely distorted pulse with a dominant low frequency component.

These characteristics are borne out in Figure 2.14 which shows such arcs recorded from a block containing side-drilled holes. The upper picture shows the signals obtained from 15 mm diameter transducers. The multiple arcs from the upper surface of the holes reduce the accuracy of depth measurement and the signals from the lower surface of the holes are obscured. A solution, for immersion probes, is to mask the transducer faces with absorbent material such as polytetrafluoroethylene (PTFE) leaving only a small aperture. The aperture can be circular or, to allow more energy through, slot-shaped, with the long axis aligned perpendicular to the plane containing the beam axes. The aperture width defines the transducer width for the calculation of near-field distance and so can be chosen to ensure that the defects of interest are effectively in the far field. The results of masking the transducers with 3 mm wide slots are shown in the lower part of Figure 2.14. The signal arcs from the upper surfaces of the holes are now single and, for the left hand hole, the signal from the lower surface is now clearly defined.

The conclusion is that, for sizing defects at short range, masking the transducer faces will bring improved sizing accuracy, equivalent to the use of smaller diameter transducers. We can go further and state as a general principle that, for best accuracy, the smallest diameter transducers that will provide adequate signal strength should be used.

## 2.4 Alternative Methods of Crack Depth Estimation

Various methods of determining the crack depth based on time-of-flight information are available and do not rely on a symmetrical disposition of the probes around the crack. Curtis and Hawker [1983] and Hawker [1983] used the information from up to 42 combinations of transducer and receiver pairs, out of a total possible 64 combinations, to locate the tips of cracks in all three dimensions by finding the common intersection of the elliptical loci, as shown in Figure 2.12.

Mak [1985] described several theoretical approaches to the identification of the depths of defect features. For a pulse-echo configuration with two transducers separated by an amount $2S$, the depth of the crack tip is found from

$$d = C\sqrt{P_1^2 - \frac{1}{4}\left(\frac{2S}{C^2} + \frac{P_1^2 - P_2^2}{2S}\right)}$$

where $P_1$ and $P_2$ are the pulse-echo travel times from each transducer to the tips of the crack, and $C$ is the propagation speed of elastic waves in the test material. In another method the two transducers are used with one as transmitter and the other as receiver. The travel time around the crack is measured and then the transducers are moved — or more than one pair of transducers is used, and the travel time recorded. If $p_{11}$ and $p_{12}$ are the original locations of transducers, then the crack tip lies on an ellipse with foci $(p_{11}, 0)$ and $(p_{12}, 0)$. If the new locations of the transducers, or the locations of another pair, are $(p_{21}, 0)$ and $(p_{22}, 0)$, then the crack depth is obtained

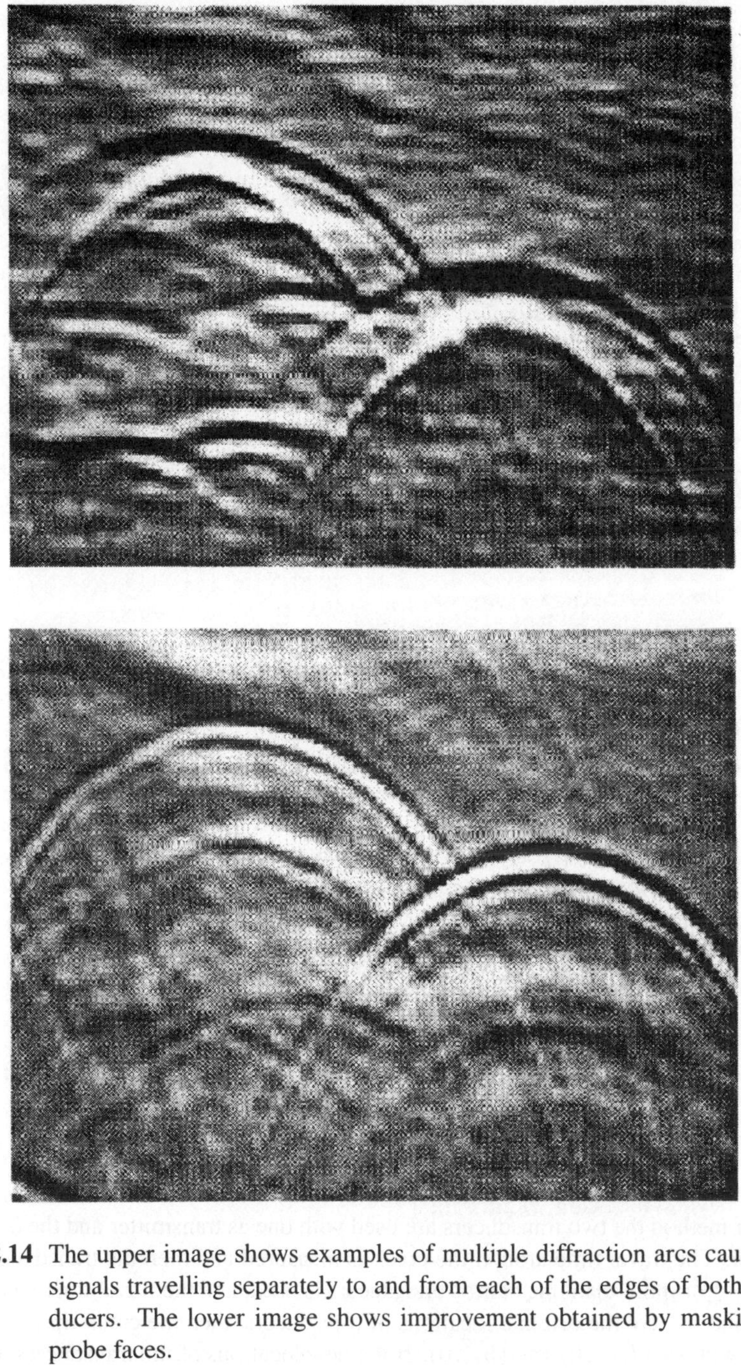

**Fig. 2.14** The upper image shows examples of multiple diffraction arcs caused by signals travelling separately to and from each of the edges of both transducers. The lower image shows improvement obtained by masking the probe faces.

from [Mak, 1985]

$$d = \pm b_1 \sqrt{1 - \frac{(x - x_1^2)}{a_1^2}}$$

where $a_1$ and $b_1$ are the semi-major and semi-minor axes of the ellipse of travel times for the first probe positions. $x_1$ is the centre of the first ellipse (obtained by averaging the locations of the probe centres) and $x$, the location of the crack tip, is obtained as a root of the equation

$$x = \frac{-M_2 \pm \sqrt{M_2^2 - 4L_2N_2}}{2L_2}$$

where

$$L_2 = (a_2b_1 + a_1b_2)(a_2b_2 - a_1b_2)$$

$$M_2 = -2a_2^2b_1^2x_1 + 2a_1^2b_2^2x_2$$

and

$$N_2 = (a_2b_1x_1)^2 + (a_1a_2b_2)^2 - (a_1b_2x_2)^2 - (a_1a_2b_1)^2$$

So far the beam entry points into the material being inspected have been assumed to be fixed on the acoustic axis, that is, on the axis of maximum amplitude in the beam profile. Since use is made of divergent beams to detect cracks which are not on the acoustic axis, it is useful to be able to correct for the actual beam entry points. These will not usually correspond to the acoustic axis marked on the transducers and the error can be large especially for immersion testing. Mak [1986] has presented a numerical scheme for making the necessary correction for either contact or immersion measurements. The numerical scheme is iterative with only five iterations being required in a computer experiment to obtain an accuracy of 0.0001 mm. The model assumes that the sound beam radiates from the centre of the transducer crystal but in practice, experimental errors will depend on how accurately the transducer has been manufactured. For focused probes the sound waves can be considered to radiate from the focal point and time measurements should be made relative to this focal point. Note that while focused probes provide a way of creating a more intense wide angle beam than can be obtained by merely reducing the diameter of a conventional probe, edge-of-beam effects like those discussed in Section 2.3.2.7 can still be expected at angles beyond the beam width.

## 2.5 Single probe techniques

We do not wish to enter into discussion about whether a single-probe technique can properly be called Time-of-Flight Diffraction. In the vast majority of situations, the optimum probe arrangement for efficient deployment of TOFD will involve at least two probes. However, a single probe technique which still aims to rely on diffracted signals can be regarded as a rather special case of TOFD. We report here some early examples of work of this kind, without attempting to give a comprehensive survey.

Early work on single probe techniques was carried out by Hunt [1975] and Miller, Fujczak and Winters [1973] where it was commonly referred to as 'crack-tip reflection' and was reviewed by Silk [1979b], along with some early results obtained at Harwell. Lidington and Silk [1975] used a single surface wave probe to measure crack depth. With these early results Silk obtained an accuracy of about ±1mm although this was less consistent than with two, or more, probes.

Two factors can make accurate depth measurement more difficult with a single probe than with a TOFD probe pair. First, if there is an error in the marking of the probe index point, the calculated depth will be affected more for a single probe than for a TOFD pair, at commonly used beam angles. This is because the probe separation error for a TOFD pair is partly compensated by the effect on the calibration signal (usually the lateral wave). Secondly, with a single probe, the angle from which the signal is coming needs to be accurately known whereas it is irrelevant in a TOFD measurement. Although the beam angle of the probe may have been accurately measured, the variation of diffraction amplitude with angle may mean that the effective beam angle is somewhat different for a crack tip signal.

During inspections of the test-block plates 3 and 4 of the UKAEA Defect Detection Trials (discussed in Section 8.4), both Time-of-Flight Diffraction and 2 MHz twin crystal 70° compression-wave probes were shown to be effective at detecting and sizing a variety of under-clad defects in austenitic-clad ferritic steel. Such an arrangement of materials is commonly found inside steel pressure vessels, particularly in the nuclear industry. However, difficulty was experienced using Time-of-Flight Diffraction to size defects extending less than about 5 mm below the interface between the austenitic cladding and the ferritic base. This is due to the presence of the lateral wave which obscures the tip diffracted signals for defects close to the surface and also to the inherent lack of time resolution near the surface. For defects near the surface, but buried, the defect size was known only to within about 5 mm, although an upper bound was given. If the defect breaks the surface, or for clad plates the interface, then the lateral wave is perturbed and bounds can also be given for the crack through-wall size. One way forward with Time-of-Flight Diffraction is to use just a single probe and make use of the back-diffracted waves from the defect extremities. This has been tried by Bann and Rogerson [1984] and results compared with a twin-crystal 2 MHz 70° compression wave technique. The test block was a ferritic steel block containing a range of elliptical, surface-breaking spark-machined slots simulating under-clad cracks. The slots were all smooth and varied in through-wall extent from 1 mm to 5 mm in four groups with aspect ratios (ratios of length to height) of 1:1, 3:1, 6:1 and 12:1. The test-block was strip clad with a double layer of austenite, the first layer of type 309L and the second layer of type 308L to allow for dilution of the alloy content of the first layer. The final cladding thickness was about 8 mm (±0.5 mm) with an error of form (waviness) to within 0.5 mm over 50 mm and

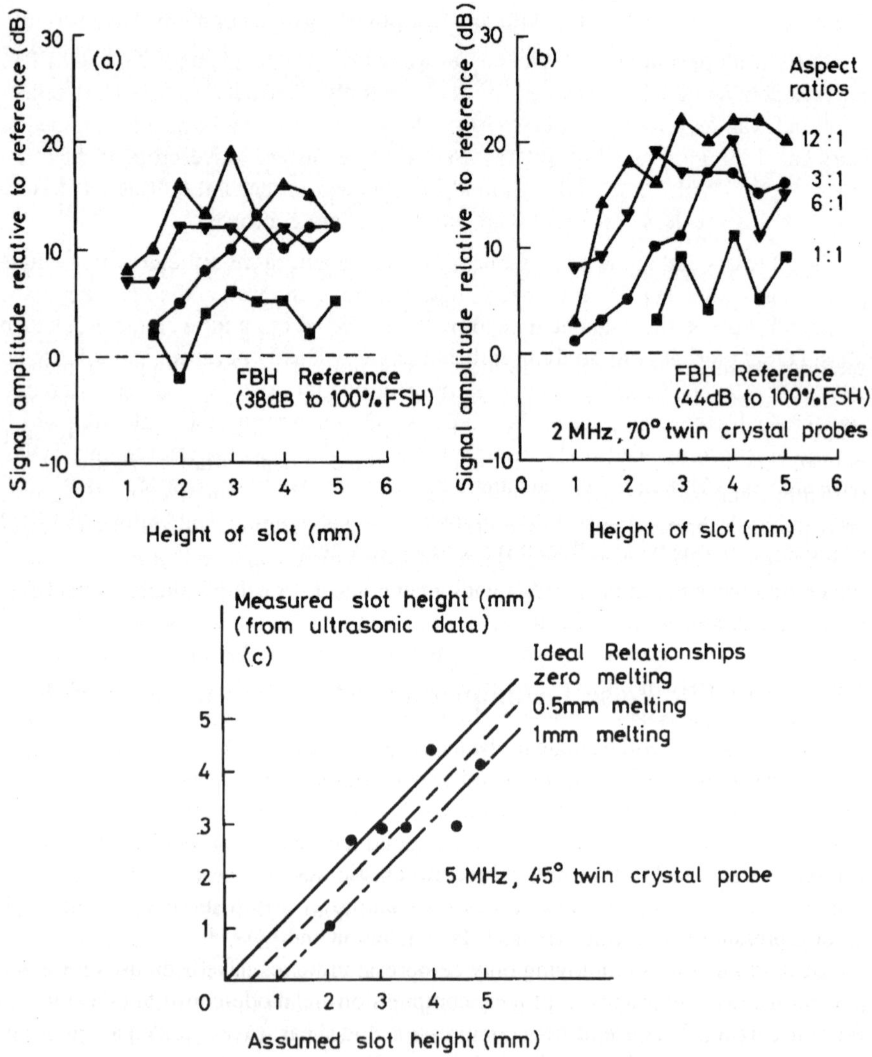


**Fig. 2.15** Comparison of pulse-echo and a single-probe Time-of-Flight technique for sizing under-clad cracks: (a) pulse-echo with a 70° longitudinal wave probe with a focal length of 18 mm, (b) as for (a) but with a focal length of 33 mm, (c) single probe Time-of-Flight Diffraction [from Bann and Rogerson, 1984].

with a surface roughness of 250 CLA (centre-line average in microinches), i.e. about 6.3 μm Ra (average roughness).

The single Time-of-Flight probe used was a twin-crystal 45° compression-wave probe operating at 5 MHz. This probe had a 6 dB beam width of about 3 mm, over the depth range 5 – 15 mm, and a pulse length short enough to enable spatial resolution of crack tip diffracted signals from slots extending both into the cladding and into the parent plate.

Initial results from the single probe showed that the as-clad surface finish introduced spurious signals and the surface finish was, therefore, hand ground to an improved finish. Results for measured versus intended defect depth, for the different techniques, are presented in Figure 2.15.

Bann and Rogerson [1984] reported only the intended defect sizes, as the actual defect sizes had not been determined at that time by destructive examination. It is possible that the actual slot heights differ from those intended due to base metal melting, so in Figure 2.15(c) the ideal correlations for fixed amounts of melting of 0.5 mm and 1 mm are shown along with the ideal correlation for zero melting. Another factor not taken account of in the results is a possible variation in water gap between the immersion probe and the clad surface. Local variations in this gap of 0.25 mm could lead to variations in the estimated crack tip depth of 1 mm. Ultrasonic velocity variations and path length variations in the cladding can add further errors (see Section 7.1.5). Nevertheless, Bann and Rogerson concluded that sizing of small under-clad flaws might be possible with greater accuracy using a single probe Time-of-Flight technique.

## 2.5.1 Satellite Pulse Techniques and SLIC transducer modules

An improvement over the single probe techniques discussed above is to use two crystals, or two transducers, both mounted on a common perspex (lucite) shoe. This is the basis of the patented SLIC transducers developed by Southwest Research Institute, Texas. SLIC stands for Shear and Longitudinal Inspection for Cracks. Separate transducers are used to transmit and receive elastic waves. These multi-beam detection and sizing tools have been successfully employed for in-service inspections of reactor pressure vessel components [Flach, Clayton and Lagleder, 1985].

SLIC-40 modules employing only compression waves have been used for crack detection and novel probes employing compression and mode-converted shear waves for crack sizing. This use of both compression and shear waves yielded a larger separation between the pulses and hence better resolution. Other designs tested included modules employing only shear waves.

The SLIC-50 sizing module has been successfully used to size near-surface and under-clad fatigue cracks in clad pressure vessel test-blocks [Gruber and Hendrix, 1984]. Compression waves were used to insonify the cracks. A diffracted compression wave is received from the top of the crack and a mode-converted, shear wave is diffracted by the bottom of the crack. The through-wall size of the crack can be derived from the time difference between these two pulses. The signals from the SLIC modules are displayed as a plot of colour-coded signal amplitude against transducer

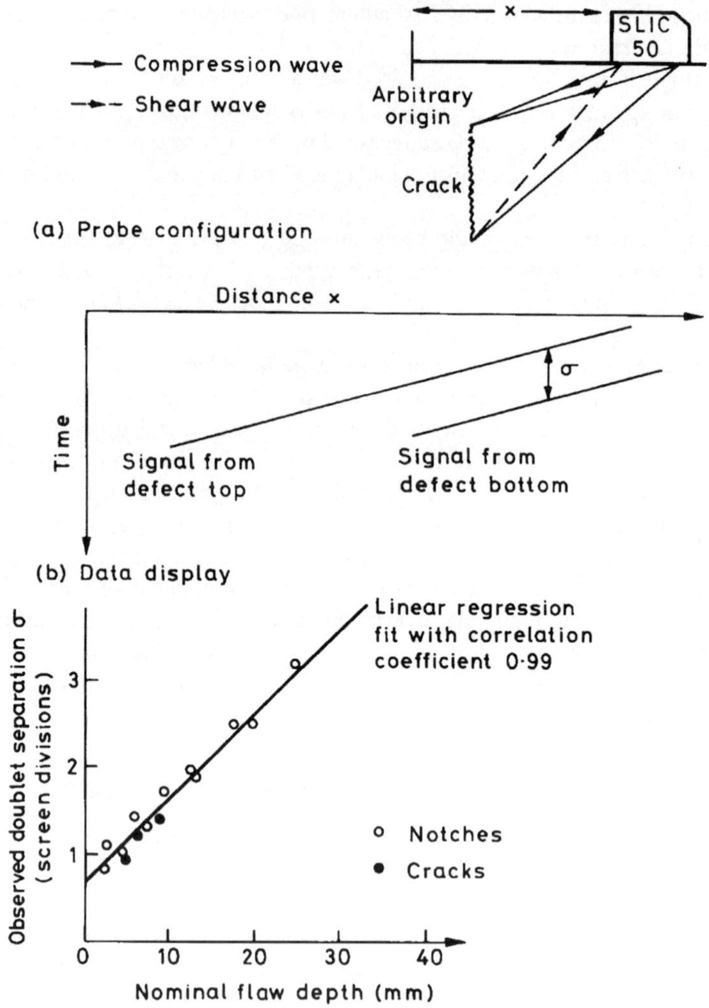


**Fig. 2.16** Typical display from an inspection with SLIC-50 ultrasonic probes.

position and time-of-flight as illustrated schematically in Figure 2.16. The separation a between the two pulses is almost independent of the probe scan position relative to the crack although the value used is that when the pulse from the crack bottom attains its peak amplitude.

Automated interpretation of the images produced with automated scanning equipment employing the SLIC modules has also been performed [Gruber, Hamlin, Grothues and Jackson, 1986]. This opens up the real possibility of automated detection and assessment of cracks during an in-service inspection.

### 2.5.2 ALOK evaluation of time-of-flight data

Time-of-flight information is used in a different way in the ALOK method of extracting information on defects. ALOK, or *Amplituden und Laufzeit Orts Kurwen* (amplitude and transit time locus curves), relies on the simultaneous storage of signal amplitude from conventional 45°, 60°, or 70° probes, together with the time of flight of the signals in pulse-echo or tandem scans. The time domain information is used to eliminate some noise signals by filtering to retain only those time-of-flight locus curves which are hyperbolae. This can lead to a signal-to-noise ratio improvement of up to 20 dB [Barbian, Engl, Grohs, Rathgeb and Wüstenberg, 1984a]. Two methods are used within ALOK for reconstruction of flaws. First, a simple geometric method employing pulse-echo information is used. The locus of the time of flight is assumed to be a circle with centre the beam entry point whereas in the tandem technique the locus is an ellipse. The intersections of all such loci derived from scanning the probe or probes over the component surface yields a reconstruction of the defect extremities. Inversion is carried out by comparison of these loci with calculated loci from postulated defects whose parameters are varied until coincidence is achieved. More detail is given by Barbian, Grohs and Kappes [1984b] and by Grohs, Barbian and Kappes [1983].

# Chapter 3

# Signal Amplitudes and Comparison with other Techniques

As we have already discussed, Time-of-Flight Diffraction makes use of the signals diffracted by the extremities of defects, in particular by crack tips. Although, unlike pulse-echo ultrasonic techniques, signal amplitude is not used as a measure of defect size, signals must be large enough to be observable. It is also useful to understand: how this amplitude might be affected by a variety of factors, such as the angle of the incident ultrasonic beam with respect to the plane of the crack; what happens if the crack is skewed so that the plane of the crack is not normal to the line joining transmitter and receiver transducers; and how large are the signals relative to more familiar signals such as those from a small flat bottomed hole. We can build this understanding through a mathematical model of the underlying physical processes.

In this chapter we present predictions, based on just such a mathematical model, of the magnitude of Time-of-Flight Diffraction signals, compared with those from a reference reflector. We use a model for two reasons. First, it is much easier to vary the parameters of defects within a model than it is experimentally with test-blocks. Secondly, it is possible to isolate the different factors influencing the outcome in a more straightforward way. The theoretical predictions are compared with experimental data as appropriate.

The results of these calculations illustrate how the signals from a variety of crack-like defects are expected to vary with the shape, size and orientation of the defect and highlight one of the strengths of the technique: its relative insensitivity to the orientation of cracks.

The first results we shall present are for the case in which the centre of a planar crack and the centres of both transmitter and receiver lie in the same plane, normal to the inspection surface. This is not a severe restriction, since in almost all cases the probes will be scanned over the defective region and this configuration will be passed through during the scan. Sometimes the shape of the component may preclude reaching such a position and so we later present results applicable to less restricted geometry.

## 3.1 Time-of-Flight Diffraction signals from smooth flat cracks

The model is based on the Geometrical Theory of Diffraction first propounded by Keller [1957, 1962]. This is a high frequency theory in which elastic wave energy propagates along rays which are reflected, refracted and transmitted at boundaries between media according to the usual laws of ray theories familiar from optics. At the edges of boundaries (e.g. on a crack edge) diffraction occurs and this too can be treated in ray theory with diffraction coefficients replacing the reflection and transmission coefficients. The Geometrical Theory of Diffraction applied to elastic wave propagation is discussed by Karal and Keller [1959, and references therein]. The theory uses the solution to a canonical problem to derive the coefficients from an expansion, in inverse powers of $ka$, of the amplitude of waves diffracted from an edge of a defect of arbitrary shape; here $k$ is the ultrasonic wavevector and $a$ is the characteristic dimension of the scatterer. The usefulness of this model is apparent if we consider ultrasonic NDT, where a typical crack size will generally be larger than a wavelength or two, often much larger, making $ka > 1$, and often $ka \gg 1$, so that only the first few terms are important. Often the first term in this expansion, known as an asymptotic expansion, gives the readily observable effects.

Since we shall present the results of some model calculations using this theory, it is outlined in Section A.3 of the Appendix, but only the results are given in this present chapter.

### 3.1.1 Optimum beam angles

The radiation pattern of the diffracted sound field was referred to in Section 2.2.1 and is given in detail in the Appendix (Section A.4). In this section we consider optimisation of the technique in terms of the angle of the beam required in the component to achieve the best trade-off between signal amplitudes and depth resolution.

The equipment will normally be set up so that any cracks will pass midway between at least one pair of transmitter and receiver transducers at some point in the scan. This is easy to achieve if any cracks are likely to be confined to a well defined region such as a weld. To achieve adequate coverage of regions with large depth or width, several transmitter- receiver pairs may be needed. The design of multiprobe arrays is discussed in Section 4.1.2 and the results obtained with such arrays in the Defect Detection Trials are described in Section 8.4.

Although amplitude is not used explicitly to determine the through-wall depth and extent of cracks, nevertheless it is essential to have sufficient amplitude for the signals to be detectable above the noise level. It is desirable, therefore, to use the maximum signal, subject to any constraints on component geometry and access. In Figure 3.1 the variation in amplitude from the top and bottom of a strip-like crack located midway between two transducers is shown as a function of the beam angle of the transducers. As this beam angle approaches 90°, so the transducers approach infinity and the depth of the crack tips from the inspection surface vanishes. This seems, at first sight, to be a rather questionable procedure, but it mimics the actual situation in a flat component and it makes the optimisation a function of a single variable, the beam angle, and hence mathematically simpler. From Figure 3.1, we see that the amplitude does exhibit a definite maximum at around 70° in steel. On the same figure the resolution of the technique for 5 MHz ultrasound in steel, copied from Figure 2.9, is plotted as a dashed line, and this rises sharply for a beam angle of about 75° or greater. This shows that beam angles of between about 60° and 75° produce good resolution and adequate amplitude. Design of the flat plate scanners in the Defect Detection Trials was based on this result [Charlesworth and Hawker, 1984; Curtis and Hawker, 1983; Stringfellow and Perring, 1984] and is discussed in Chapter 4.

The corresponding results for shear waves were found to be an optimum angle, in steel, of between 50° and 55° for the top and bottom of a vertical planar crack [Ogilvy and Temple, 1983].

Measurements, with a specially designed goniometer, of the amplitude of compression waves diffracted into compression waves have been carried out by Golan [1981]; Golan, Adler, Cook, Nanstad and Bolland [1980], who found that the amplitude peaked when the angle between the incident and diffracted beams approaches 180°. This is expected, since it corresponds to the straight-through signal. For other dispositions of the probes around the spark cut slit Golan found evidence of signal peaks around a beam angle of 60°.

### 3.1.2 Magnitude and variation of diffracted signal amplitudes

Techniques, such as ultrasonic pulse-echo or tandem, which have been used traditionally for detection and sizing of cracks are based on specular reflection from the face of the crack. With point transducers and a perfectly smooth planar defect of infinite extent, a specular reflection would occur only at the unique angle where the angles of incidence and reflection at the defect are equal. In practice, because of the finite aperture and broad bandwidth of the transducers and the finite size and imperfect smoothness of the defect, a 'specular' reflection will occur over a small range of angles, though still with a well defined central maximum. However, once the orientation of the crack is a few degrees away from the specular orientation the amplitude at the transducer will fall rapidly as the amount of misorientation increases.This is illustrated in Figure 3.2, taken from Toft [1987], which shows experimental values of signal strength in pulse-echo inspections of circular defects as a function of both tilt and skew of the defect. It can be seen that a misorientation of the defect of about 15°, of either tilt or skew, or a combination of the two giving a similar angle between the normal to the defect and the transducer beam axis, gives a signal strength reduced by 6 dB from the perfect orientation. Time-of-Flight Diffraction signals, as

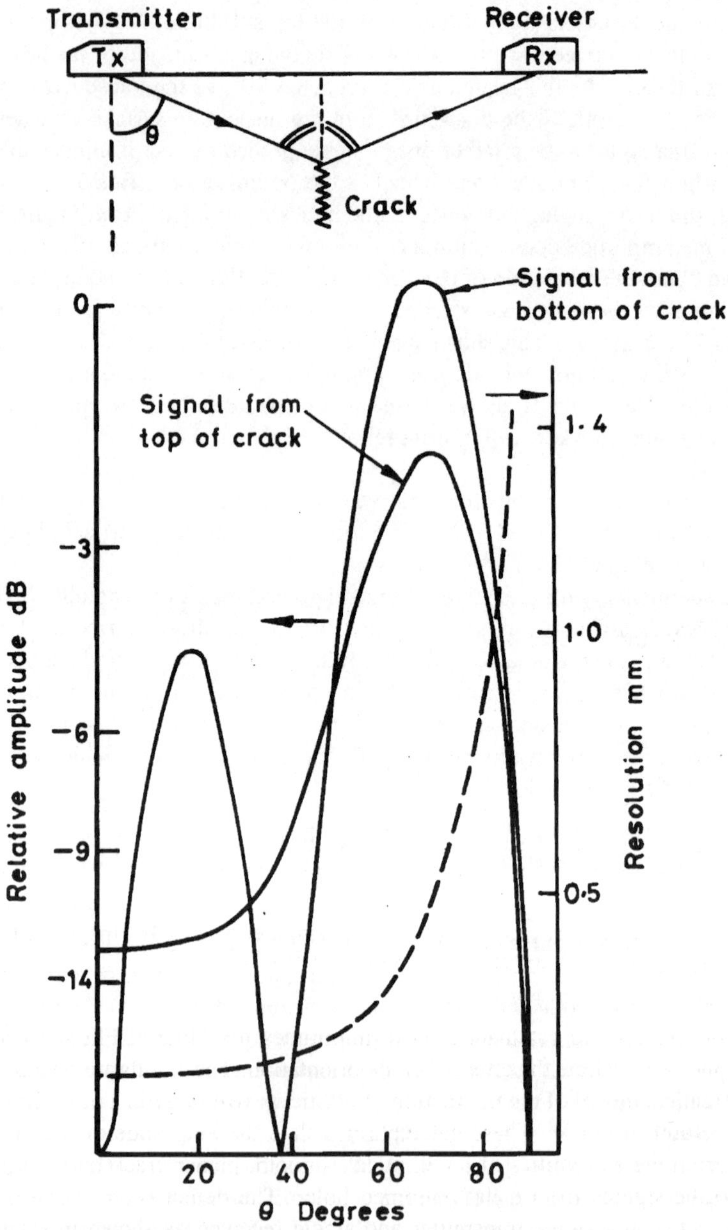


**Fig. 3.1** Optimisation of transducer beam angles for Time-of-Flight Diffraction in steel using compression waves. The effects of beam angle on resolution are also shown. At $\theta = 90°$ the transducers are infinitely far apart.

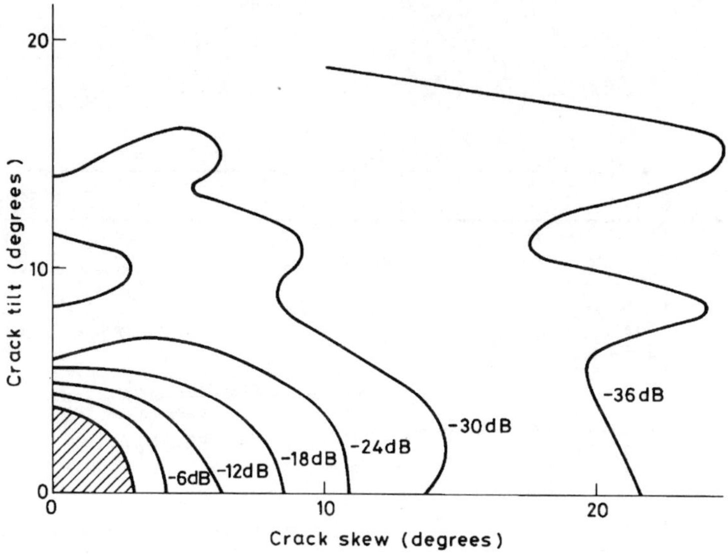


**Fig. 3.2** The effect of crack tilt and skew on signal amplitudes from a 25 mm diameter circular defect with pulse-echo inspection. The hatched region has a signal level of at least 36 dB above 10% DAC (distance-amplitude correction). The other contours are relative to this level. [After Toft, 1987].

we shall see in Section 3.3, drop by 6 dB after only 45° – 60° of skew, and often increase rather than decrease with crack tilt. To ensure adequate sensitivity, using pulse-echo techniques, when inspecting a component which may contain defects at a range of angles, it is necessary to use several probes at different angles. This is the basis of the American Society of Mechanical Engineers (ASME) inspections which require inspection at 0°, 45° and 60° [ASME, 1974,1977,1983] and which are often supplemented by 70° probes.

In this section we calculate typical amplitudes for Time-of-Flight Diffraction signals and demonstrate the effect of crack orientation. The results are obtained from a mathematical model of the interaction of elastic wave energy in a transducer beam with an elliptical crack. These calculations relate the amplitude of the diffracted signals from the extremities of an elliptical, smooth, planar crack buried in a steel plate, to the signals from a flat-bottomed hole. The defect centre is taken to lie midway between a single transmitter and single receiver, as shown in Figure 3.3, and the amplitude of diffracted signals is calculated as a function of the tilt of the crack. This tilt $\varepsilon$ is measured away from the normal to the inspection surface so that $\varepsilon = 0$ corresponds to a crack in a vertical plane in Figure 3.3. The Time-of-Flight Diffraction signal amplitudes from this geometry are compared with those obtained when the same probes, with the same separation $S$, are positioned over a

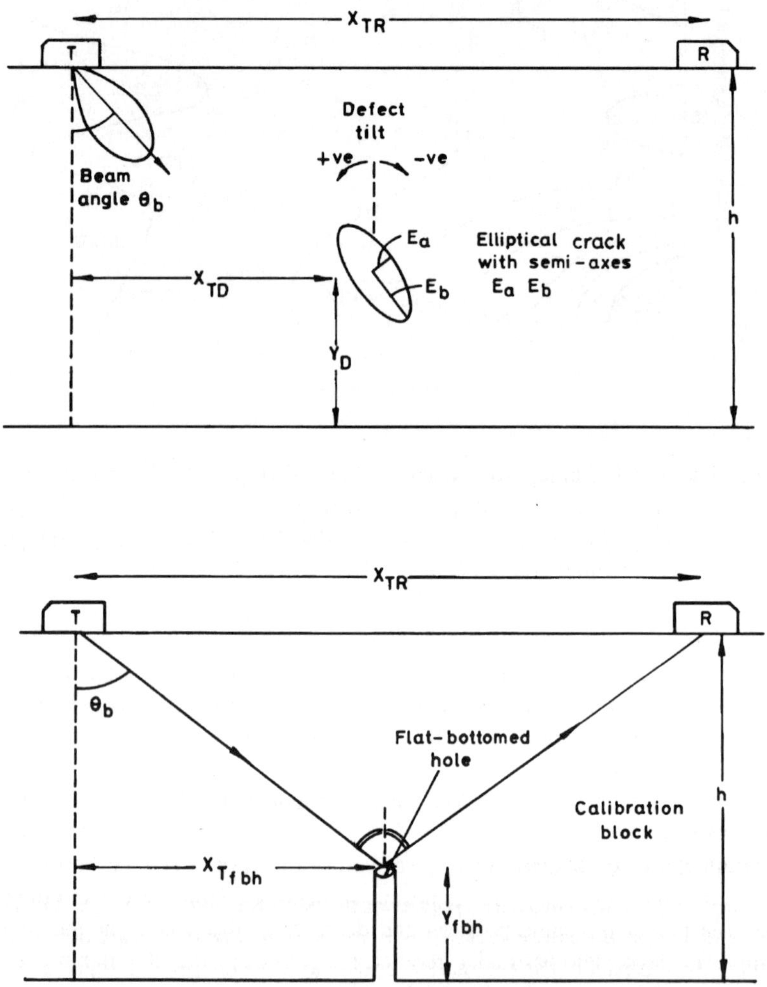


**Fig. 3.3** Geometry used in the mathematical model to predict Time-of-Flight Diffraction responses from elliptical, planar cracks.

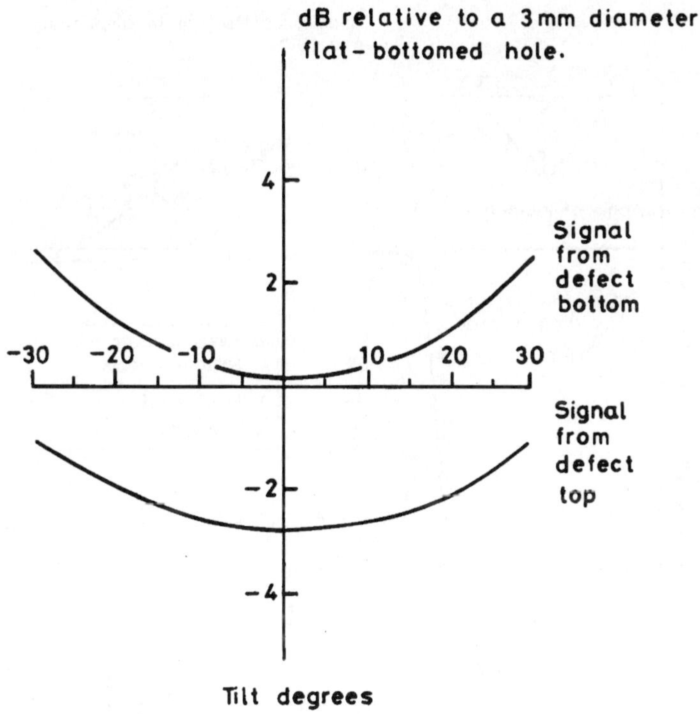


**Fig. 3.4** Variation of Time-of-Flight Diffraction signals with tilt for an elliptical defect 24 mm by 60 mm, located 220 mm below the inspection surface. The calibration reflector is a flat-bottomed hole located midway between transmitter and receiver and 220 mm deep, with the flat end parallel to the inspection surface.

flat-bottomed hole, as shown in the lower part of the figure. The flat-bottomed hole is assumed to have an axis which is normal to the inspection surface and the centre of the hole lies at the same position and depth from the surface as the centre of the elliptical crack. The particular geometry is chosen so that the maximum signal possible from the flat-bottomed hole is used in the comparison, i.e. the calibration signal is obtained by specular reflection at the flat-bottomed hole.

The transducer beam has a central maximum lying along a direction at angle $\theta_b$ to the normal to the inspection surface, and spreads out with the usual Bessel function form appropriate for a circular piston source (see Section A.3.2 of the Appendix). Details of the calculations are given in Temple [1984a] and some typical results are presented in Figure 3.4. In this figure, the crack is taken to be a smooth, planar, elliptical crack with through-wall extent $2a = 24$ mm and length, parallel to the inspection surface, of $2b = 60$ mm, buried at a depth of 220 mm from the inspec-

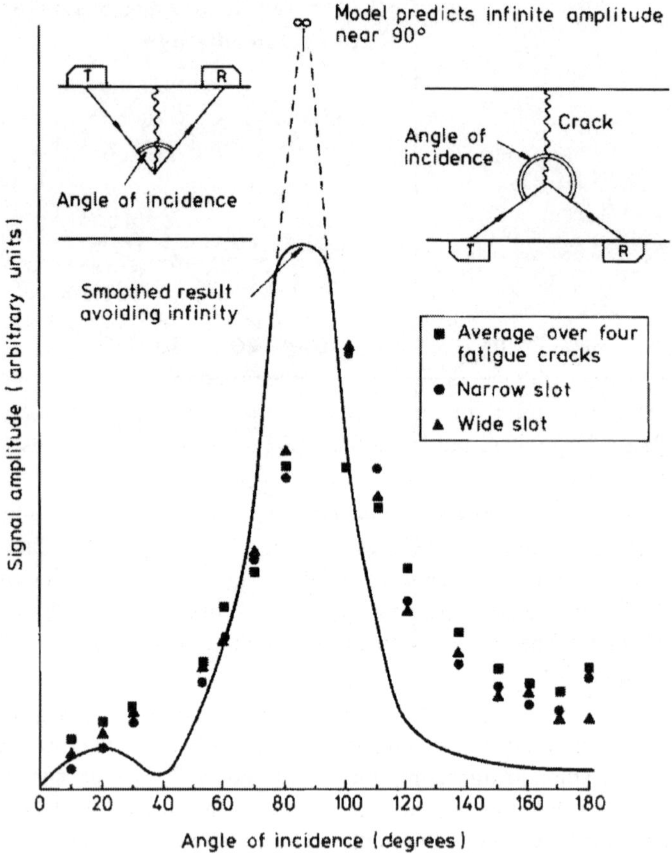


**Fig. 3.5** Comparison of experimentally determined Time-of-Flight Diffraction signal amplitudes with theoretical predictions. The experimental results (from Silk [1979f]) are for narrow (0.5 mm) slits and for wide (2 mm) slits. Theoretical values for the wide slit are adjusted to have the same value as for the narrow slit for 60° incidence.

tion surface. The transducers have circular faces with diameter 24 mm and operate at a frequency of 5 MHz in such a way as to produce maximum amplitude travelling at 60° to the normal to the surface. The host material is taken to be isotropic steel and the two transducers are separated by 762 mm. The reference reflector is a 3 mm diameter flat-bottomed hole. Figure 3.4 [based on Temple, 1984a] shows how the diffracted signal varies as the tilt varies between $-30^\circ \leq \varepsilon \leq +30^\circ$. Two things are important about this figure. First, the amplitudes of the diffracted signals are both comparable with that from a 3 mm diameter flat-bottomed hole at the same range, and, second the signal improves as the tilt of the defect increases. The reason for this latter point is, of course, that the signal is at a minimum value for a vertical crack and so must increase with tilt angle. It would become a specular reflection, like that from the flat-bottomed hole, as $\varepsilon \rightarrow 90°$ and the ratio of the two signals would simply approach the ratio of their areas. For the particular crack chosen in this example, this would yield a maximum signal of 32 dB for a tilt of 90°. This result, for crack tilts of up to 30°, demonstrates how relatively insensitive the Time-of-Flight Diffraction technique is to crack orientation.

Temple [1983a,b] also showed how the signal varies as the crack position relative to the two transducers changes. It was shown that the signals from the defect considered above, and shown in Figure 3.4, would only have fallen to 10 dB below those from a symmetrically placed 3 mm diameter flat-bottomed hole even if the crack were 30 mm off the symmetric position between the probes. This result also demonstrates the versatility and utility of the Time-of-Flight Diffraction technique. Calculations similar to these but for different defect parameters have also been presented [Temple, 1983b].

In the model, the crack is taken to be a cut in the material of zero width but with non- interacting faces on which the stress vanishes. This is an idealised model and it is obviously interesting to compare the predictions of the model with experimental evidence. To do this we use experimental results of Silk [1977, 1979b] on both saw cuts and real cracks. The saw cuts were of two widths, 0.5 mm and 2 mm. The results are given in Figure 3.5.

In the top part of the figure the experimental geometry is defined. Results for diffracted signal amplitudes from the two saw cuts are given in the lower part of the figure and the variation in signal amplitude averaged over four cracks is also shown. The model is not valid at angles close to specular, that is near 90°, but gives fairly good agreement over the remaining range. The experimental signal amplitudes are higher than those predicted, over a good deal of the angular range, especially for diffraction by the top of a crack, and this may be a result of the blunt tips of the slit defects used. According to theory, the amplitude from the bottom of the defect should go to zero and the phase of the signal change by $\pi$ at an angle which depends on Poisson's ratio for the material and would be about 38° for steel (see Section A.4). However, neither a zero nor a minimum signal was observed experimentally and if any change of phase was present, it was not recorded. It has proved very difficult to detect this phenomenon, using conventional broad-band, finite size transducers and artificial defects. With a laser beam as the source of ultrasound and a capacitance transducer as receiver, however, Scruby and Newton [1986] were able to confirm the change of phase and hence the mathematical zero in amplitude.

Using the same laser technique, Ravenscroft et al. [1991] carried out a very detailed investigation of the diffraction response of both slots and cracks in steel blocks and were able to explain why previous experiments had usually not detected a minimum. Using an open fatigue crack, they obtained a very clear minimum amplitude at 38°, with a phase change of close to 180°, and excellent agreement with theoretical amplitudes at all angles in the ranges 20° – 80° and 120° – 160°. These results are

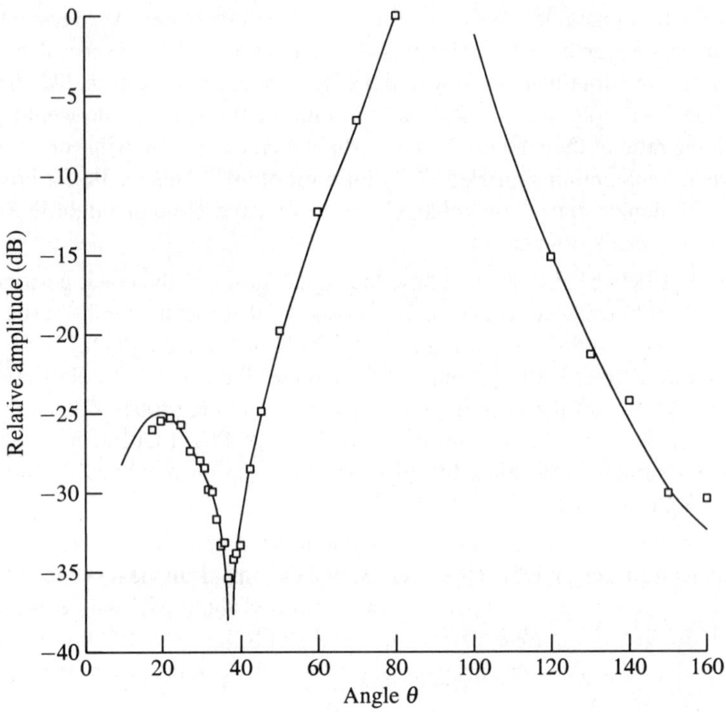


**Fig. 3.6** Comparison of theoretical predictions with measured signal amplitudes from an open fatigue crack, using a laser beam as the source of ultrasound and a capacitance transducer as a detector. Reprinted from *Ultrasonics* **29**, F. A. Ravenscroft, K. Newton and C. B. Scruby, 29–37, Copyright 1991, with permission from Elsevier Science .

reproduced in Figure 3.6. They also showed that the phase change is obscured if the defect tip is blunt, which may explain why earlier attempts to confirm it failed.

### 3.1.3 Calibration reflector

For Time-of-Flight geometries, and for the calculations used here, the signals are measured relative to those from a flat-bottomed hole situated symmetrically between the transmitter and receiver and with the flat surface of the reflector horizontal so that the maximum signal is transferred by the calibration reflector to the receiver [Temple, 1984a]. To complete our description of the model used, we outline in Section A.3.3 of the Appendix how the amplitude from the calibration reflector is calculated.

To convert the signal amplitudes from those relative to a flat-bottomed hole calibration reflector to those measured relative to a side-drilled hole reflector, we use the relationship [Bowker, Chapman and Wrigley, 1985] that the signal strengths differ by a factor of:

$$Signal_{sdh} = Signal_{fbh} + 20\log_{10}\left[\frac{2\pi a_{fbh}^2}{\lambda\sqrt{ra_{sdh}}}\right] \tag{3.1}$$

where $a_{fbh}$ and $a_{sdh}$ are the radii of the flat-bottomed and side-drilled holes respectively, the range from the transmitter is $r$ and the signals are measured in dB. The wavelength of the ultrasound is $\lambda$. Note that as $r$ is greater than the dimensions of the calibration reflectors, the correction is actually negative so that the signals measured relative to a side-drilled hole are smaller than those measured relative to a flat-bottomed hole. Typical values of this difference in these calculations are about 10 dB. Results are given in Temple [1987] for signal amplitudes from some typical defects, taken from the PISC II parametric studies [see Oliver, 1984, for the background to PISC II]. The signals from the defects are compared with those from flat-bottomed hole reflectors and results are given for conventional pulse-echo techniques as well as for Time-of-Flight Diffraction.

## 3.2 Signal amplitudes compared with those generated by other techniques

In Section 3.1.2, variations of Time-of-Flight Diffraction signals with parameters of the defect, such as tilt or position, were considered. In this section we shall compare predicted amplitudes of Time-of-Flight Diffraction signals with those from conventional pulse-echo techniques.

### 3.2.1 The defects

The most serious defect in a stressed component is a crack oriented perpendicular to the principal stress. Many cracks, for example lack of weld fusion and some fatigue cracks, are smooth in an ultrasonic sense; that is, with roughnesses which are much less than the ultrasonic wavelength. A root mean square roughness less than $\lambda/20$ is ultrasonically smooth (i.e. it produces negligible diffuse scattering) while a roughness greater than $\lambda/5$ is very rough [Ogilvy, 1987]. Roughness on the faces of certain fatigue cracks is on a scale less than $\lambda/20$ at typical frequencies of 2 to 5 MHz and, therefore, hardly affects the ultrasonic signal from the defect. The simplest mathematical model of such a crack is of a completely smooth planar cut in the material properties. The surfaces of this model defect are taken to be stress-free and non-interacting.

As a part of the PISC II international collaboration, model defects, of certain specific sizes, were inserted into steel blocks and the ultrasonic response from them determined experimentally with a number of scans using differing ultrasonic probe configurations. These experiments have been directed towards testing existing theoretical models. The cracks used have through-wall extents in the range 10 to 25 mm, and most are oriented in planes normal to the inspection surface. Since in laboratory experiments such as these the inspection surface will be horizontal, the defect planes are vertical. One defect is tilted by $\pm 7^\circ$ away from this vertical direction.

The plates into which these defects have been inserted are about 200 mm thick and so are representative of the pressure vessel of a pressurised water reactor. The shapes of defect chosen correspond to what can be easily modelled: thin parallel edged ribbon cracks and thin, circular cracks.

In what follows, we present model predictions for the behaviour of the ultrasonic response from certain of these types of defect.

### 3.2.2 The transducer scans

The transducers parameters selected are 2 MHz probes producing shear (SV) waves at angles of 45°, 60° and 70° respectively. The crystals in the probes are rectangular, 20 mm wide by 22 mm high. Probes with such typical parameters used in practice might be Krautkrämer WB 45 N2, WB 60 N2, and WB 70 N2 which have near-field lengths of 90 mm and a far field resolution of about 4 mm. The 45°, 60° and 70° probes are scanned in pulse-echo mode along a single scan line which passes directly over the centre of the defect and in the same plane as the normal to the defect surface.

### 3.2.3 The calibration signals

The signals from the defects are compared with those from a 3 mm diameter flat-bottomed hole oriented normal to the transducer beam profile maximum. The geometry of the two calibration calculations is shown schematically in Figure 3.7. The peak amplitudes are recorded for pulse-echo and Time-of-Flight Diffraction inspections in Table 3.1.

In the table, signal amplitudes are in decibels relative to those from a 3 mm diameter flat-bottomed hole at the same depth below the inspection surface as the centre of the defect. For Time-of-Flight Diffraction the flat surface of the calibration reflector is parallel to the inspection surface, and for pulse-echo the flat face of the calibration reflector is normal to the transducer beam centreline. The pulse-echo inspections are all SV waves.

### 3.2.4 Resolution of diffracted signals in pulse-echo

For short pulse operation, the signal amplitudes in Table 3.1 are thought of as being those appropriate to the part of the frequency spectrum in which there is maximum amplitude. The calculations reported here for pulse-echo examination of ribbon and circular cracks are for signals returned to the transducer at angles well away from specular reflection at the defect, and because the ray paths from the transmitter to the defect extremities differ by more than about 2 wavelengths, the signals observed will be resolved in time and will not, therefore, suffer from interference.

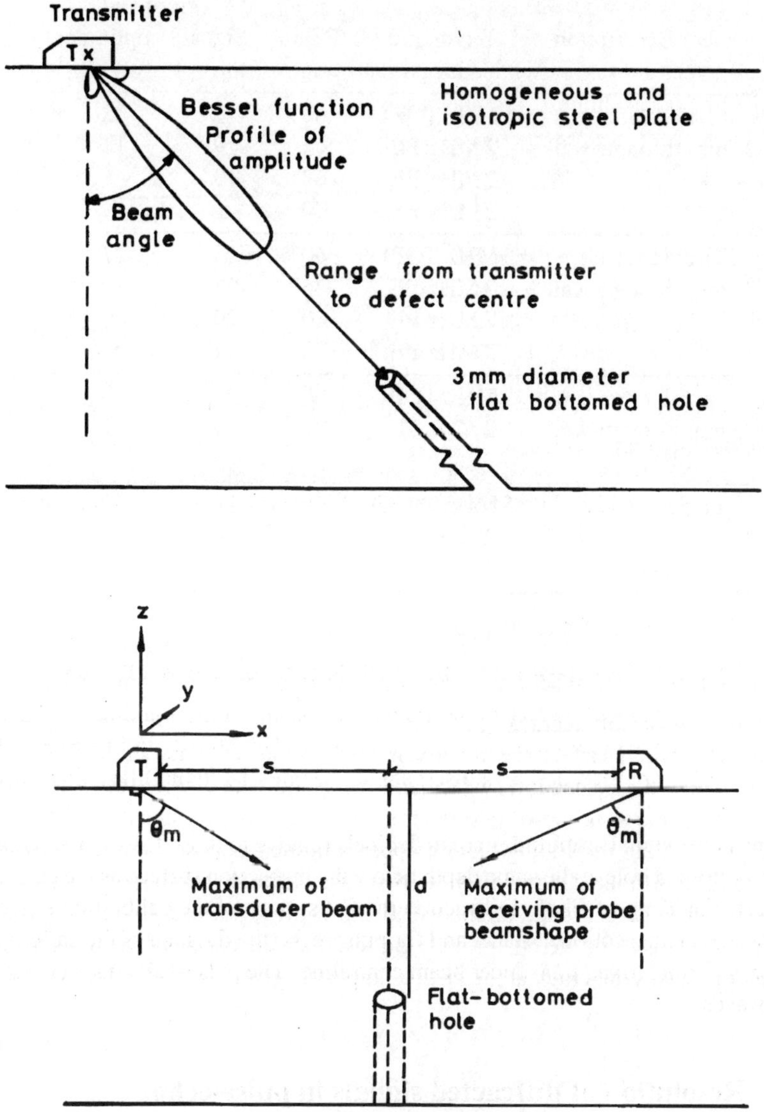


**Fig. 3.7** Geometry of calibration reflectors for pulse-echo and Time-of-Flight Diffraction inspections.

**Table 3.1** Predicted time-of-flight and pulse-echo amplitudes

| Defect Description | Technique | Beam angle | Predicted Signal Amplitudes top | bottom |
|---|---|---|---|---|
| vertical ribbon | 5 MHz TOFD | 60° | -18 | -22 |
| 25 mm through-wall | 2 MHz PE | 45° | -19 | -11 |
| | 2 MHz PE | 60° | -13 | -3 |
| | 2 MHz PE | 70° | -6 | -1 |
| circular crack | 5 MHz TOFD | 60° | -25 | -27 |
| 25 mm through-wall | 2 MHz PE | 45° | -28 | -19 |
| | 2 MHz PE | 60° | -20 | -10 |
| | 2 MHz PE | 70° | -14 | -8 |
| circular crack | 5 MHz TOFD | 60° | -27 | -30 |
| 25 mm through-wall | 2 MHz PE | 70° | -19 | -11 |
| tilted 7° | | | | |
| circular crack | 5 MHz TOFD | 60° | -27 | -30 |
| 25 mm through-wall | 2 MHz PE | 70° | -7 | -4 |
| tilted 7° | | | | |

### 3.2.5 Pulse-echo inspection of ribbon and circular cracks

We consider first a ribbon crack of 25 mm through-wall extent, lying in a plane normal to the inspection surface (i.e. a vertical crack in the geometry shown) at a depth of 82 mm below the inspection surface and inspected with 2 MHz, 60° shear-wave probes. The geometry is shown in Figure 3.8 together with the signal amplitudes.

In Figure 3.8, an interesting feature appears in the response from the bottom of the defect. The diffracted signal in these two cases is predicted to have a small lobe at a transducer to defect range of about 140 mm. This is marked A in the figure. At this particular range, for the 60° probes, the ray from the centre of the transducer to the crack tip strikes the crack at the critical angle, $\theta_c$ given by Snell's law as

$$\theta_c = \sin^{-1}\left[\frac{C_s}{C_p}\right] \tag{3.2}$$

where $C_s$ and $C_p$ are the speeds of shear and compression waves in the test piece. For steel $\theta_c$ is about 33°. Below the critical angle, an incident shear wave is reflected into compression and shear components at different angles. Above this critical angle, however, while the reflected shear wave is still present, the compression wave cannot propagate and is said to be *evanescent.*

For a circular defect of the same through-wall extent, all the signals are decreased by 8 – 10 dB from those from a vertical ribbon defect.

The vertical orientation of the previous defects is well away from the ideal ori-

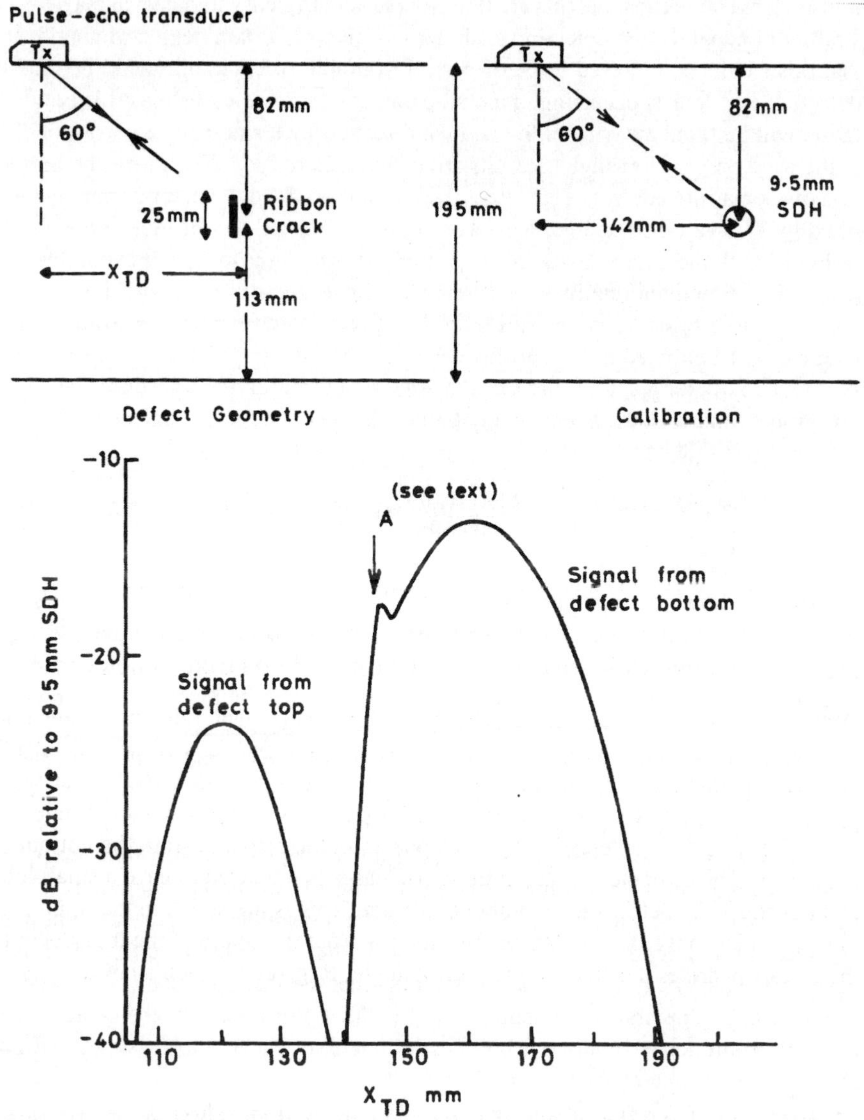


**Fig. 3.8** Pulse-echo response with 2 MHz 60° shear-wave probes for a vertical ribbon crack 25 mm high located 82 mm below the inspection surface. Results are relative to 100% DAC.

entation for effective pulse-echo inspections. Ideally, the crack should be normal to the interrogating ultrasonic beam in order to return a large specular signal to the transducer. The vertical defects are thus not particularly easy to detect and a demonstration of capability in detecting such defects gives a certain degree of confidence that other defects, believed to be of more favourable orientation, would be readily detected. For defects occurring in the preparation of a V-weld, the most likely orientation will be tilted away from the vertical direction by a small angle corresponding to the weld preparation angle. Results are included here for a 70° pulse-echo inspection of such a tilted defect. The defect is a circular crack of diameter 25 mm and it is tilted by 7° away from the vertical. The signals predicted for this defect are shown in Figure 3.9 and Figure 3.10, corresponding to scanning in the unfavourable and favourable directions relative to the sense of tilt respectively. Peak signals from the favourable orientation are still only −4 dB compared with those from a 3 mm diameter flat-bottomed hole. For this defect the maximum pulse-echo signal would be about 25 dB for a defect tilted by 20°, that is, normal to the transducer beam for 70° probes, and with the beam centre directed at the centre of the defect.

### 3.2.6 Time-of-Flight Diffraction signals for ribbon and circular defects

In order to draw comparisons between the Time-of-Flight Diffraction signals expected from typical defects with those expected with pulse-echo techniques, we have presented some results which are for similar defects. Because the two techniques do not share a common geometry, some assumptions had to be made. In the previous calculations for pulse-echo inspections the scan over the defects produced an optimum signal from both the top and bottom of the defect, and so the depth of the defect was largely irrelevant (except to make the signals stronger as the defect is brought nearer the transducer, in general). However, for the Time-of-Flight geometry, the probes are usually optimised for a particular defect depth as indeed they are in the tandem technique — this being a general feature of two probe techniques. Thus we have assumed that the beam centrelines of the transmitter and receiver transducers intersect at a depth equal to the centre of the defect. Other assumptions would have been equally valid, for instance assuming that the intersection of the two beam centres was at a depth corresponding to either the top or bottom of the defects. The present assumption is unbiased in the sense of not particularly emphasising the Time-of-Flight Diffraction signals.

The calibration reflector is a 3 mm diameter flat-bottomed hole drilled vertically from the bottom of the plate such that the flat end surface is at the depth of the defect centre. The flat surface of the calibration reflector is situated midway between the transmitter and receiver transducer centres, thus giving an ideal specular reflection for the calibration signal.

The transducers used are compression wave probes generating 5 MHz ultrasound at an angle of 60° (beam maximum) to the normal to the inspection surface. The probes have a diameter of 25 mm. The Time-of-Flight Diffraction amplitudes are

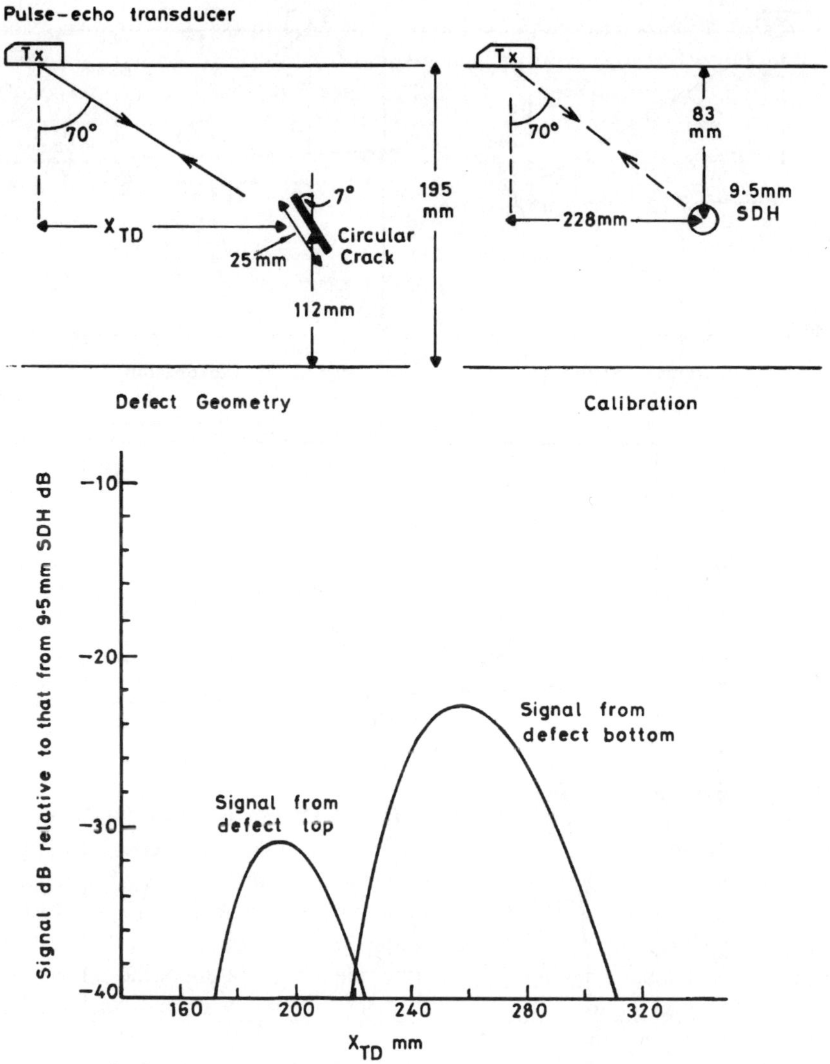


**Fig. 3.9** Pulse-echo response with 2 MHz 70° shear-wave probes for a 25 mm diameter circular crack tilted by 7° from the vertical. Signal amplitudes are relative to 100% DAC.

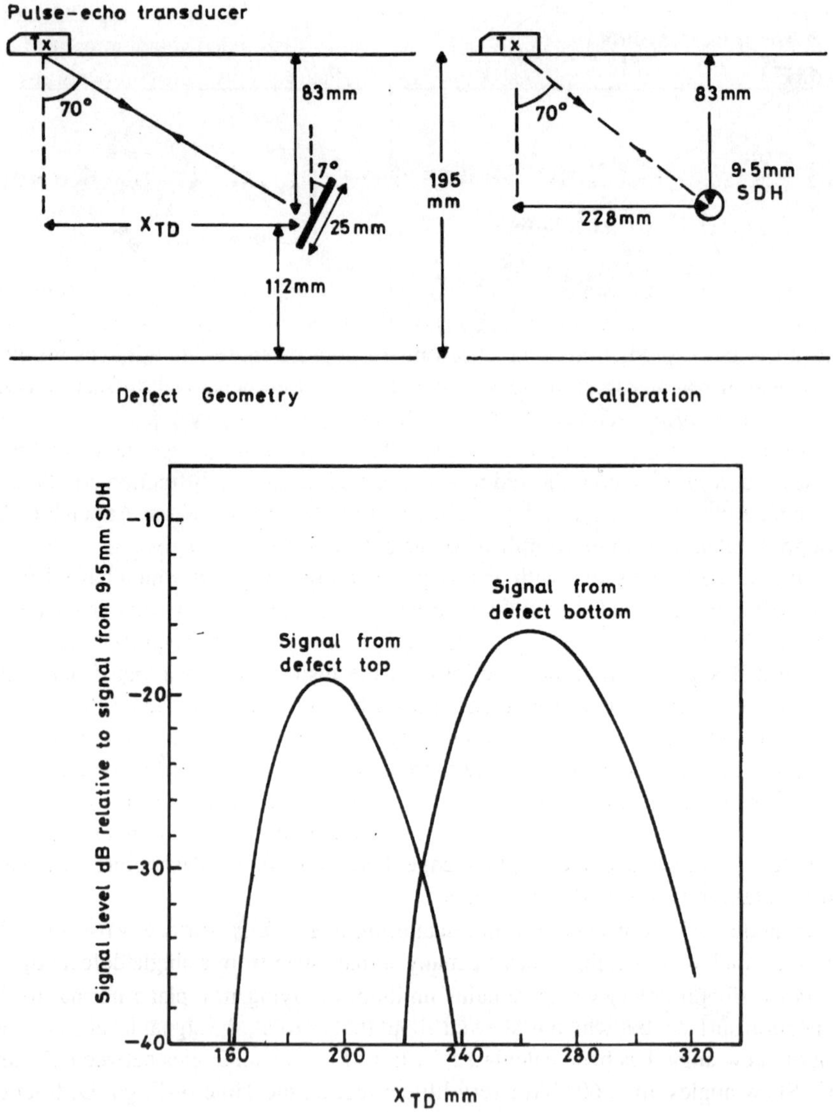


**Fig. 3.10** Pulse-echo response with 2 MHz 70° shear-wave probes for a 25 mm diameter circular crack tilted by −7° from the vertical. Signal amplitudes are relative to 100% DAC.

given for comparison in Table 3.1. From these results, we conclude that the relative signal amplitudes from Time-of-Flight Diffraction tend to be of the same order of magnitude as those from a poorly oriented reflector in pulse-echo inspections, i.e. comparable to those for a 45° probe and a vertical defect, but are less than those from 60° or 70° probes. For pulse-echo inspections, the added signal strength from the higher angle probes is the reason for their inclusion in inspection procedures.

## 3.3 Time-of-Flight Diffraction signals from skewed, planar cracks

For defects which do not lie with one axis perpendicular to the line joining transmitter and receiver, or for defects which do not lie immediately under the scan line of the transducer pairs, prediction of the ultrasonic response is more difficult. The problem becomes intrinsically three-dimensional and the three-dimensional diffraction coefficients are required. These have been calculated by Achenbach et al. [1982] and, in a different format, by Ramsdale [1983]. We shall not reproduce the results here as they are even more complicated than the two-dimensional diffraction coefficients referenced in Section 2.2.1 and given in detail in Section A.4 of the Appendix. Although the algebra is more complicated, the outline of the model given in Section 3.1 is still essentially the same, with energy propagating along rays which have diffraction coefficients associated with interactions at crack edges. The points on the defect edge which contribute to the signal observed at some position are called flashpoints. The term flashpoint would be descriptive if the inspection was a visual one using light; with the transmitter producing a pencil beam of light; replacing the receiver by the human eye; and the defect consisting of a shiny reflective rim and optically transparent faces. Bright spots would then be seen on the defect rim, corresponding to the flashpoints. These flashpoints are a function of the position of the transmitter and receiver relative to the defect centre and depend on the orientation and shape of the defect edge. For a single elliptical edge there may be four flashpoints for a wave which retains a single mode throughout.

If mode conversions and multiple scattering of Rayleigh surface waves over the crack are included then there may be many signals seen from a single defect edge.

For a ribbon defect which remains untilted, i.e. lying in a plane normal to the inspection surface, but which is skewed about that normal, the signal level as a function of skew angle has been calculated for transducer beam angles between 20° and 65°. Skew angles up to 60° have very little effect on the Time-of-Flight Diffraction signal strength. As the skew approaches 90°, the signal from the bottom edge falls to zero, while that from the top edge remains finite. However, in this orientation the result is affected by the assumption of an infinite defect length.

An experimental comparison with these results was carried out using a plate with a spark cut slit running the full width of the plate and penetrating vertically to half the plate thickness. The slit was 0.4 mm wide with a semicircular tip. It was found that the Time-of-Flight Diffraction signal amplitude decreased by only 1 dB for skew

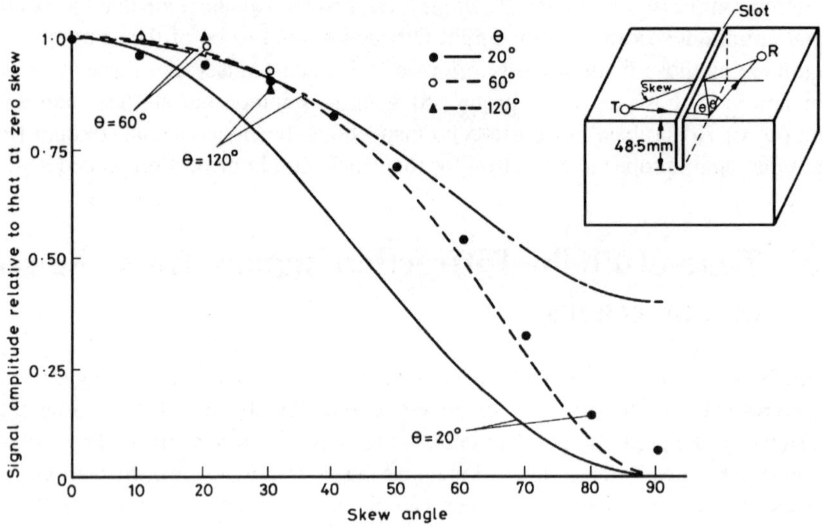


**Fig. 3.11** The effects of crack skew on Time-of-Flight Diffraction signals from an untilted ribbon crack 48.5 mm through-wall. Points are experimental values and the lines are predictions based on the Geometrical Theory of Diffraction.

angles up to 30°. A comparison of these results with the theoretical predictions has been given by Stringfellow and Temple [1987] and the results are shown in Figure 3.11. In this figure the diffraction coefficients used in the calculations are from Achenbach et al. [1982].

Although results have been presented here only for skew or tilt alone, but not for both present simultaneously, the response surface as a function of both angles is quite smooth so that the general conclusion is expected to remain valid even in the presence of both tilt and skew. Coupled with the intrinsic capability for accurate determination of the through-wall extent of cracks, this insensitivity of Time-of-Flight Diffraction to defect orientation shows that the technique has an obvious and useful role to play in inspections.

# Chapter 4

# Design of Time-of-Flight Diffraction Equipment for Simple Geometries

During the early stages of the development of the Time-of-Flight Diffraction technique on samples less than 90 mm thick, little theoretical modelling had been done and the design of TOFD inspection systems was largely empirical. When the Defect Detection Trials (DDT) were planned, in which plates up to 250 mm thick were to be inspected, the scale of the task, the short timescale and the weight which would be attached to the results made it imperative to use a more systematic approach to achieving optimum experimental design. This process has been described in detail for the two girth weld simulation plates (Plates 1 and 2) by Curtis and Hawker [1983] and for the near surface defect plate by Charlesworth and Hawker [1984]. That part of the work related to design of probe arrays and scanning processes is described in this chapter, while information on data display and analysis techniques appears in Chapter 5. The results of the Defect Detection Trials are discussed in Chapter 8. The additional design problems associated with more complex geometries are discussed in Chapter 6. Although the DDT work was done a long time ago, it is still of historic importance because exercises on this scale have not been repeated in recent times. There have however been some advances in inspection design and instrumentation which will be presented to bring the picture more up to date.

## 4.1 Coverage design for buried defects

One of the principal advantages of ultrasound over other crack detection and sizing methods is the ability to detect and size buried defects in thick opaque materials. The Time-of-Flight Diffraction technique can be applied to either surface-breaking or buried defects. In this section we consider the approach to detecting and sizing buried defects, such as those implanted in the Plates 1 and 2 of the Defect Detection Trials. These two plates were each formed from two 1500 by 750 mm plates, 250 mm thick, which were butt welded to form a square plate. One 1500 mm square surface of each plate was covered with an 8 mm thick layer of austenitic strip cladding.

### 4.1.1 Choice of frequency

Since the Time-of-Flight Diffraction technique reduces defect depth and size determination to a time measurement on the recorded waveform, the accuracy of measurement may be expected to improve with increasing frequency. However, there were two constraints on the use of higher frequencies. First, for reasons of economy and convenience, the signals were to be digitised at a sampling rate of 20 MHz, limiting the usable bandwidth to 10 MHz. Secondly, the presence of austenitic cladding, giving scattering which increased markedly with frequency, set a similar limit. The use of short pulse probes with a 5 MHz centre frequency met both these criteria. Digitisation at much higher frequencies is now readily available but would not have been useful in DDT because of the effect of the cladding.

### 4.1.2 Arrangement of probes

#### 4.1.2.1 Coverage from a single probe pair

The dependence of depth measurement accuracy on defect depth and probe separation has already been explained in Chapter 2, and it has been shown in Chapter 3 that combining this geometrical factor with the dependence of diffracted amplitude on angle of incidence leads to a usable range of 45° to 80° for the beam angle in the steel. These angular limits define, in the vertical plane through the beam axes, a quadrilateral zone where the beams cross; the inspection design for DDT was based on the assumption that defects anywhere in this quadrilateral would produce adequate signal amplitude. While that approach demonstrably produced good results in DDT, it is clearly far too simple as it stands. The 45° to 80° angular range is based on the range-corrected diffraction amplitude calculated for a vertical strip-like crack in the symmetry plane (see Figure 3.1 in Chapter 3). It takes no account of the actual beam characteristics of the probes which result from their beam axis angles and the finite size of their radiating faces. It also ignores the effect of changes in range from the probe index points with movement away from the symmetry plane. Figure 4.1, taken from Hawker and Burch [1999], shows the product of the beam spread functions for a pair of 15 mm diameter 60° probes at 100 mm separation, calculated from the beam model of Coffey and Chapman [1983]. This can be treated as a plot of signal amplitude from a diffraction source, assuming the diffraction coefficient to be reasonably constant, as discussed below. Even if a signal amplitude range of 24 dB is allowed, the sensitive area falls somewhat short of the quadrilateral zone, especially in the near surface region. A zone defined by the angles 45° to 74° would fit the calculations with reasonable accuracy. The major cause of the reduced coverage is the restricted beam width of the probes; the sensitive region can be enlarged by

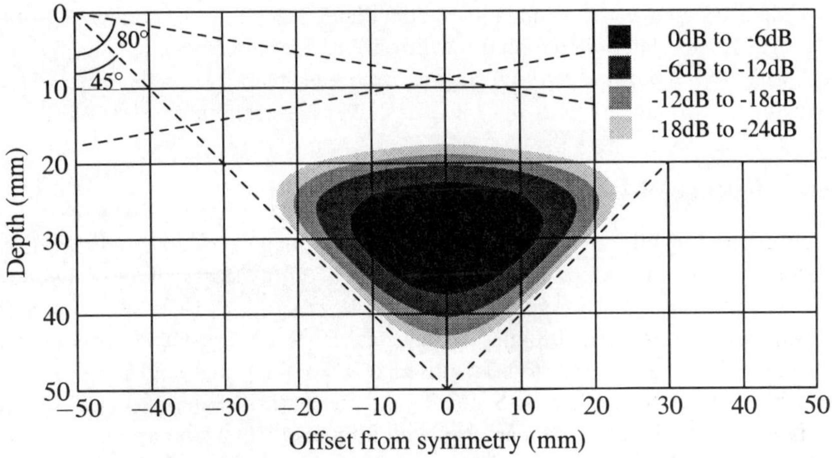


**Fig. 4.1** Beam spread at 3.5 MHz for 15 mm diameter 60° probes separated by 100 mm. The dashed lines mark the 45° to 80° zone used by Curtis and Hawker [1983].

using smaller probe-face diameters and of course can be biased more towards the near surface region by using, say, 70° probes instead of 60°.

Hawker and Burch [1999] also discuss the effect of the variation of the diffraction coefficient of the upper and lower edges of a crack-like defect, based on the work of Lewis, Temple, Walker and Wickham [1998]. Figure 4.2 shows their plots of diffracted signal strength for a straight crack edge, corrected for range but ignoring any absorption effects. From these it can be deduced that:

- The assumption of a constant diffraction coefficient in the coverage calculation is not unreasonable.
- Defect tilts of 45° or more can be tolerated without drastic loss of signal strength.
- The optimum sensitivity is achieved when 68° probes are used.

Once the size of the sensitive zone for any given probe pair has been determined, the next stage of coverage design is to determine how the full inspection volume can be swept out by the sensitive zone of one or more probe pairs. It will often be necessary to specify several different probe separations to cover different depth zones. Where probe pairs with small separation are used to inspect a near-surface region, the small width of the sensitive zone may mean that multiple probe pairs at different displacements from the inspection volume centre line are required.

Where defects may lie very close to the back wall but displaced from the centre line, there is a risk that their signals may be masked by the back-wall echo unless additional laterally displaced probe pairs are provided. There is always a trade-off

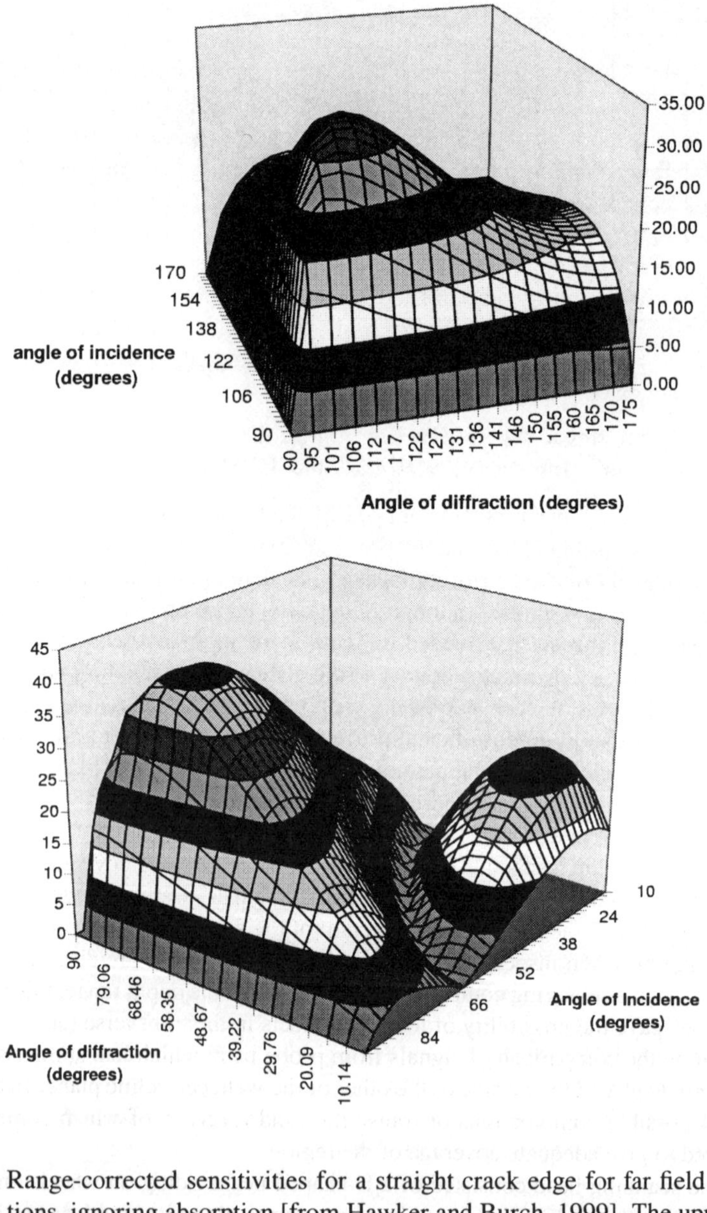


**Fig. 4.2** Range-corrected sensitivities for a straight crack edge for far field conditions, ignoring absorption [from Hawker and Burch, 1999]. The upper figure is for the top edge of the defect and the lower figure for the bottom edge.

between the number of probe pairs and the amount of scanning and the arrangement chosen will depend on the number of data collection channels available, the capabilities of the scanning equipment and the time available for the inspection. For simple inspection geometries, such as butt welds in flat plates or girth welds in cylindrical vessels, working out a probe set and scanning sequence to give adequate coverage is fairly straightforward but in more complex geometries, such as nozzle to shell welds, K-nodes etc., it may be a complex process. In such geometries, unless probe mounting arrangements, probe placements and scanning patterns are carefully analysed, inadequate coverage can arise from probe skewing, causing loss of sensitivity from loss of beam overlap or displacement of the sensitive region from its expected location. In inspections where a high degree of confidence is required, it is usually necessary to model the geometry of the system mathematically to prove that all parts of the inspection volume will be covered. In addition, it is often wise to provide calibration specimens of appropriate geometry, with deliberately induced defects, to demonstrate that coverage has been achieved.

#### 4.1.2.2 Probe arrangement for DDT Plates 1 and 2

The primary aim in the inspection of DDT Plates 1 and 2 was the detection and sizing of longitudinal weld defects and the probe array was designed with this in mind, although it was also used to inspect for transverse defects. The description of scanning arrangements below applies to longitudinal defects, except where otherwise stated. The zone to be inspected extended in depth from approximately 10 mm below the cladding interface down to the bottom of the plate and in width for a distance of half the plate thickness on each side of the weld centreline. Because the inspection had to be done in a short time, sufficient probe pairs were provided for all the ultrasonic data to be collected in a single pass of the probe array along the plate surface in the direction of the weld axis. Figure 4.3 illustrates how the probes were arranged to give complete coverage.

The bulk of the inspection zone, from the bottom up, was covered by three symmetrically placed pairs of probes but a further five pairs were needed to achieve adequate coverage in the remaining top section of the zone. Further complications arise in this region when inspecting from the clad side and these are discussed in Chapter 7. As well as ensuring complete coverage through the depth range, this large array of probes gave the possibility of locating defects in the transverse (across-weld) direction by the comparison of signals from probe pairs which had similar separation but were displaced to one side or the other of the weld centreline plane. In total there are 64 possible combinations of transmitter and receiver, of which some 33 were required to give adequate coverage of the region.

The scanning head consisted of a U-shaped beam riding on wheels on the plate surface with the probes distributed in a linear array along its length as can be seen in Figure 4.4.

As there were no spring mounts or gimbals for the probes, they were mounted with sufficient clearance to avoid touching the plate surface at any point, coupling being provided by a sufficient depth of water. One consequence of this method

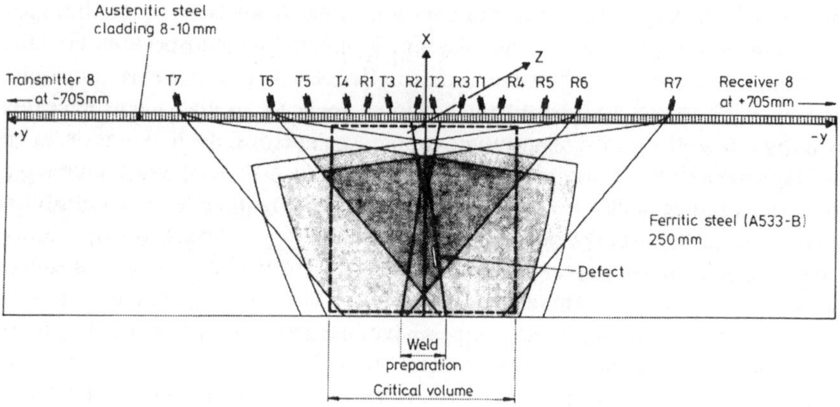


**Fig. 4.3** Weld volume inspected with the design of flat-plate scanner used in the Defect Detection Trials.

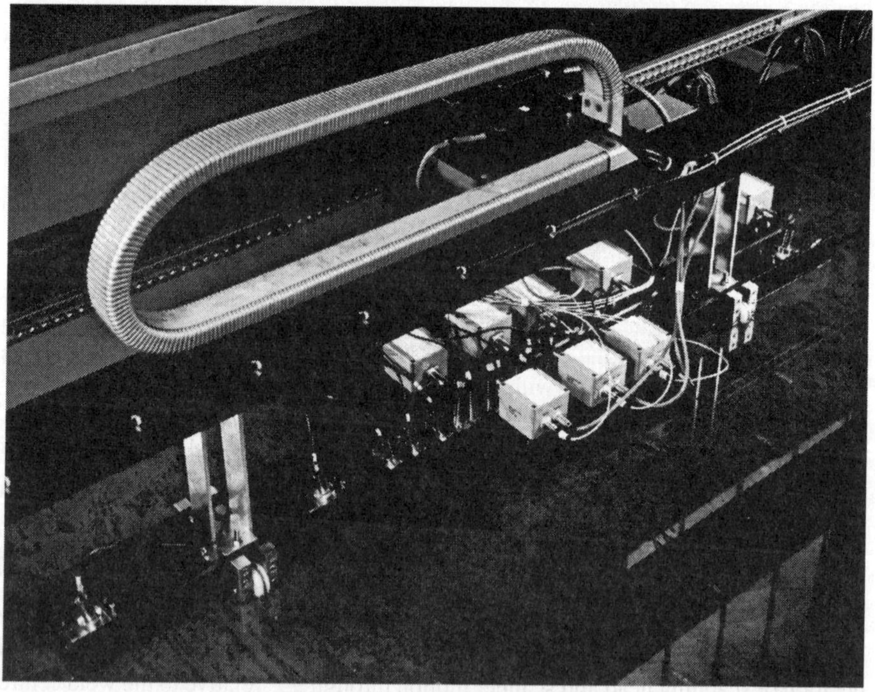

**Fig. 4.4** The flat plate scanner head used in the Defect Detection Trials.

of mounting was that bowing of the plate and undulations in the surface caused variations in that part of the ultrasonic path which was in water, giving substantial variations in signal timing. The techniques for handling this problem are described in Chapter 5. The required incidence angle in water was 12.5° and was achieved in most cases by tilting the probes at that angle. However, in the centre of the probe array there was insufficient space between adjacent probes for this to be done and the angled beams were produced instead by attaching polystyrene wedges, coupled to the faces of the probes with a thin layer of grease. To allow for the possibility of some slight misalignment between the mechanical and ultrasonic axes of the probes, a small range of angular adjustment was provided on each probe mount. The beam angles were optimised before the inspections by setting up the array on a calibration block and adjusting each probe angle for maximum amplitude from an appropriately located side-drilled hole.

### 4.1.3 Scanning arrangements

The scanning head was attached to the crosshead of a 2 metre square x-y scanning frame developed by Risley Nuclear Power Development Laboratories, driven by computer-controlled stepping motors (Figure 4.4). The attachment allowed the head to follow the undulations of the plate surface in the vertical plane while being constrained to follow the scanning frame in the horizontal plane. The head was set up with the plane of the probe array parallel to the $y$ motion, the workpiece being set up with the weld parallel to the $x$ motion, with the surface as near as possible horizontal. The centre of the scanning head was set on the centreline of the weld as near the edge of the plate as possible for the start of the complete traverse of the weld and a sequence of probe firing and signal recording carried out as described above. At the end of each sequence of data collection from all appropriate probe pairs the scanning head was moved along the weld to a new position and the sequence repeated. The distance moved between sequences, 2.5 mm, was a compromise between obtaining accurate information about defect length and minimising the volume of data collected. The data from the complete pass along the weld were recorded on a 730 m reel of magnetic tape, starting with a header describing the details of the run and the data format and followed by the complete set of records of the ultrasonic signals. Analysis of the signals was carried out on a computer interfaced to image analysis and display devices and is described in Chapter 5.

### 4.1.4 Transverse defects

Although signals from transverse defects were obtained during the inspection for longitudinal defects, thorough inspection for such defects required changing the orientation of scanning head and scanner motion through 90° relative to the weld centre line and scanning across the weld. Complete coverage of the length of the weld then required several scans, the scanning head being moved about 250 mm along the weld between scans.

## 4.2 Near-surface defects

Plate 3 of the Defect Detection Trials contained defects which could be anywhere in a 30 mm deep zone beneath the cladding over the whole surface of the plate. This change in the shape of the inspection zone, compared with Plates 1 and 2, required a redesign of the probe array and the method of scanning.

### 4.2.1 Probe arrangement

It was clearly not practicable to construct a probe array which could inspect the whole near surface zone in one pass. It was necessary, therefore, to do a raster scan of the plate surface to ensure complete coverage. In principle this could have been done with one or at most two probe pairs, scanned over the complete surface; however, since eight signal channels were available, eight pairs of probes of identical separation were simultaneously scanned over separate areas of the plate, a small overlap being provided between the areas scanned by adjacent probe pairs. The same probes, electronics and digital data acquisition system were used as on DDT Plates 1 and 2 but, because the zone of interest was only 30 mm deep, digital records of only 256 samples were adequate. The records did not include the back-wall echo, so it was necessary to measure the compression wave velocity in the plate.

It was anticipated that the variations in water path length experienced with the fixed probes in the inspection of DDT Plates 1 and 2, which can distort the characteristic signal curves, would make the detection of the very-near-surface defects in Plate 3 more difficult. The probes were therefore mounted at the appropriate angle in cylinders which could slide vertically in a housing. The bottom of the cylinder carried a hollow shoe which rode on the plate and so maintained the probe-to-plate-surface distance constant, within the small scale roughness of the surface. A photograph of the probe array used in this inspection appears in Figure 4.5. Improved near-surface resolution could, in principle, have been achieved by the use of higher frequency probes but because the scattering in the cladding layer increases strongly with frequency, there was nothing to be gained by a change from the 5 MHz probes used for Plates 1 and 2.

The choice of probe separation for optimum near-surface detection and sizing is complicated by the presence of the anisotropic austenitic cladding. This matter is dealt with in detail in Chapter 7 and will not be further discussed here but it should be noted that, at the probe separations used, the lateral wave travels along the interface between cladding and base material and depth measurements are related to that interface, which plays much the same role as the physical surface on an unclad plate. Two sets of scans with probe separations of 60 mm and 120 mm were used to ensure complete depth coverage but the results indicated that a single set of scans at 80 – 100 mm would have been adequate.

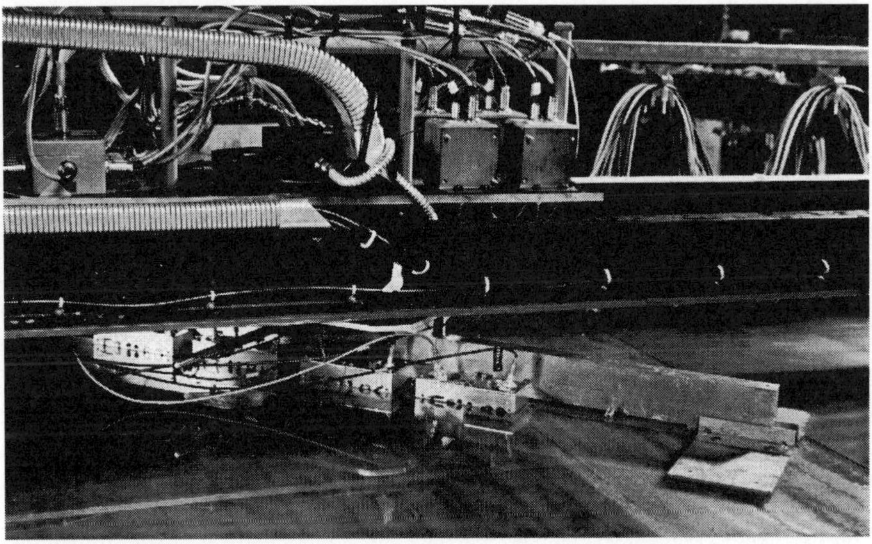

**Fig. 4.5** The DDT scanner head used for near-surface defects, deployed in the 45° position.

### 4.2.2 Scanning technique

The amount of skew of the defects relative to the principal axes of the plate was not known, so two sets of scans were required with the probe array turned through 90° for the second scan. To provide more comprehensive information about the dependence of defect signal strength on skew angle, scans were also carried out at the two intermediate 45° angles but this was not necessary for detection or sizing.

The main problem with applying the Time-of-Flight Diffraction technique to near surface defects is the fall-off in depth resolution as the depth decreases. At the frequencies and probe separations used on Plate 3, the signals from defects within 5 mm of the surface tend to merge with the lateral wave and even for deeper defects interference effects with the lateral wave can make estimation of signal timing difficult. As discussed in Chapter 5, recognition of signals in the Time-of-Flight Diffraction technique is greatly facilitated by the characteristic change in signal timing as the probe pair passes the defect. When the scanning motion is perpendicular to the plane of the probes (variously referred to as *longitudinal,* or *perpendicular,* or *non-parallel* scan) the signals persist only for the relatively narrow beam width and the curved signal tails, while usually easily seen for deep lying defects, may scarcely appear for very shallow defects. If, however, the scanning motion is in the plane of the probes (known as a *transverse* or *parallel* scan), the overlap region of the transmitter and receiver beam is larger in the scan direction, so adequate signal strength can be expected for a much longer scan distance and signal tails appear even for very near surface defects. This longer overlap is partly a result of the oblique crossing angle of the beams and partly of the increased beam width in the vertical plane which results from the refraction at the plate surface. The data from a raster scan can be organised to represent either type of scan but it is advantageous to collect them in the transverse scan mode so that initial inspection for significant signals can be carried without reordering the data.

With the data displayed in this manner, it is possible to recognise defect signals from the presence of tails, even when the minimum delay part of the signal merges with the lateral wave. Accurate depth measurement should then be possible by measuring the width between the signal tails at an appropriate time delay and comparing with a set of calculated curves such as those in Figure 5.5. In the inspection of DDT Plate 3 only one defect was so shallow as to require this type of treatment.

## 4.3 Data acquisition system

We describe here the data acquisition system used for DDT but, in view of the advances in instrumentation technology in the intervening years, we follow this description with some information on more recent forms of data acquisition equipment.

### 4.3.1 The DDT instrumentation system

At the time of the Defect Detection Trials, commercially available ultrasonic inspection equipment was almost universally designed exclusively for application of amplitude-based techniques. Rectified signals were generally displayed on a screen where their characteristics could be measured manually by the operator but there was generally no provision for digitisation of the signals and linkage of the instruments to computers for permanent recording of data was in its infancy. The DDT equipment had to be available at short notice, which precluded major instrumentation development, so it was assembled largely from existing instrumentation modules, some commercial and some built in-house at Harwell, and integrated with a general purpose mini-computer.

A schematic layout of the data acquisition system for DDT is given in Figure 4.6. Each transmitter probe had its own pulser unit (Harwell Model 0870) giving a 200 V 0.1 s pulse on command from the computer. The receiver probes were connected to preamplifiers (Harwell Model 81E09) mounted on the scanning head and, from there, the signals were taken via coaxial cables to the main amplifiers (Harwell Model 0187) in the computer room. These amplifiers have a broad-band response (0.7 – 30 MHz) so, to avoid aliasing in the digitisers, the signals passed through 10 MHz anti-aliasing filters before reaching the input of the eight LeCroy 2256A 8-bit Waveform Digitisers operating at a sampling frequency of 20 MHz. These digitisers were triggered from the computer via Sension 1351A Delay Generators so that the start of the recorded signal from each receiver probe occurred just before the arrival of the lateral wave. This time depended, of course, on which transmitter probe the signal had come from and so had to be altered by the computer whenever a different transmitter probe was fired. The length of each recording was chosen to cover the depth

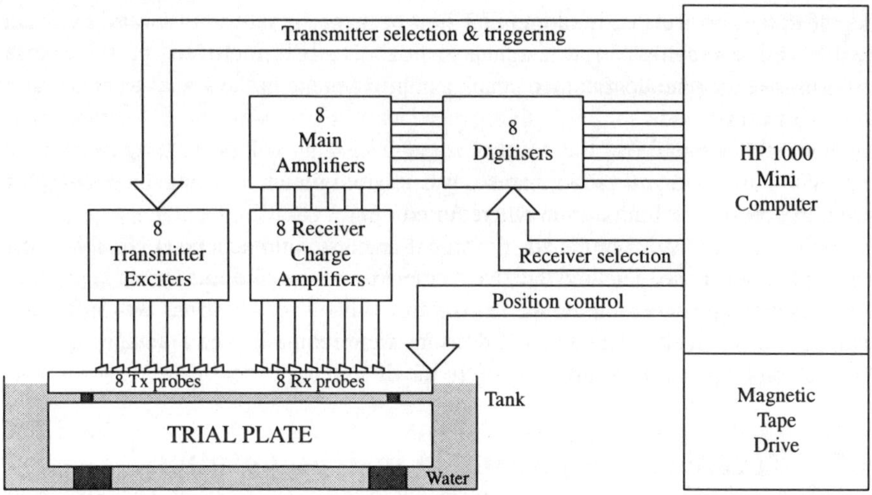


**Fig. 4.6** Schematic layout of the data acquisition system used for the Defect Detection Trials.

range from which adequate signals could be expected. There is always an advantage in including the echo from the back surface of the plate, if this can be done without excessively lengthening the record, since it allows a check to be made that its timing is consistent with the assumed values of probe separation, ultrasonic velocity, plate thickness etc. Record lengths of either 512 or 1024 samples were chosen, to give compatibility with the 512 byte block length of the computer files.

# 4.4 Signal Averaging

Specular reflections from defects of structural significance usually give large signal amplitudes over the narrow range of angles for which they can be received and enhancement of the ratio of signal amplitude to random noise is rarely necessary. In contrast, the energy from diffraction at a defect edge is spread over a large range of angles, allowing detection from a wide range of probe positions; however, because of the angular spread, the amplitude is generally smaller than would arise from a specular reflection. The position of the defect relative to the ultrasonic probes, the shape of the defect, its roughness and whether it is under compressive stress are factors which all affect the diffracted signal amplitude. These factors are discussed elsewhere in this book (see, for example, Section 3.2, and Figures 3.5, 3.6, 3.11 and 7.7).

Although the amplitude of Time-of-Flight Diffraction signals is not used for estimation of the important through-wall dimension of defects, reliable detection of such signals at long range (e.g. in a thick pressure vessel) may often be enhanced by averaging a number of repetitions of the signal. The theoretical basis of signal averaging is given in the Appendix (Section A.6). Averaging 64 signals which are degraded by uncorrelated random noise improves the signal-to-noise ratio by about 18 dB, while averaging 256 such signals gives about 24 dB improvement. If the noise is correlated to some degree then smaller improvements in the signal-to-noise ratio will be obtained.

It should be noted that this form of signal averaging will do nothing to improve the ratio of signal to grain scatter noise. Where grain scatter is strong, more complex signal processing techniques may be required.

In the Defect Detection Trials, the signal-to-noise ratio depended chiefly on the range of travel in the plate and thus was a function of the particular probe pair used. For the closest pairs, averaging the signals from only 4 repeat firings was sufficient, whereas for the most distant pairs 128 firings were required. The averaging process for each probe pair was completed before moving on to the next pair.

## 4.5 Recent developments in instrumentation

After the success of the trials, as TOFD began to be considered for a wider range of inspections, the cumbersome and expensive nature of the equipment was a serious hindrance and effort was therefore put into producing an integrated test set which more closely resembled a conventional flaw detector. Digital signal acquisition is not essential to the practice of TOFD but was felt to be a vital feature of the new approach to ultrasonic inspection which TOFD typified. The period between the time of the DDT trials and the present day has been characterised by a very rapid development of computer technology and it took some years for the design approach to stabilise. However, the ubiquity of the PC and its consequent low price has ensured that development fairly quickly became concentrated on instruments which are essentially customised PCs, usually running some version of Microsoft Windows, containing a number of special purpose modules such as probe drivers, amplifiers, digitisers and digital signal processors to handle the generation and reception of signals, their conversion to digital data and subsequent analysis. As a result of these developments, TOFD equipment can now be made extremely portable and, in comparison with the era of DDT, very inexpensive in real terms.

As an illustration of a very portable system, we quote here the specification of ***μinUT**-tofd* (pronounced MinUT-TOFD), a miniature dedicated TOFD version of the MicroPlus inspection instrument produced by AEA Sonomatic. The core of the system is a single ISA bus card which needs to be hosted by a ruggedised laptop computer containing a 75 MHz Intel Pentium processor (or better), with at least 32 MB RAM, and a 1024 × 768 display with at least 256 colours, running Microsoft Windows NT 4.0. The specification of the card is set out in Table 4.1.

The user interface is, of course, provided by the PC system. Table 4.2 lists the data collection functions which can be accessed. Data analysis functions are discussed in Chapter 5.

The majority of TOFD applications are much less complex than the DDT trials, which were simulating the inspection of a PWR pressure vessel. For most purposes a portable instrument with a small number of data collection channels, similar to the

**Table 4.1** Technical specification of TOFD inspection system

| **Probe Driver** | | **Receiver/Amplifier** | |
|---|---|---|---|
| Number of probes | 2 | Number of inputs | 2 |
| Probe type | Single/twin crystal | Input impedance | 50 Ω |
| HT pulse voltage | 0–400 V in 2 V steps | Bandwidth | 20 MHz |
| HT pulse width | 20–500 ns in 1 ns steps | Gain range | 0–80 dB |
| Maximum p.r.f. | 1 kHz | | |
| **Filtering** | | **Distance/Amplitude Correction** | |
| High/Low pass filter | 1–20 MHz in 100 kHz steps | Number of curves | 16 |
| Rectification | None/Full wave | Gain range | 0–80 dB |
| Rectifier time constant | 0–10 ms in 100 ns steps | Points in curve | 8 K |
| **Digitiser** | | **Encoders** | |
| Resolution | 8 bits (256 levels) | Number of encoders | 2 |
| Digitiser rate | 80, 40, 20, 10 MHz | Interface | Single/differential |
| Collection memory | 64 K | Count range | 32 bits |
| Number of gates | User definable | maximum count frequency | 1 MHz |
| Digitiser delay | 0–3.2 ms | | |
| Points in gate | up to 32 K | | |

**Table 4.2** Data collection functions of TOFD inspection system

| | |
|---|---|
| **Setup** | Real time A-scan Display<br>Channel parameters: Pulse width, gain, material velocity, probe delay, angle.<br>System parameters: PRF, averaging, HT voltage.<br>Collection parameters: parallel, non-parallel, height, separation, scan start, scan end, scan step, free-run or encoder<br>Advanced hardware diagnostics.<br>Stick values. |
| **Data Collection** | Live A-scan and B/D-scan scrolling display.<br>600 kbs throughput. |

one described in Tables 4.1 & 4.2, is all that is required. Such a system is not, of course, capable of supporting an inspection on the scale of DDT but it lacks only extra data acquisition channels and perhaps a suitable bulk storage medium such as a CD writer for archiving data. Probe driver units and signal preamplifiers mounted close to the probe assemblies would still be used whenever there was a need to operate the data acquisition system more than a metre or two from the probe assemblies.

There are some applications which have such unusual requirements that it is still necessary to design special purpose systems. To give only one example of such a system, the Snorre Tether Inspection Equipment (STINE) is an inspection system for the tension leg welds of the Norwegian Snorre oil platform in the North Sea. It embodies a remotely controlled vehicle which travels up and down the bores of the tubular tethers, stopping at particular welds as programmed and carrying out a scanning sequence with multiple ultrasonic probes, some of which are used to collect TOFD data. The ultrasonic equipment is split between the vehicle and the control room system, the probe selection and firing units and receiver preamplifiers being on the vehicle with a control computer (a single board PC system) and the main amplifier, digitiser and data storage and display equipment in the control room. This equipment is capable of carrying out a complete inspection schedule, on a specified set of welds on a tether, without operator intervention.

# Chapter 5

# Processing, Display and Analysis of Time-of-Flight Data

In Chapter 4, we discussed the design of signal acquisition equipment for the Time-of-Flight Diffraction technique. In this chapter we shall describe the remainder of the inspection system, devoted to processing the signals and extracting information from them. The use of novel techniques of display and analysis has been one of the marked features of the development of Time-of-Flight Diffraction but many of the techniques have subsequently proved applicable to pulse-echo data.

In this chapter we shall confine ourselves to analysis techniques which are generally applicable and sufficient for a full analysis in simple geometries like butt welds in flat plates or girth welds in cylindrical vessels. When the geometry is more complicated, the analyst needs some geometrical assistance from the system to help locate the sources of defect signals and this will be described in Chapter 6.

At the time of the Defect Detection Trials, it was the common practice to collect TOFD data on systems which had few or no facilities for data analysis, the data being transferred, for analysis, to other computer systems containing what were then very expensive image display systems. As the cost and size of computers and image display equipment decreased, the analysis functions for TOFD tended to be more and more integrated into the data collection system, so that, now, it is usual for the whole process of collection and analysis to be carried out on one portable instrument.

## 5.1 Simple forms of display

Because the phase of the diffracted signal contains information about the position and orientation of the edge from which it came, Time-of-Flight Diffraction signals are usually displayed in unrectified form. Although some traditional flaw detectors had a facility for displaying the signals without rectification, many did not. The time base on a flaw detector was usually calibrated in terms of range, because, for the pulse-echo technique, the range is proportional to the time of flight and the combination of range and probe angle provides an estimate of defect location. For the two probe Time-of-Flight Diffraction technique, the defect depth information is related to the time differences between signals in a non-linear way, so a simple range based display is not very useful. As a result of these factors, conventional flaw detectors were unsuitable for use in Time-of-Flight Diffraction work and new forms of analysis equipment had to be developed.

The simplest type of data display, used in the early development work on the Time-of-Flight Diffraction technique, is an oscilloscope, on which the received waveform may be displayed without any processing. To be most useful, the oscilloscope should have a delayed trace facility with a calibrated delay setting so that the portion of the signal which is of interest (for a flat plate, that from the lateral wave to the back-wall echo) may be expanded to occupy most of the screen and the time of occurrence of any signals from defects may be accurately measured. Such a display is adequate for manual measurements, in ultrasonically clean material, of the depth of visible surface-breaking cracks, or of buried defects detected by some other method. As a search technique or for sizing in less clean materials, this simple equipment leaves something to be desired, since judging the significance of a small signal in a single A-scan may be difficult.

## 5.2 Two-dimensional displays

For the best detection and sizing capability, it is necessary to record A-scans as the probes are moved over the workpiece and display them in suitable form. Such displays are analogous to well known methods of displaying pulse-echo data. For instance, if we define a vertical plane containing the beam of an angled pulse-echo probe, then a two-dimensional display of A-scans resulting from motion within the plane is called a B-scan, while a similar display from motion perpendicular to the plane is a D-scan. Time-of-Flight Diffraction scans with probe motion parallel to and perpendicular to the line joining them are analogous to pulse-echo B- and D-scans respectively, apart from the inherently non-linear depth scale in the Time-of-Flight Diffraction case. In the past, the term B-scan has often been applied to both directions of motion and, in the remainder of this chapter, references to B-scans may be taken to apply equally to D-scans, unless otherwise stated.

In this type of display, the information has three dimensions, voltage, time and position, and must be displayed in two-dimensional form; a variety of different representations have been tried.

### 5.2.1 Line drawing displays

One method, which was fairly widely used in the early days of TOFD, is to draw the A-scans with some line drawing device (pen plotter, storage cathode ray tube display etc.), with the base line for each successive A-scan slightly shifted to form a stack. In essence, time and voltage are displayed in the two orthogonal directions

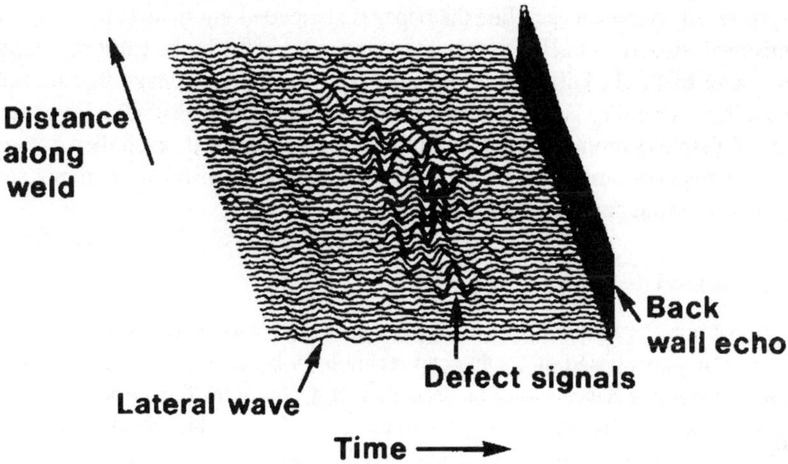


**Fig. 5.1** Time and voltage displayed in two orthogonal directions, with a small offset on each axis between successive traces to represent displacement in the scanning direction.

and position represented by an offset which may either be in the same direction as the voltage, or in an intermediate direction between the voltage and time axes. A modification of the method, which may be used on devices capable of blocking in areas (e.g. matrix printers), is to block in either positive or negative half cycles to draw attention to the areas with significant signals. Figure 5.1 illustrates how such a display enables the coherent pattern formed by the position of a defect signal in successive traces to be recognised. This form of display was rapidly abandoned as grey-scale images became available and is mentioned here only because some of the references quoted use this kind of presentation.

## 5.2.2 Grey scale and colour displays

### 5.2.2.1 Analogue displays

The most satisfactory form of display is one where the voltage dimension can be represented by a change of intensity or tone, leaving the two spatial dimensions for time and position. This type of display may be produced in crude form by the use of a boxcar integrator and a facsimile recorder. In the boxcar integrator, a narrow gate samples a small portion of the waveform and passes the sampled voltage to an integrating circuit and a low pass filter. By delaying the gate a small extra amount on each firing of the transducer, the sampling point is swept along the whole length of the waveform. The output thus becomes a representation of the signal transformed to a lower frequency. This low frequency signal is then used to draw a line on a facsimile recorder in such a way that the amplitude of the signal determines the depth of tone produced. Between each line the paper is stepped along so as to produce a two-dimensional display. This type of display was much used in the early development of the Time-of-Flight Diffraction technique and has the advantage that it requires only analogue circuitry and does not necessitate storage of the signals. However, the quality of displays produced was not high, the equipment was, even then, rather expensive and is now probably unobtainable, and, because the signals were not stored, no post-processing could be done.

#### 5.2.2.2 Digital displays

As digital computers became less expensive and video display technology developed, grey scale displays based on raster scan technology became widespread. The set of A-scans forming a B-scan may be recorded in a computer file, usually with 8-bit precision, and transferred to a digital frame store for display. Early frame stores typically had a resolution of 512 points per line and 512 lines, split between two interlaced half-frames, and used long persistence monochrome monitors to remove the unpleasant flicker caused by the interlacing. With 8-bit data, 256 levels can be displayed, far more than can be distinguished by eye. There is usually some means of dynamically changing the mapping between the signal level and the displayed intensity, so that the contrast may be adjusted to bring out desired features of the data. Colour displays soon became available but experience showed that the fine details of a B- or D-scan could be better appreciated in shades of grey (obtainable on a colour system by mapping all three colours to the same intensity).

The main use of colour is for graphics overlays and annotation to aid interpretation, or to highlight features or particular amplitude levels in, for example, amplitude based sizing after SAFT processing (see Section 5.8.1). Figures 2.2, 2.14, 5.3, 5.4, 5.6, 5.7 and 5.8 are good examples of grey scale images.

As a result of developments in video display technology in the last few years, even inexpensive PC video cards are now typically capable of displaying 16, 24 or 32-bit colour with screen resolutions of at least $1024 \times 768$ pixels, non-interlaced, on compatible colour monitors. A typical TOFD data analysis screen would require 256 grey levels for B-scan display and some other colours for other parts of the display. This would normally require 32-bit colour capability, although a fairly satisfactory display could be created with 24-bit colour by sacrificing a few of the high intensity grey levels. Figure 5.2 shows a fairly typical inspection analysis display taken from AEA Technology's $\mu$PIPELINE system, a combined pulse-echo and TOFD system for pipeline inspection.

### 5.2.3 Hardcopy output

In the early days of TOFD, much ingenuity went into the production of grey-scale hardcopy on such devices as electrostatic matrix printers. Records of screen displays were produced by photographing the screen or by the use of a special device with a small high quality display tube and built in camera. Now, very inexpensive color inkjet printers can produce accurate copies of screen displays and can also produce

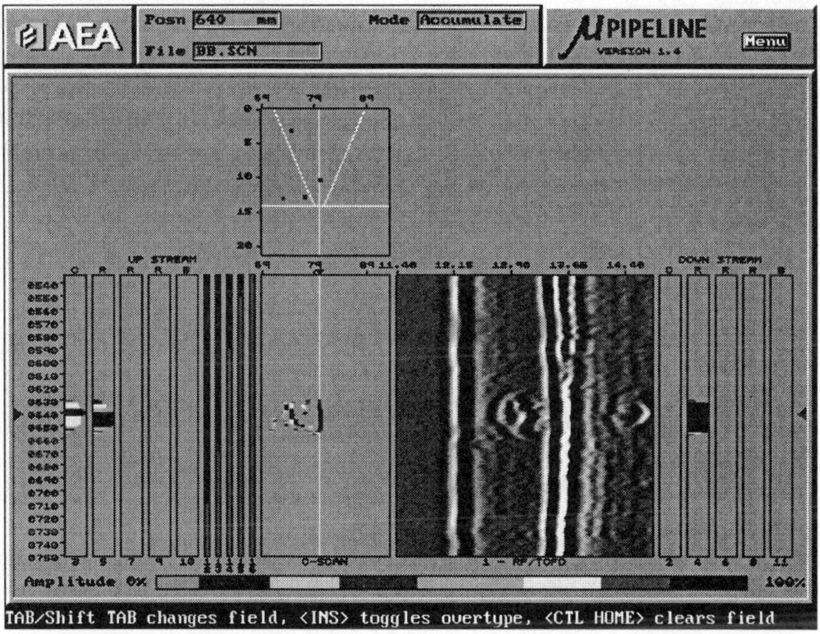


**Fig. 5.2** Typical analysis screen of a modern digital inspection system (AEA Technology's $\mu$PIPELINE system).

output of much higher resolution (typically at least 600 dots per inch) than available on current screen displays.

## 5.2.4 Storage and exchange of raw and analysed data

Long term storage of screen displays on computer media has become practicable with improvements in storage technology, especially with the advent of writable compact discs. By the use of such storage methods, both the raw inspection data and all details of the analysis can be archived on very robust and long-lasting media, and this is immensely useful for long term integrity monitoring of safety-critical components.

Early TOFD data was stored using file formats invented specially for the purpose which were incompatible with any used by other image display software. With the vast increase in the availability of commercial software for image display and analysis, the advantages of using standard file formats have become more obvious. There are many such formats and it is not the purpose to review them exhaustively here; GIF (graphics interchange format) and TIFF (tag image file format) files are widely used and TIFF is especially useful as it can be extended by the definition of additional tags to accommodate extra data which can be understood by specially designed software, without preventing display by standard TIFF image display programs. The other file format of interest is the JPEG (Joint Photographic Experts Group) format which accommodates images which have been compressed by an efficient but lossy compression technique. For storage of an analysis display, the reduction in storage space is worthwhile and the corruption of data implicit in the use of JPEG may be hardly detectable by eye and be of little significance provided the original TOFD data has been archived elsewhere.

## 5.3 Analysis of A-scan data

The analysis of a single A-scan is straightforward provided the various signals can be easily identified. To carry out the depth calculation as detailed in Chapter 2, it is only necessary to measure the time of occurrence of the signals, taking care to choose corresponding points on each wave packet, allowing for possible phase reversal. The first well-defined zero crossing is a convenient point to choose for timing each signal, since it can be accurately measured, for instance, by use of a superimposed cursor with continuous readout of position. However, the lateral wave, being generated by the off-axis part of the ultrasonic beam, usually has a different pulse shape and lower centre frequency than the defect signals and this can lead to errors in estimating the time interval between the lateral wave and the defect signal. The problem has been discussed at greater length in Section 2.3.2.7 where recommendations can be found for minimising the errors.

As we have already pointed out, however, a single A-scan is of rather restricted value and it will generally be necessary to analyse a two-dimensional B- or D-scan constructed from many A-scans. This requires some additional aids. The B-scan presentation is particularly useful in aiding data interpretation since the human eye is very good at detecting correlations between adjacent traces. The following sections describe the processing and analysis of these two-dimensional images.

## 5.4 Data flattening

Water coupling is often the most convenient way of ensuring that the signal amplitude is not unduly affected by surface condition. However, it is not always possible, with water coupling, to maintain the water path precisely constant throughout a scan and this can produce substantial variations in signal timing because the wave velocity in water is only about one quarter of that in a steel workpiece. This effect is illustrated in Figure 5.3 with signals from a probe pair scanning at constant height over a plate with an undulating surface.

The resultant distortion not only makes accurate depth measurements more difficult but also affects the recognition of defect signals and the measurement of defect length. In addition, it complicates the application of further digital processing. This type of distortion of the B- or D-scan may be minimised by the use of hollow shoes which maintain a constant distance between probe and surface but even then, small

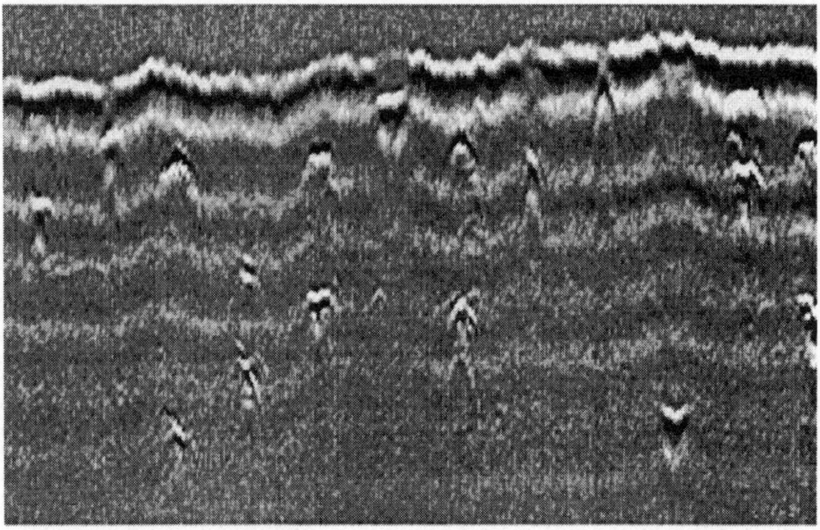

**Fig. 5.3** Signals from a probe pair scanning immersed in water at constant height over an undulating surface.

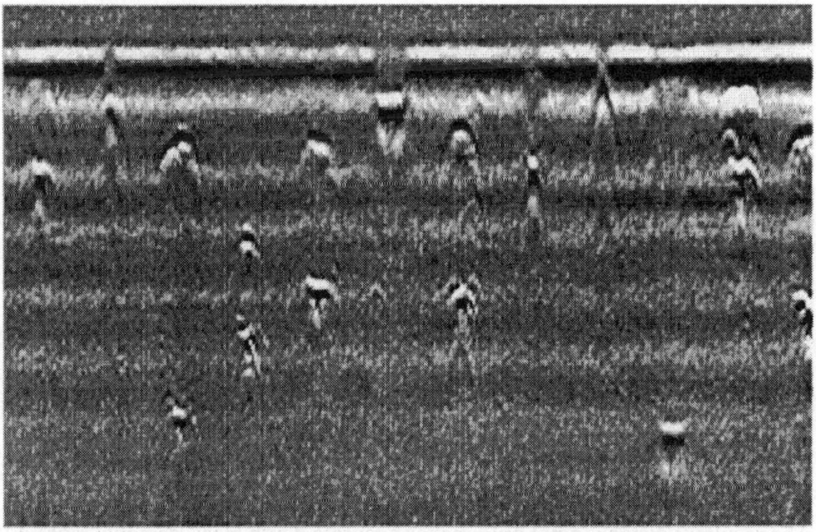

**Fig. 5.4** The B-scan image after data flattening to remove the variations in water path due to the undulating surface. Compare this with Figure 5.3.

scale roughness can produce sufficient fluctuation in signal timing to render the analysis of signals from near-surface defects more difficult.

Fortunately, provided there is a reference signal, either a lateral wave, or a backwall echo, of adequate amplitude, simple processing algorithms can be used to *flatten* the image so that it appears as if the water path had been constant. The B-scan from Figure 5.3 is shown after flattening in Figure 5.4.

If the reference signal is of large amplitude, a 'digital trigger' algorithm is convenient. In this method, the point at which the recorded A-scan crosses a particular voltage level is found and used to time shift the recorded signals to bring the reference signal to a constant position in the traces. The voltage level and the starting point for the search must be chosen so that the trigger will occur on the corresponding part of the reference signal on every waveform and this is easiest to arrange for the first or second half cycle of lateral wave since there should be no larger voltages occurring earlier in the trace. In favourable circumstances, this flattening process can be accurate to a fraction of a sampling interval, and, to take advantage of this, the method of time shifting the signals should be capable of doing shifts of a fraction of a sampling interval. This can be done by transforming to the frequency domain, applying a phase shift proportional to frequency and transforming back to the time domain.

Where the signal amplitude is weak or fluctuating, the simple trigger algorithm may not work well and better performance may be achieved by using the peak cross correlation between a model reference signal and the recorded signals to correct the timing. The model signal can be obtained from a single trace or by averaging several traces in a region where the timing is nearly constant. When the lateral wave is used as a reference, the functioning of the algorithm is aided by the fact that the lateral wave is usually far from the beam axis and so has a lower centre frequency than the defect signals.

If the above methods fail at some points in the scan, for instance where the reference signal amplitude is very low, or where it suffers interference from a defect signal, the time shifts for the failed region may be based on interpolation between neighbouring successful regions or may be derived interactively by shifting individual traces to give the most satisfactory appearance.

It will be apparent, from the discussion of errors given in Chapter 2, that variations of the lateral-wave time arising from changes in coupling thickness imply some small variations in the geometry of the TOFD process. Consequently, while data flattening techniques remove the primary problem arising from such variations, there is still some degradation of the accuracy which would have been achieved if the coupling thickness had been kept constant. It is desirable, therefore, to design probe mountings so as to minimise coupling thickness variations and to use flattening only to remove residual effects.

In the following description of analysis techniques, it is assumed that flattening will have been done where necessary.

## 5.5 Signal recognition

In many circumstances, the defect signals of interest will be the only signals of significant amplitude occurring between the lateral wave and the back-wall echo and no recognition aids will be needed, However, this is not always so. In large-grained anisotropic materials or in materials containing inclusions or other inhomogeneities, there may be a background clutter of amplitude comparable with that of the defect signals. Even when the defect signals are clear, the presence of mode-converted signals cannot always be excluded because there may be physical constraints on the choice of probe separation. In these circumstances, some aid to recognition of the signals of interest is desirable.

Little can be done to assist in signal recognition on a single A-scan trace and this is one of the chief disadvantages of such displays. On a B- or D-scan display, however, the effects of beam spread give the defect indication a characteristic shape which can be used as an aid to recognition.

### 5.5.1 Arcs and curve fitting

The way in which the time-of-flight of a defect varies with transducer position during a scan leads to characteristic arcs appearing in the data displays which can be used to enhance defect detection and to give more accurate sizing capability. Consider a single point on a diffracting edge in a block of uniform thickness. When that point lies in the vertical plane defined by the probe beam centrelines and is equidistant from the two probes, the transit time will be a minimum. If the probe assembly is moved a little in any direction, the signal will still be present because the point still lies within the beams but the distance will have increased and the indication will therefore appear a little later on the display. A continuous scan across the location of the edge will therefore produce an indication having characteristic downward-curving tails as we saw in Figures 2.2 and 2.14 and can also be seen in Figure 5.4. Figure 5.5 shows the shape of the diffraction arcs as a function of the depth below the surface of the diffraction point for a probe separation of 62 mm and a cladding layer thickness of 7 mm (see Chapter 7 for a discussion of the effects of cladding). The displacement in this case is parallel to the line joining the probe index points. For displacements perpendicular to that line, the arcs are all hyperbolae (see Section 2.3.4), broadening as the defect depth increases.

When the argument is extended to all points on a continuous horizontal edge, the tails from interior parts of the edge cancel, so that the resultant indication is horizontal over the length of the edge with the characteristic tails still appearing at each end. An example of such a signal from a rectangular patch defect appears in Figure 5.6.

Since the shape of the tails depends only on the defect depth, probe separation and direction of probe motion, it is predetermined for any given depth on a B- or D-scan display. The prediction of the shape has already been discussed in Section 2.3.4. It is a simple matter to provide a means of displaying the correct shape as a cursor on a digital display and to allow it to be moved interactively to check its fit to any

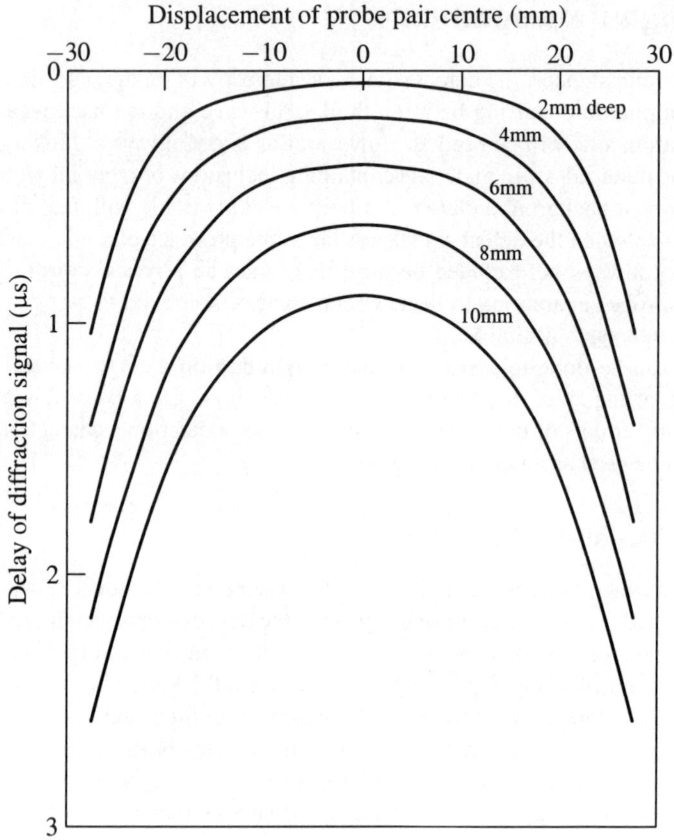


**Fig. 5.5** Theoretical curves of signal delay versus probe displacement for 62 mm probe separation and 7 mm thick cladding. The displacement is parallel to the line joining the probe index points.

suspected defect indication. An example of an overlay display is given in Figure 5.7, taken from Slesenger, Hesketh and Silk [1985].

Where the pattern of signals is very complex as a result of mode conversions, it may be necessary to make a judgment as to which are the unconverted compression wave signals from the top and bottom of the defect and then calculate the positions and curve shapes of all possible mode converted signals. By overlaying the set of curves so produced on the B-scan image, the hypothesis that all signals arise from a single defect can be thoroughly tested. Figure 5.8 is an elegant example of such an overlay used on a complex pattern of signals [Ramsey, 1987].

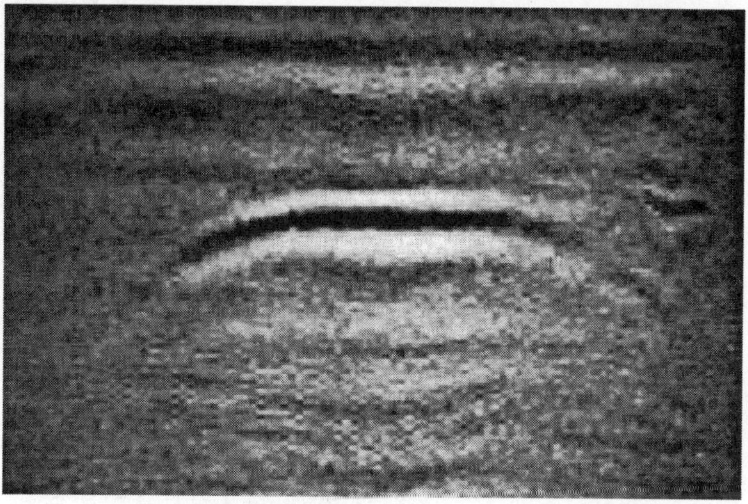

**Fig. 5.6** Experimental signals from a crack with an extended horizontal edge.

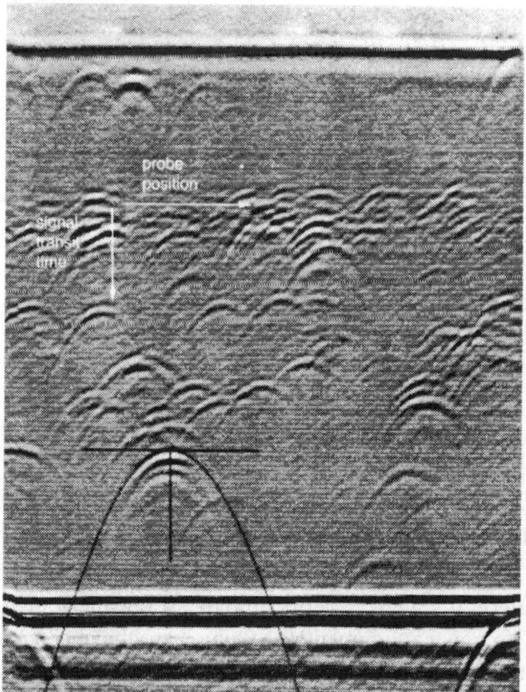


**Fig. 5.7** Hyperbolic cursor superimposed on the signal from a pointlike defect (from Slesenger et al. [1985]).

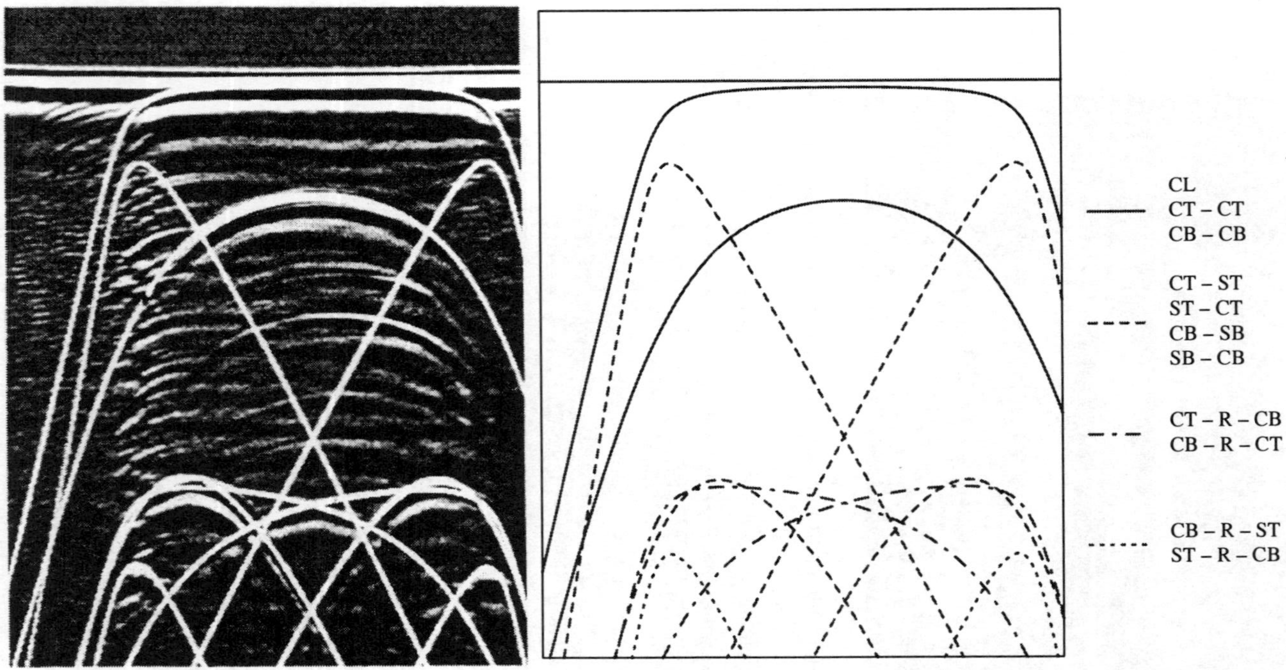


**Fig. 5.8** The left-hand figure is reproduced from Ramsey [1987] and shows a TOFD B-scan from a test block with the signal arcs marked with loci calculated on the basis of assumptions about the presence of a smooth planar defect. The right-hand figure provides an explanatory key. In the key codes at extreme right, each group of characters indicates a leg of the ultrasonic path. The first character indicates the wave mode, C, S and R representing compression, shear and Rayleigh wave modes respectively. For the second character, L indicates the lateral wave, while T and B indicate that the source or destination of that particular leg of the path is the top or bottom of the defect respectively. The Rayleigh wave leg is on the defect surface, from top to bottom or *vice versa*.

## 5.6 Measurement of defect location

In simple geometry, such as a flat plate, locating the source of a defect signal involves measuring its depth from the inspection surface, its distance from the start of the scan along the scan line and its lateral displacement from the scan line. By *scan line*, we mean the line on the inspection surface followed by a point equidistant from the probe index points during the inspection scan. The lateral direction is parallel to the the line joining the index points. The extra complications arising from more complex inspection geometries are dealt with in Chapter 6.

### 5.6.1 Depth from the inspection surface

The interactive cursor may also be used for depth measurement. The cursor is first located on the start of the lateral wave and the equivalent time logged. Then the cursor is located on the defect indication and the time logged again. The remarks in Section 5.3 about choice of timing point apply equally here. The computer, previously loaded with velocity and probe separation figures can then display the defect depth. In the case of defects very near the surface, interference between the defect signal and the lateral wave may make time measurements on the central portion of the curve difficult but the tails may be clearly visible. The tails are more likely to be visible if the scan is a true B-scan (i.e. transducer beams and probe movement in the same plane). Depth measurement may then be done by choosing the depth for which the cursor best fits the tails of the indication. As already mentioned in Section 5.5.1, this will require recalculation and redisplay of the cursor shape at each depth adjustment, since the shape is very depth-dependent in the near-surface region.

An alternative way of displaying depth information is to transform the whole image to give a true depth scale. First, the range of depth to be displayed is selected and divided up so as to give (say) 512 equally-spaced depth values. The sample number in the digitised records which corresponds to each depth value may then be calculated. Finally, a complete new set of A-scans is constructed by selecting from the original set those samples which correspond most closely to each of the equally-spaced depth values. A B-scan constructed from these new A-scans provides an image which is linearly related to a cross section of the workpiece and from which approximate depths and sizes may be read by eye. It also indicates clearly, from the apparent sharpness of the defect signals, how the depth resolution varies as a function of depth.

### 5.6.2 Position along the scan line

Estimating the position of the defect along the scan line is inseparable from estimating its length in that direction; this measurement is dealt with in detail in Section 5.7.

### 5.6.3 Lateral position

It is not possible to estimate the lateral position from a single scan of one pair of probes. The path length derived from a single pair defines an ellipsoid of revolution, with the probe index points as foci, on which the signal source lies. There are two ways of getting unambiguous information about the lateral position of the source. The first is to use two or more probe pairs with scan lines laterally displaced and to derive the source location from the crossing of the ellipsoids. This is the method used by Hawker [1983] to locate defects in the Defect Detection Trials (see Figure 2.12 on page 38). The second method is to do an additional scan over the defect in a direction perpendicular to the primary scan. When the time of flight of the defect signal is at a minimum, the source is located symmetrically between the probes.

## 5.7 Measurement of defect length

If a defect has straight horizontal upper and lower edges, its length in the scan direction can be measured by first fitting the shaped cursor to the left-hand tail of the indication and then to the right-hand tail and noting the movement between these two positions. This technique is particularly effective for near-surface defects, because the hyperbolic signal arcs are narrow in the scan direction, so there is little ambiguity in positioning the cursor. For defects at considerable depth, the arcs are broader and the measurements consequently less accurate. In this case, more accurate length measurements may be derived from data processed by the synthetic aperture focusing technique (SAFT) (see Section 5.8.1).

If the defect edges are curved or sloping, good length measurements may still be obtained in many cases, provided the procedure described in the next section is followed. If the defects are very irregular in shape, it may be that SAFT processing would deliver better accuracy of length measurement but no convincing systematic demonstration of SAFT on this type of defect has been published thus far.

### 5.7.1 Using the shaped cursor for defect length measurement

To demonstrate that good results can be obtained on realistic defect shapes, we include here in Figure 5.9 a simulation due to Hawker and Burch [1999], showing successive steps in measuring the profile of a far-surface crack by careful matching of the shaped cursor against the signal indication. The point to emphasise here is that where the cursor curve touches the signal indication curve, the slopes must match. For all such points, the position of the centre of the cursor is marked (being the position of the diffracting edge which produced that portion of the signal). The locus of the marked points traces out the profile of the diffracting edge and, if it is sensibly complete, gives an accurate indication of the whole extent of the defect. Another useful technique illustrated here is that of fitting the cursor to the tails on the back-wall echo at each end of the region where it is obscured. This allows one to estimate the full length of the crack where it opens to the back surface.

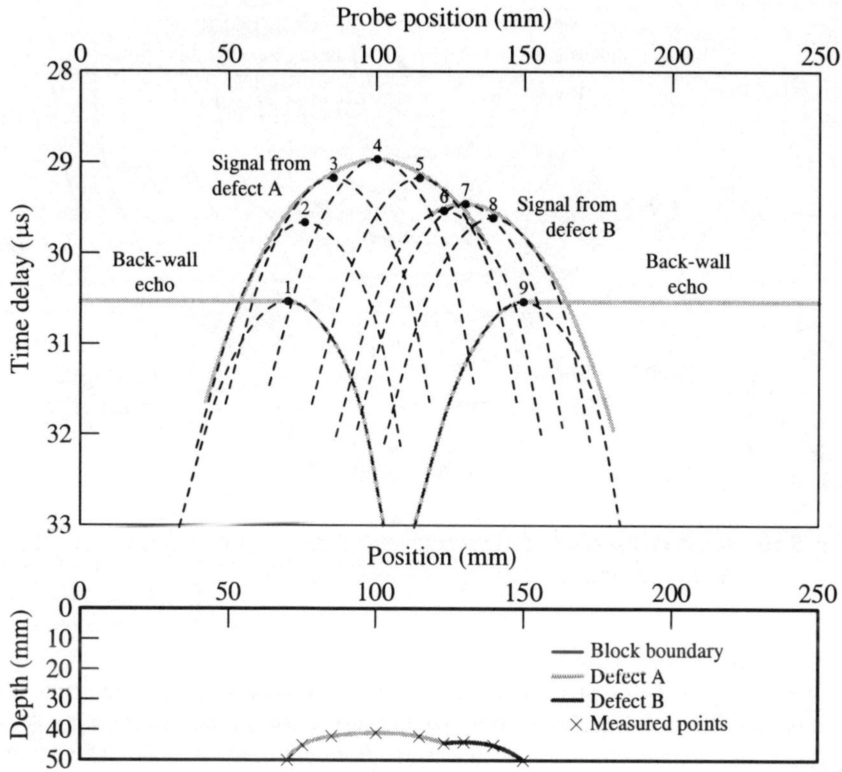


**Fig. 5.9** Simulated derivation of a defect profile using shaped cursor. The upper figure shows the successive positions of the hyperbolic cursor used in derivation of the profile. At each point, the cursor touches a defect signal or back-wall echo at a point where the slopes match. The lower figure shows the actual defect shape in the block with the measured points superposed.

The defect used in this demonstration was such that it gave a continuous signal indication over its whole length and every part of the diffracting edge contributed to the indication. The majority of real defects would fall into that category but it is possible to imagine 'pathological' defects which would be much more difficult to profile. How this may arise is described in the next section.

### 5.7.2 Effects of defect shape on apparent defect length

Diffracted waves arise from all the insonified parts of the edges of a defect but signals will be detected only when the contributions from different parts are sufficiently close in phase for constructive interference to occur. From Fermat's principle, this will occur whenever the path length from the transmitter to the receiver via a point on the defect edge is approximately stationary with respect to variations in the position

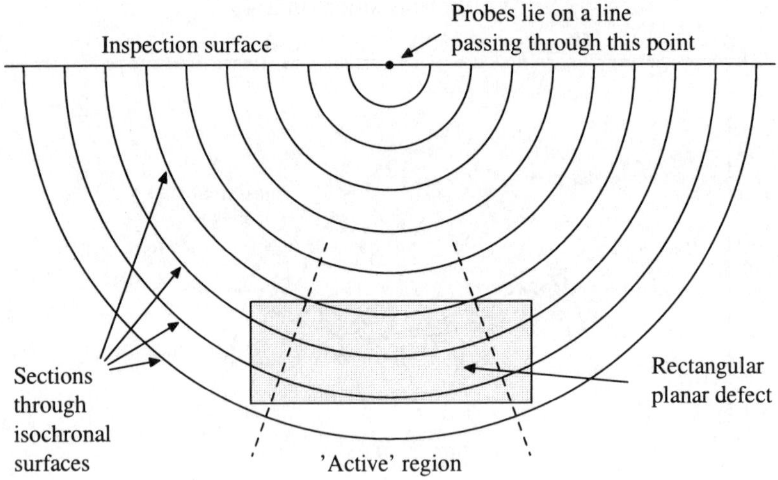


**Fig. 5.10** Isochronal surfaces for a rectangular defect located midway between the transmitter and receiver.

of the point on the defect edge.

Let us consider the standard Time-of-Flight Diffraction probe arrangement of two probes facing each other on a horizontal inspection surface and, further, let us suppose that the pulse is a single half cycle. For contributions from different edge points to add, they must have transit times which differ by less than the pulse duration. Let us divide transit time into units of one half cycle and associate an isochronal surface or isochrone with each integral time point. The isochrones are then ellipsoids of revolution with the probe indices as foci. The only regions of these isochrones relevant to signal production (active regions) are those which lie within both ultrasonic beams. A particular defect edge will produce a noticeable signal if it follows the active region of an isochrone closely.

Consider a planar defect lying in the vertical plane which is equidistant from the two probes; this plane cuts the isochrones in a set of circles centred on the point in the inspection surface which lies on the line joining the probes. If a long rectangular defect lies directly between the probes, and perpendicular to the line joining the probe centres, its top and bottom edges pass through a horizontal active region of the isochrone and thus produce strong signals, while its outside vertical end edges are either nearly normal to the isochrones, or are outside the active region, and so produce a negligible resultant signal. This situation is illustrated in Figure 5.10.

Suppose now that the probes are scanned parallel to the defect plane so as to approach and pass over the defect. The top and bottom signals will remain constant over most of the defect length, falling by 6 dB at the points where the defect ends are aligned with the beam centreline. At these points the signals should be showing slight extra delay and this will increase, giving rise to the characteristic signal curves, as the scan passes beyond the defect. Thus, for a rectangular defect, the length of the

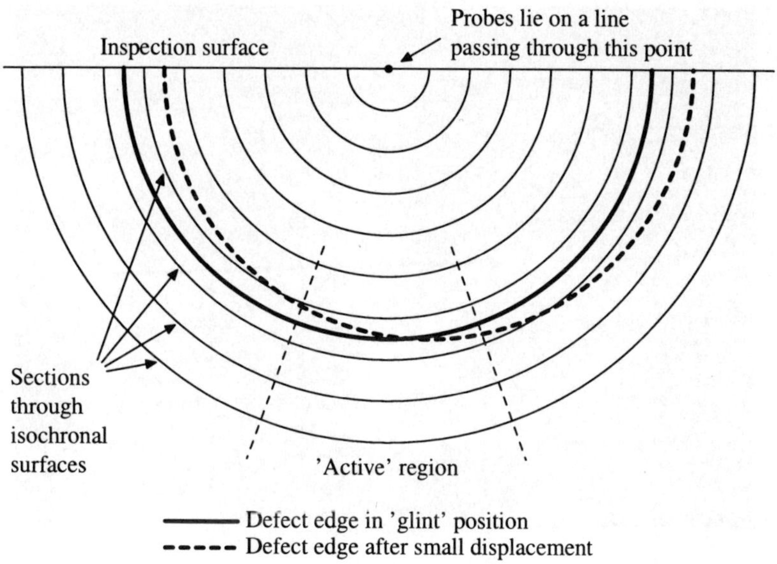


**Fig. 5.11** Isochronal surfaces for a semi-circular defect located symmetrically between the transmitter and receiver (solid line) and with its centre laterally displaced (broken line).

top and bottom signals in the D-scan image will give a good indication of the defect length and length measurements made either by 6 dB drop or cursor fitting should be reasonably accurate.

Let us replace the rectangular defect with one of a rather special shape, a surface-breaking semi-circular crack. As Figure 5.11 shows, at almost every scan position the defect edge crosses several isochrones and the signal will be destroyed by destructive interference. When the centre of the semi-circle lies on the line joining the probes, however, the whole defect edge lies parallel to an isochrone and a very large signal will result. This effect is most clearly demonstrated for very wide-beam probes but even for conventional probes the effect is striking, as shown in Figure 5.12.

This tendency to produce a strong glint or flashpoint at the symmetrical position and weak or negligible signals elsewhere applies whenever a section of the lower edge of a defect approximates a portion of a semi-circle centred on the inspection surface. Typical defects showing this effect are semi-elliptical surface-breaking cracks. Note, however, that the total length of a surface-breaking crack can be estimated from the scan distance over which the lateral wave is blocked. For a defect of elliptical shape, in an arbitrary orientation with respect to the transmitter and receiver, there are up to four flashpoints on the defect edge, generally three on the lower edge and one on the upper edge of the defect. The curvature of the edge causes focusing of the diffracted rays, described in the theory by caustics — regions of (theoretically)

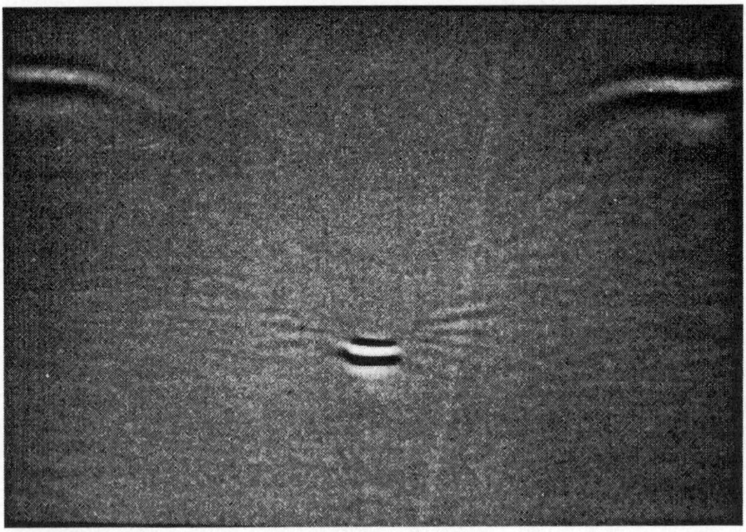

**Fig. 5.12** A glint or flashpoint from a semi-circular defect edge.

infinite amplitude.

The signal patterns produced by defects of other shapes can be worked out by similar arguments to those used above. A buried crack with irregular edges would tend to produce top and bottom signals appearing intermittent on the scan image. In attempting to characterise the defects from the appearance of such signals, it must be borne in mind that discontinuous signals do not necessarily arise from discontinuous defects.

One method of obtaining additional detectable signals in a conventional scan is to carry out further scans with the probes skewed so that the active region moves out to the side of the vertical plane through the probes [Atkinson, Birchall and Plevin, 1989; Highmore and Rogerson, 1988]. SAFT processing of data collected with wide-beam probes should also be effective.

# 5.8 Signal Processing

## 5.8.1 Processing techniques for improving the accuracy of defect length measurement

The conventional method of sizing defects larger than the beam width is to measure the probe movement between points where the defect signal amplitude is 6 dB below its maximum value. This technique achieves adequate accuracy on large defects at moderate ranges and has been used for measuring the length of defects from Time-of-Flight Diffraction signals, as an alternative and more easily automated method than the cursor fitting technique described in Section 5.7.1. In general, it is not necessary, for integrity assessments, to know the length of a defect as accurately as its through-wall extent. However, for small defects in areas of high stress or for defects at long range where the beam spread is considerable, the 6 dB drop technique may not give acceptable accuracy. Without some form of processing the width of a reflector measured using the 6 dB drop method will be systematically oversized for reflectors smaller than the diameter of the transducer. This applies equally to the length measurement of a defect made with Time-of-Flight and to both through-wall extent and defect length when measured with conventional pulse-echo techniques.

The most commonly applied method of improving the accuracy achievable by the 6 dB drop method is to process the data first by means of the Synthetic Aperture Focusing Technique (SAFT) and apply the 6 dB drop method to the processed signals.

The essence of synthetic aperture focusing is that the unrectified radio frequency data from different transducer positions are combined with the correct phases to synthesise the effects of a single transducer having a large aperture. This aperture can be focused accurately at all depths. Data taken during an ultrasonic scan of the transducer along a line are combined to give a theoretical lateral resolution of one half the transducer width. The difference between processed and unprocessed data depends on the ratio $r/N$, where $r$ is the distance of the defect from the transducer and $N$ is the transducer near-field distance given by $D^2/4\lambda$, where $D$ is the transducer diameter and $\lambda$ is the ultrasonic wavelength. The oversizing from unprocessed data is worse for larger values of $r/N$, that is, as the defect goes further into the far field. For $r/N = 2$, there is very little difference between unprocessed data and that processed using SAFT [Burch, 1987], but by $r/N = 4$ the limiting ratio of the 6 dB drop defect width to the transducer diameter for a small defect (with length, say, 0.2 times the transducer diameter) is about 0.8 for unprocessed data and about 0.5 with SAFT processing. At $r/N = 7$, and for defects of length 0.2 times the transducer diameter, the unprocessed 6 dB drop width is 1.6 times the transducer diameter, that is eight times the actual value, whereas with SAFT the value becomes 0.6 times the transducer diameter, or three times the actual value.

Other forms of processing, such as Wiener filtering or the maximum entropy method, can be applied instead of SAFT to enhance lateral resolution. They have been compared in effectiveness by Burch [1987] who concluded that these deconvolution techniques were practical on B-scan images provided the appropriate point spread functions were known. However, these functions vary with range to the defect so that, where images contain defects at significantly different depths, these would need to be deconvolved separately. The lateral resolution achieved by Wiener filtering was higher than that by SAFT processing by a factor of from 1.3 in the far field to about 2 at twice the near-field distance. Wiener filtering is not adversely affected by phase differences between the point spread function and the signal to be deconvolved, whereas the maximum entropy method is. This suggests that Wiener filtering would probably be the optimum processing technique where the highest resolution is required. However, while SAFT achieves less good resolution, it requires no knowledge of the pulse shape, it is not sensitive to changes in the pulse shape and it is convenient to apply. The heavy computing requirements of the maximum entropy method and its sensitivity to phase ruled it out in the early development history of the Time-of-Flight technique but sufficiently powerful computers now reside on almost every desktop.

### 5.8.2 Derivation of signal phase

When a simple defect is detected there is usually no ambiguity about which signal arises from the top and which from the bottom of the defect. When the defect breaks one surface, this will be apparent from the effects on either the lateral wave or the back-wall echo. With a single defect of complex shape or a number of defects in close proximity, it may not be immediately obvious whether a given indication arises from a top or a bottom edge. As we have seen from Chapter 3, the phase of top and bottom edge signals differs but judging phase by eye is not always easy. Burch and Ramsey [1986] describe a Fourier transform processing method of deriving phase information and and a way of displaying the results to facilitate interpretation. This method also provides an unambiguous way of measuring the difference in time-of-flight of two signals, irrespective of any phase difference.

### 5.8.3 Other signal processing methods

Silk [1994] reviews signal processing methods which have been applied to both TOFD data and data from other ultrasonic techniques. While some of the methods cited have shown promise, it is fair to say that only SAFT is in reasonably widespread use and even that is not exploited to the extent that its capability would justify, perhaps because the technique is not understood by NDT practitioners and is often not provided as standard on the equipment used for analysis.

In another field, where the same type of signal processing techniques are required as in ultrasonic TOFD, the Hough transform has been used to find the best fit to hyperbolic diffraction arcs in the B-scan images of ground penetrating radar [Capineri, Grande and Temple, 1998] and a similar approach using Hough and Oja transforms has been applied to ultrasonic TOFD data [Capineri, Grande, Masotti, Temple and Windsor, 1997].

Time-of-Flight Diffraction tomography has also been considered as a possible processing tool and its potential demonstrated using synthetic data [Capineri, Tattersall, Temple and Silk, 1992; Capineri, Tattersall, Silk and Temple, 1993].

## 5.9 Defect characterisation

The state of the art of defect characterisation with conventional ultrasonic techniques, *circa* 1980, was reviewed by Rogerson and Murgatroyd [1980]; more recent advances in characterisation methods for conventional techniques have been discussed by Burch and Bealing [1986, 1987]. Highmore and Rogerson [1988] and Atkinson et al. [1989] explored scanning with skewed probes as a means of obtaining additional information for defect characterisation, but there has been no concerted study of characterisation by means of the Time-of-Flight Diffraction technique. The strength of TOFD lies in its ability to reveal the location of defect edges, whereas the pulse-echo technique is sensitive to the presence of planar features. The most complete characterisation is therefore likely to require the application of both techniques. A combination of the TOFD technique and tandem probe inspection was used on samples from the PISC II Parametric Study on Flaw Characterisation [Murgatroyd, Highmore, Burch, Bann and Ramsey, 1988]. Some of these blocks had several defects in close proximity in such a way that complex patterns of signal arcs on the B-scan could arise from the ultrasound skipping between the defects. To interpret such complex signals, it is usually necessary to consider a number of model defect configurations and to calculate the expected signal patterns, comparing the calculated pattern with the observed one to eliminate model defect configurations which produce poor matches to the experimental data. Several steps of refinement of the model may be necessary. Figure 5.8 illustrates this technique.

Planar defects with complex shapes will give rise to several distinct diffracted and backscattered signals. The backscattered or diffracted signals consist of a series of pulses as has been shown theoretically by Friedlander [1958], Freedman [1962] and Lam and Tsang [1985]. Consider a rigid, impenetrable and convex defect having dimensions and radii of curvature which are large in terms of the ultrasonic wavelength. The shape of the defect can be projected along the line joining its centre to the receiver. The envelopes of the returning pulses for backscattered radiation are copies of the transmitted pulse and originate from those parts of the defect where a change in the projected cross-sectional area occurs. The pulses arrive with a time dependent on the range of the transducers from the discontinuities in defect area. Each echo amplitude is governed by the size and type of discontinuity in the projected area of the defect. The mathematical description of this is included in Section A.7 of the Appendix. Making use of this type of information on arrival times only, Lam and Tsang [1985] demonstrated that a microcomputer system could be used to reconstruct the shape of unknown planar, straight-edged, flaws from diffraction echoes of short ultrasonic pulses.

## 5.10 Modelling studies on analysis of TOFD data

Silk [1996a] used synthetic data to investigate the sensitivity of the detection capability of TOFD to the noise level in the ultrasonic signals. Because the theoretical TOFD response from "ideal" flaws is well understood (see Chapters 2 and 3), it is easy to synthesise the B-scans from such defects. To these artificial B-scans, which have been used in TOFD training courses, realistic noise can be added in the digital images. Silk created 50 B-scan simulations representing either cracks or slag lines. Each simulation had a scan length of 500 mm and the notional probe separation was 100 mm. From this study, which involved five TOFD inspectors, Silk concluded that at noise levels typical of TOFD inspections, the probability of detection was 100% with no false calls. At moderately elevated noise levels the trial produced a

3% chance of reporting a false call while maintaining the 100% detection rate. At higher noise levels the probability of detection fell and the probability of false calls increased, as expected.

Silk [1996b] also used simulated data for investigating the sizing capability of TOFD. This simulation of 26 flaws was used to show that the theoretical through-wall sizing capability should be close to 0.25 mm. In addition, five procedures for estimating the length of the defects were tested. Several procedures gave good results on simulated flaws with straight profiles, but most were ineffective on flaws with curved profiles, so that errors of 10 mm might arise. However, more recent work by Hawker and Burch [1999], described in Section 5.7.1, shows that accurate defect lengths can be derived for quite complex defect profiles by using a hyperbolic cursor facility in the correct manner.

# Chapter 6

# Complex Geometries

Much large industrial plant contains pipes and nozzles welded to thick cylindrical components, often working under high pressure. The welds tend to be in regions of high stress and therefore require inspection for weld integrity during manufacture and possibly for crack initiation and propagation during service. As we have already seen, ultrasonics is the most useful nondestructive test, since it can give information on which fracture mechanics assessments of component integrity may be based.

Where two cylinders intersect, for instance, two cylindrical components of an offshore structure or a nozzle attached to a pressure vessel, the weld forms a three dimensional saddle shape. Probes with a given, fixed, beam angle placed on any one of the surfaces cannot always cover the entire weld volume which needs to be inspected. Thus, design of scanners for such geometries necessitates even more care than is taken with scanners for the simpler geometries of flat plates.

The Time-of-Flight Diffraction technique opens up new alternatives for inspection of complex geometries compared with pulse-echo techniques because of its insensitivity to the relative orientation of probes and defect. With pulse-echo techniques relying on specular reflection it often proves very difficult to arrange for probe beams to illuminate areas of concern, such as welds, at near normal incidence. Tandem techniques also prove difficult because the back wall of the specimen is very often not parallel to the inspection surface in nozzle to shell welds or offshore nodes, for example.

## 6.1 T-butt welds

The Welding Institute, the Harwell Laboratory and the Central Electricity Generating Board carried out a programme of collaborative work on the ultrasonic detection, sizing and characterisation of cracks and other defects in steel components. The work was in four phases, the results from the first three of which, on flat plate specimens, are discussed later, in Section 8.3. Phase 4 was aimed specifically at extending the work on flat plates to more complex geometries. Material to BS 1501 grade 223-

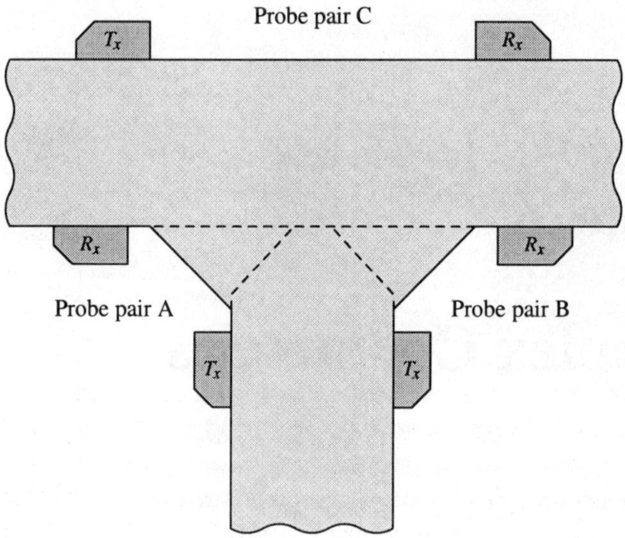


**Fig. 6.1** Arrangements of probes for Time-of-Flight Diffraction inspection of a T-butt weld in phase 4 of the Welding Institute programme.

32B was welded into six specimens with deliberately created defects and two other specimens were used from scrapped structures. In the made-up specimens, the defect types were cracks, linear slag, lack of fusion, porosity, and lack of penetration, while in the other two specimens the defects were lamellar tears. Time-of-Flight Diffraction was applied to detection and sizing of the lack of fusion, cracks and porosity in two T-butt welds formed from two plates, each 38 mm thick, welded together with a full penetration weld. The geometry and locations of the Time-of-Flight Diffraction probes are shown in Figure 6.1. A B-scan obtained with probe pair B of Figure 6.1 is shown in Figure 6.2. The first signal, equivalent to the lateral wave in a flat plate, is a wave which follows the surface from the transmitter probe to the receiver probe, undergoing diffraction at the edges of the weld fillet. Clear signals from defects in the weld metal can be seen both ahead of and behind the strong continuous signal arising from reflection at the far surface of the web. While the detection of defects by this means is straightforward, locating and sizing them require a careful analysis of possible wave paths, reflection points, diffraction from geometrical features, mode conversions, etc.

Once experience had been gained in interpreting the B-scan images with the probe arrangements which were novel at that time, Time-of-Flight Diffraction demonstrated an accuracy on T-butt welds similar to that obtainable on flat plates. Initial accuracy obtained was a mean sizing error of 1.7 mm with a standard deviation of 4.0 mm but this improved to a mean error of 0.1 mm with a standard deviation of 1.1 mm after progression up the learning curve. To quote the conclusions of the report [Cameron, Jessop, Mudge, Charlesworth, Silk, Bowker, Wrigley and

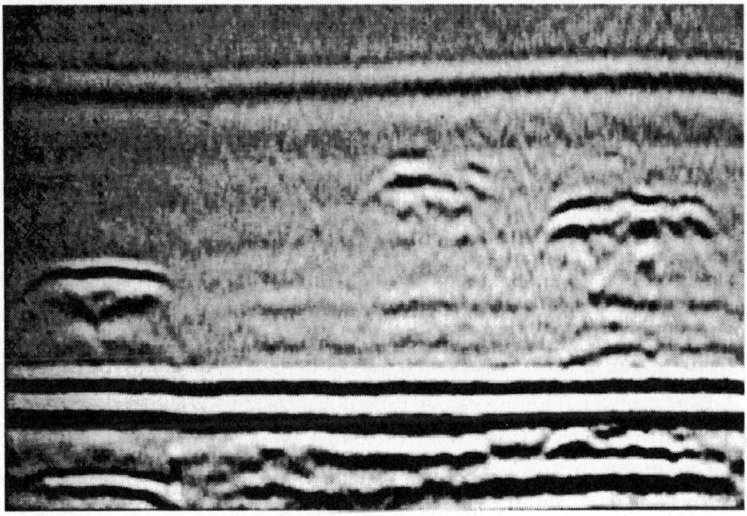

**Fig. 6.2** Signals observed with Time-of-Flight Diffraction on Welding Institute T-butt weld.

Denby, 1983], '... *The Time-of-Flight Diffraction appears to have been successfully adapted to allow the inspection of complex joints. The ability of conventional ultrasonics to accurately predict defect character has again been shown to be insufficient to allow high confidence to be placed in the prediction.*'

Cecco and Carter [1983] also studied T-welds containing volumetric flaws and a tight fatigue crack. The T-weld containing a fatigue crack consisted of two plates welded together; one plate, 22 mm thick, formed the web while the other plate, 50 mm thick, formed the base. The weld was 130 mm long and cracked along its entire length. They concluded that the volumetric weld flaws and fatigue crack were detectable from the surfaces forming the angle between the web and the web and the base even though the signals were weaker, and more difficult to interpret, than those obtained with inspection from the surface of the base opposite to the weld.

## 6.2 Inspection requirements for offshore structures

The first fixed structures for the northern North Sea, where depths of 150 m to 200 m of water are encountered, were positioned during 1974. Diving and operational difficulties for inspection are substantially greater in this area than in the southern North Sea. Exploration has continued into new areas, most of which are expected to pose no significant extra problems apart from the increasing number of structures. However, the regions such as the Western Approaches basin, the Hebrides and Rockall area and the fringes of the Shetland basin could involve structures being emplaced in up to 500 m of water and there is no doubt that these structures will require periodic underwater inspection. A noticeable characteristic of underwater inspection by divers at present is the unavoidable inefficiency compared with similar inspections on dry land. Tides, for example, may limit operation to an hour and a half per day while weather conditions may limit operations to less than 150 days per year [Bainton, Silk, Williams, Davies, Lyon and Peters, 1975]. Underwater, there are problems of manoeuvrability in a dark hostile environment with intrinsic personal danger. All these factors reduce the efficiency of underwater inspection.

Underwater, the need for rapid inspection has restricted the use of ultrasonic and radiographic techniques and emphasis has been placed on visual inspection, supplemented by magnetic particle and eddy current inspections. With the advent of thicker materials, and the availability of underwater welding repair techniques, it became more important to be able to assess the size of any cracks found, including buried defects which cannot be detected by these surface inspection methods.

Equipment designed for offshore use must work underwater at the depth required. In general the inspection routines adopted for offshore structures so far have been a regular manual inspection of the platform to include all joints over a 3 to 5 year period, with inspection of critical joints annually. Inspection normally starts with a general survey of the condition of the structure and weed growth. After appropriate local cleaning the welds are examined both visually and by nondestructive methods. The thickness of metal is checked where either the visual indications make it necessary, or in critical areas. Scour of the sea bed around the platform is normally checked during annual inspection. In 1975 no ultrasonic crack detection was used [Bainton et al., 1975], although ultrasonic thickness gauges were in use. By about 1983 various ultrasonic devices had been invented for defect detection and sizing [Anon., 1983; Fuller, Nestleroth and Rose, 1983; Rose, Fuller, Nestleroth and Jeong, 1983], although it was by no means accepted as the ultimate tool to supplant magnetic particle inspection, since others, such as photogrammetry, also gained acceptance [Anon., 1984]. Work since 1975 with Time-of-Flight Diffraction is detailed below.

## 6.3 Application to offshore structures

The use of fitness for purpose assessment to determine the severity of a defect is the most recent recommended practice for ultrasonic inspection of offshore structures both during fabrication and in-service [Gardner and Bosselaar, 1984]. Such an assessment places specific requirements on the inspection procedures employed to detect and size flaws. Fatigue is a major factor in determining the life of steel-jacketed structures in the North Sea. Many structures are now well into their third decade of operation so inspection for fatigue is becoming increasingly important. Of the several methods available for detecting defects, such as radiography, magnetic particle inspection and ultrasonics, only magnetic particle inspection and ultrasonics are applicable to complex geometries. For defect through-wall extent measurement, only alternating current potential drop (ACPD) and ultrasonics methods are suitable. Conventional ultrasonic methods, as we have pointed out elsewhere in this book, are based on interpretation of signal amplitude changes with probe movement and difficulties of interpretation can lead to inaccuracies of sizing. In order to improve the accuracy of sizing crack-like defects in offshore structures, the Time-of-Flight Diffraction technique has been evaluated in a joint industrial programme. Detailed procedures have been developed and refined in the light of practical experience, to cover all aspects of underwater application of Time-of-Flight Diffraction to the sizing of weld defects.

Time-of-Flight Diffraction was evaluated for the sizing of defects primarily because it allows accurate measurement of defect through-wall extent; the technique can be understood by ultrasonic technicians and the technical demands are simple, since adequate results can be obtained from a one dimensional scan [Gardner and Bosselaar, 1984]. Further, the ultrasonic Time-of-Flight Diffraction technique is the only ultrasonic technique not severely hindered by the signal amplitude fluctuations caused by surface roughness. For butt weld inspection, Time-of-Flight Diffraction simultaneously sizes any known defect and establishes the depth of weld penetration at that location. Finally, the sea-water provides the ideal ultrasonic coupling medium.

The welds of T-nodes, K-nodes and node connections involve more complicated geometry than flat plates. Figure 6.3 shows two examples of possible probe configurations for sizing a crack in the weld of an offshore node. Using beam angles of about 60° and 70° for transmitter and receiver respectively, the signals corresponding to six ray paths will be observed as shown on the figure. Paths 1, 2 and 5 give a good indication of the crack-tip position relative to the outer surface while path 6, the transmitted shear wave which is mode converted to a compression wave at the inner surface, provides confirmation of the geometry of the structure. This is important since measurements of crack extent are made relative to component surfaces. If these do not correspond to design drawings of the structure, then errors will be made in assessing the severity of any defects found. By using some of the measurements to check the component geometry such errors can be avoided. Paths 3 and 4 in Figure 6.3(a) provide enhanced precision in crack-tip location. Figure 6.3(b) shows an alternative arrangement in which a 45° beam is used to carry out the same inspection.

## 6.4 Signal acquisition and analysis

At least two probes are required with a mounting assembly which allows the operator to maintain predefined positions and angles for the probes with respect to the weld being inspected. A digital electronic system, located on the platform, is used to control the inspection process, to perform signal averaging in order to improve the signal-to-noise ratio, to record the data and to support the computer software used for data interpretation. A digital frame store display is used to present the data in pictorial form on a monitor as they are being collected. This allows a qualitative assessment of the results during scanning. The same display is used during signal interpretation, with the aid of the interactive modelling program, to superimpose the results on the component cross-section. The recorded data are inspected either on the

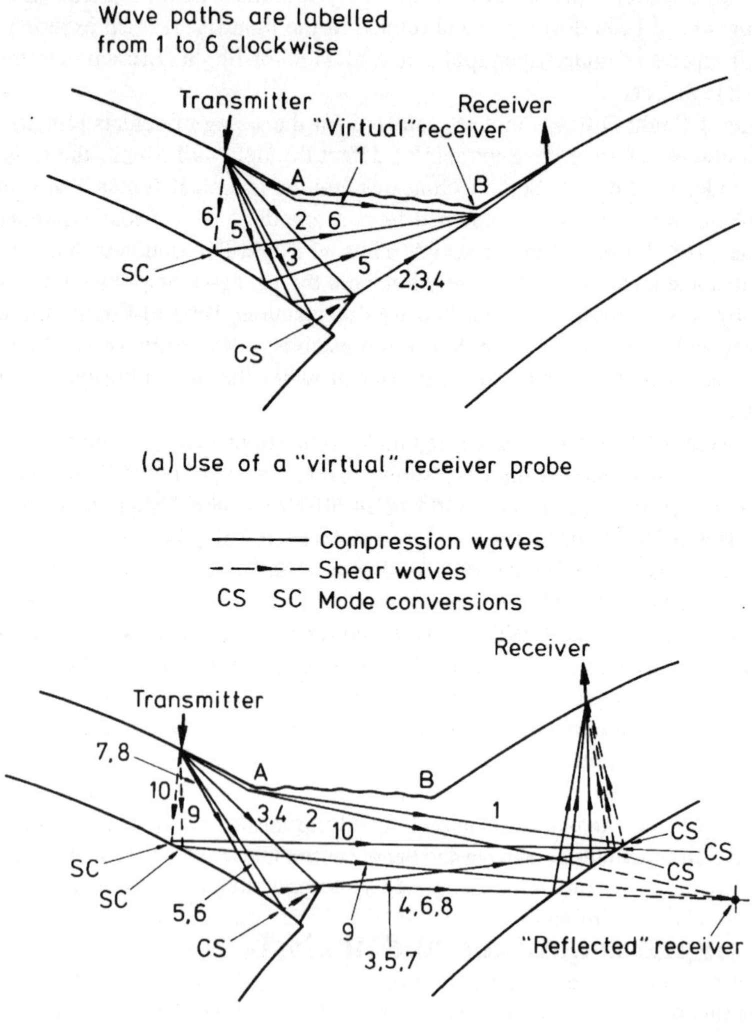


**Fig. 6.3** Examples of ultrasonic crack-sizing geometries in nodes of offshore structures (from Gardner and Bosselaar [1984]).

video display or on hardcopy output and defect indications assessed. The probe positions are determined from recorded scan speeds and operators' notes. The relative arrival times are determined using interactive graphics software or from measurements made on the hardcopy.

## 6.5 Results of trials

Gardner and Bosselaar [1984] reported on the results of applying Time-of-Flight Diffraction to the sizing of defects in samples relevant to offshore structures. Three specimens were used: a butt weld between flat plates of thickness 12.5 mm joined to 25 mm, containing a fatigue crack at one weld toe; a 90° T-butt weld containing a fatigue crack at the base toe of the weld; a section of a tubular node with member thicknesses of 32 mm and 18 mm intersecting at right angles with a fatigue crack approximately at the 3 o'clock position in the larger member at the weld toe. The results from these three samples, following destructive examination, showed that an accuracy of sizing of 1 mm was consistently achievable for features more than 5 mm below the inspection surface.

A series of trials of a complete prototype Time-of-Flight Diffraction sizing apparatus was carried out with divers in a diver training tank at facilities provided by Oceaneering International [Hawker, Newton and Wein, 1985; Newton, Wein and Hawker, 1986]. Node samples were located at a depth of 6 m in the tank. Divers who were unfamiliar with the Time-of-Flight Diffraction technique and without any NDT qualifications were required to make use of the manual scanners to move the ultrasonic transducers over the inspection surfaces. A diver operating the equipment within the tank is shown in Figure 6.4 (taken from Newton et al. [1986]).

A microprocessor-based data acquisition system was situated topside and used to collect and interpret the data. The data were displayed in real-time so that an immediate assessment of their quality could be made. Provided the data were satisfactory, they were stored on magnetic disc to provide a permanent record of the inspection. Interpretation could be carried out immediately or could be deferred until after diving operations were completed. Interpretation of data to derive a crack depth took about ten minutes. Newton et al. [1986] noted that the divers found the scanners easy to operate and were able consistently to obtain satisfactory data for crack sizing. During these trials a comfortable scanning speed of about 0.5 m/min was established.

A further series of trials was carried out at the Veritas site at the Coast Centre Base, Bergen, Norway. These open water trials were a more realistic test of Time-of-Flight Diffraction to sizing of cracks on offshore structures. Divers were required to operate at mid-depth of 10 m with all the problems associated with scanning while free floating or rigged to the structure, and coping with marine growth. The equipment itself was operated down to depths of 20 m. Some results from these two trials are presented in Figures 6.5 and 6.6.

In Figure 6.5, the destructive examination of the sample revealed that the crack had initiated at many locations along the toe of the weld, resulting in a large number

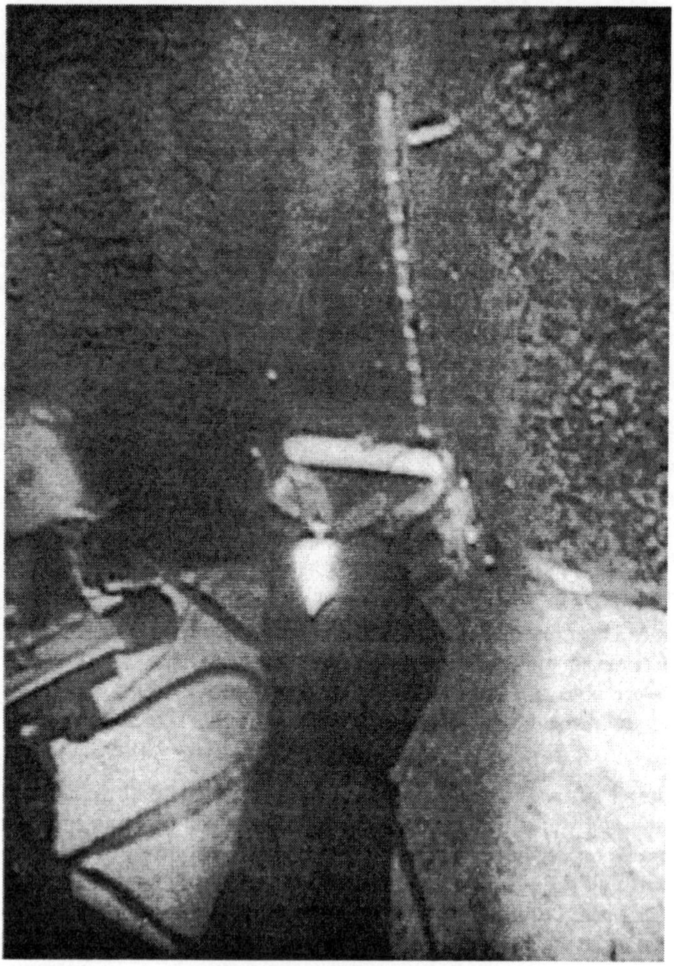

**Fig. 6.4** Underwater closed circuit television display of a diver operating ultrasonic Time-of-Flight Diffraction equipment for crack detection and sizing.

of bridges across the crack. Good agreement between the Time-of-Flight Diffraction crack profiles and those obtained during destructive examination are apparent in the figure, which is taken from Newton et al. [1986]. However, there is a clear discrepancy between the ACPD measurements and those obtained destructively, confirming that crack bridging can severely hinder accurate sizing with electromagnetic techniques. Figure 6.6 shows results obtained by a diver in open sea trials of Time-of-Flight Diffraction where the data obtained were as good as those achieved in the laboratory. The scans of this sample showed two small welding defects that had previously gone undetected.

Limitations to the use of Time-of-Flight Diffraction for offshore structures are:

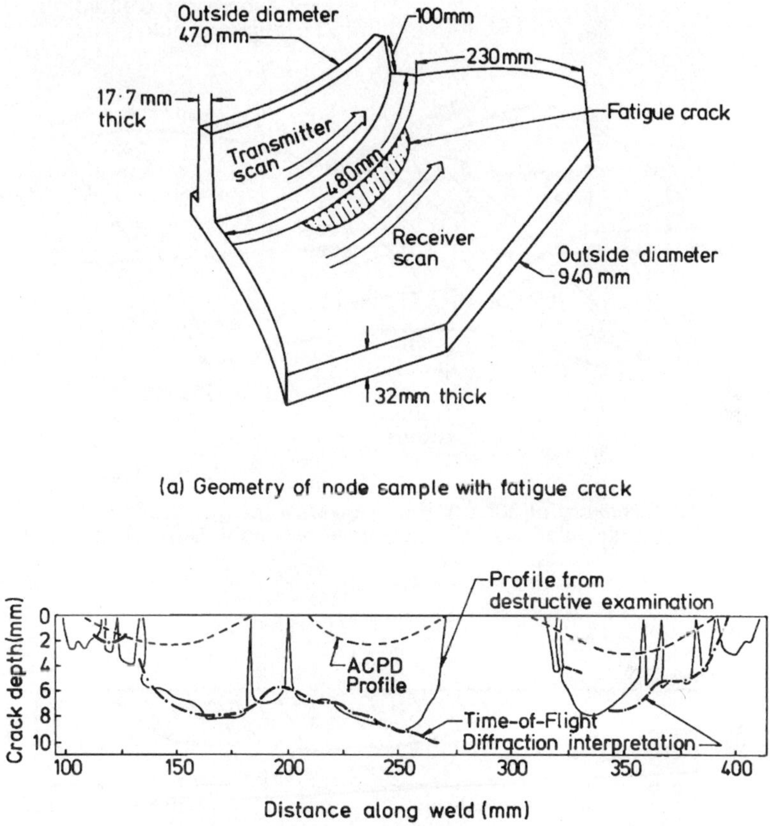


(a) Geometry of node sample with fatigue crack

(b) Comparison of crack profile obtained using Time-of-Flight Diffraction and A.C. Potential Drop with the profile obtained during destructive examination.

**Fig. 6.5** Comparison of results obtained with Time-of-Flight Diffraction and AC Potential Drop for cracks in a simulated node of an offshore structure.

the inspection surfaces must be cleared of calcareous deposits; access is required to both sides of the defect, so for a weld at the intersection of two tubular members, both of the members must be cleared of hard deposits; the steels used offshore contain more small inclusions than steels used in nuclear reactors, giving rise to ultrasonic signal clutter; some operational experience may be required to discard the signals from small, non-significant defects without a full sizing analysis. Where defects occur in welds of very acute angles (i.e. intersections of less than 45°), it can be difficult to establish the orientation of any cracks. There are of course compensating advantages: the early work, related to offshore structures, [Newton, 1987; Temple,

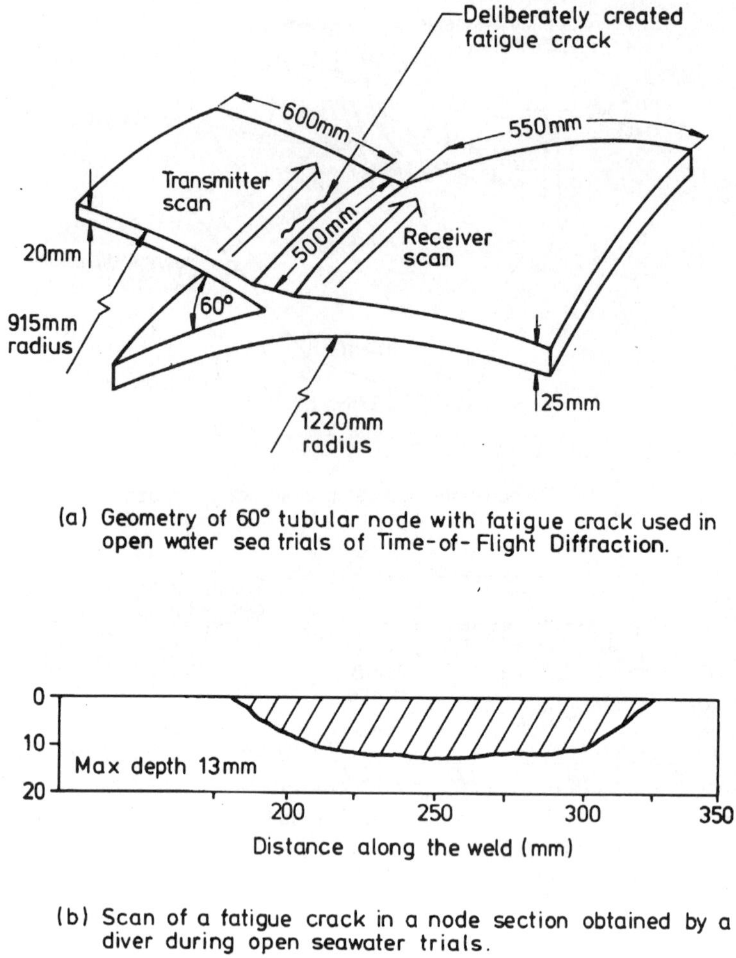


**Fig. 6.6** Time-of-Flight Diffraction result for a crack profile in a node section as obtained by a diver in open water sea trials.

1984b; Whapham, Perring and Rusbridge, 1985a], suggested that even when the crack is subjected to closing stresses the technique remains a viable way of establishing crack size. Indeed, the frequency filtering effects of cracks under compressive stress, causing preferential transmission of lower frequencies, may be used to characterise such cracks.

Another advantage of Time-of-Flight Diffraction is that it can be used for both buried defects and surface-breaking ones and can be used to give accurate location of the crack tip in three spatial dimensions. Techniques such as ACPD provide slant

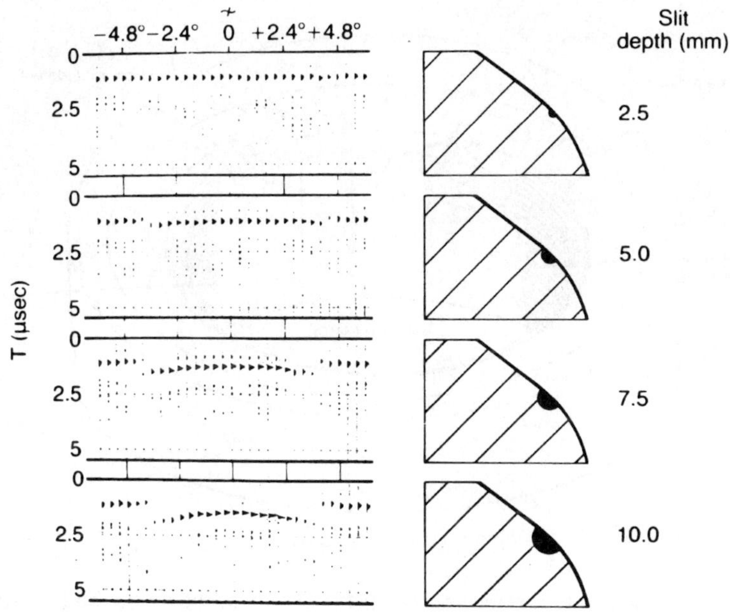


**Fig. 6.7** Variation of Time-of-Flight signals with defect through-wall size in the nozzle inner radius.

height (that is the depth of the defect measured in its own plane) but not crack orientation, so the two techniques complement each other for surface-breaking defects. Time-of-Flight Diffraction can size cracks on the inside of tubular members whereas ACPD cannot.

## 6.6 PWR nozzles

In a pressurised water reactor (PWR), the inner radius of a coolant nozzle is not normally particularly highly stressed. However, in the unlikely event of a loss-of-coolant accident, cooler water is injected and this will impose severe thermal stresses on the inner radius of the nozzle. This means that the critical defect size is small, and defects with size down to about 6mm, considerably smaller than those which might affect safety, may need to be detected and sized in a component up to over 300mm thick, to provide a handsome margin between critical sizes and targets for inspection. Defects sought are those which grow in planes containing the nozzle bore axis and these are difficult to size with conventional ultrasonic means with access limited to the inside of the nozzle.

The way in which Time-of-Flight Diffraction signals vary with defect through-wall size in the complicated geometry of a PWR nozzle inner radius is shown in

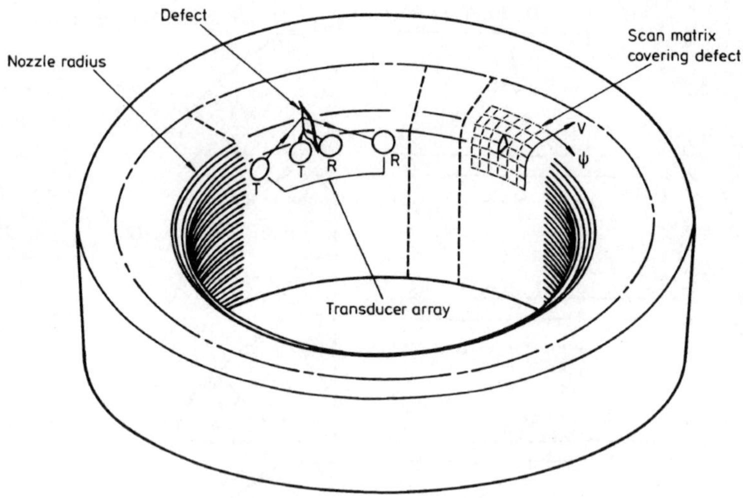


**Fig. 6.8** The nozzle radius region showing disposition of the probes and coordinates used for an azimuthal scan.

Figure 6.7. In this figure, the A-scans have been widely separated in forming the B-scan image so that individual traces can be seen more clearly. Defects less than 5 mm deep are difficult to detect by casual examination of such a plot and more sophisticated processing would be required. The larger defects, however, are clearly visible.

In the UKAEA Defect Detection Trials [Watkins, Ervine and Cowburn, 1983b], one specimen, Plate 4, was intended to represent the complex geometry of the nozzle inner radius. It was made from SA508 Class 2 specification steel purchased from a reactor pressure-vessel vendor. Spark eroded slits and welding cracks were deliberately implanted and then the surface was clad in two layers, either automatically using strip feed or manually, with wire feed, as appropriate. The surface was then ground to an Ra value of 3 μm. Details of the defects and their geometry are given in Watkins et al. [1983b].

Defects in Plate 4 were specified as extending no more than 30 mm below the surface of the base metal. Previous experience had shown that this region could be covered satisfactorily with a single pair of probes, which were mounted on gimbals 35 mm apart with their line of centres transverse to the local axial plane, as shown in Figure 6.8.

The probes were highly damped 12.5 mm diameter compression wave transducers operating with centre frequencies between 2 and 4 MHz, generating a short pulse of between 2 and 3 cycles. To provide coupling for the ultrasound, the test block was immersed in water in a circular tank. This was spanned by a specially constructed scanner, shown in Figure 6.9, having its principal vertical axis along the bore of the

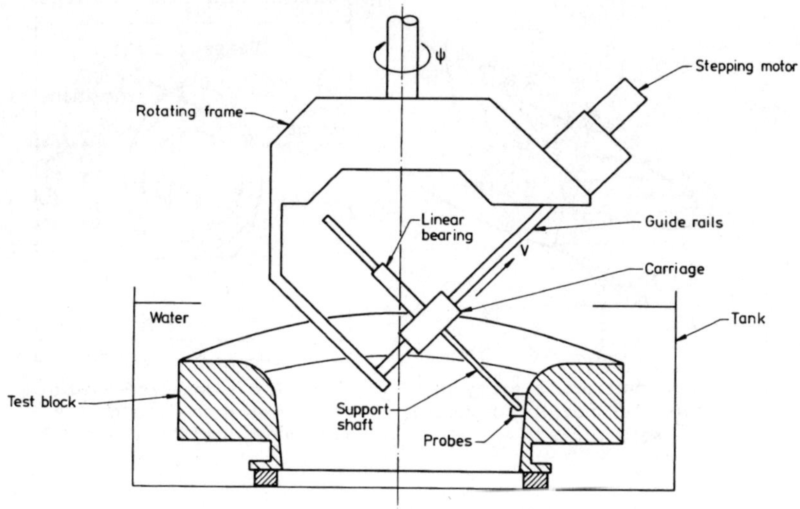


**Fig. 6.9** Schematic diagram of the scanner for inspection of the nozzle inner radius.

test block.

Data collection and control of the scanning were carried out by a computer. A rectangular scan raster of $\psi$ and $V$ coordinates (see Figure 6.8) was obtained by selecting a particular value of $V$ and then incrementing $\psi$ by equal amounts through 360°. At each point on this mesh of points a portion of the time trace, 12.5 μs long following the arrival of the lateral wave, was digitised and stored. With a digitisation rate of 20 MHz this gave 250 sample points per trace. Signal averaging was used, summing several time traces from each probe position, to improve the signal-to-noise ratio.

A search scan was first conducted with a raster spacing of 0.4° in $\psi$ and 4 mm in $V$, giving a step size on the surface varying from 2.9 mm to 4.5 mm in the circumferential direction and between 4 mm and 5.6 mm in the axial direction. Equal increments of $\psi$ and $V$ give rise to step sizes on the surface which depend on the absolute position of the probes on the surface because of the effect of the local geometry. The data from the search scan were analysed using an image processing display system linked to a computer. The B-scan presentation was used to reveal defect indications through either perturbation of the lateral wave signal or through the obvious presence of diffracted signals.

Having identified the defect locations with the coarse raster scans, a series of fine scans, in the neighbourhood of detected defects, was used with a raster of 0.2° in $\psi$ and 2 mm in $V$. Zero crossings of the time waveform following the principal positive peaks were used as the timing references and absolute travel times were used to calculate defect depths from this information [Stringfellow and Perring, 1984]. Provided the defect edge nearest the surface was more than 5 mm below the inter-

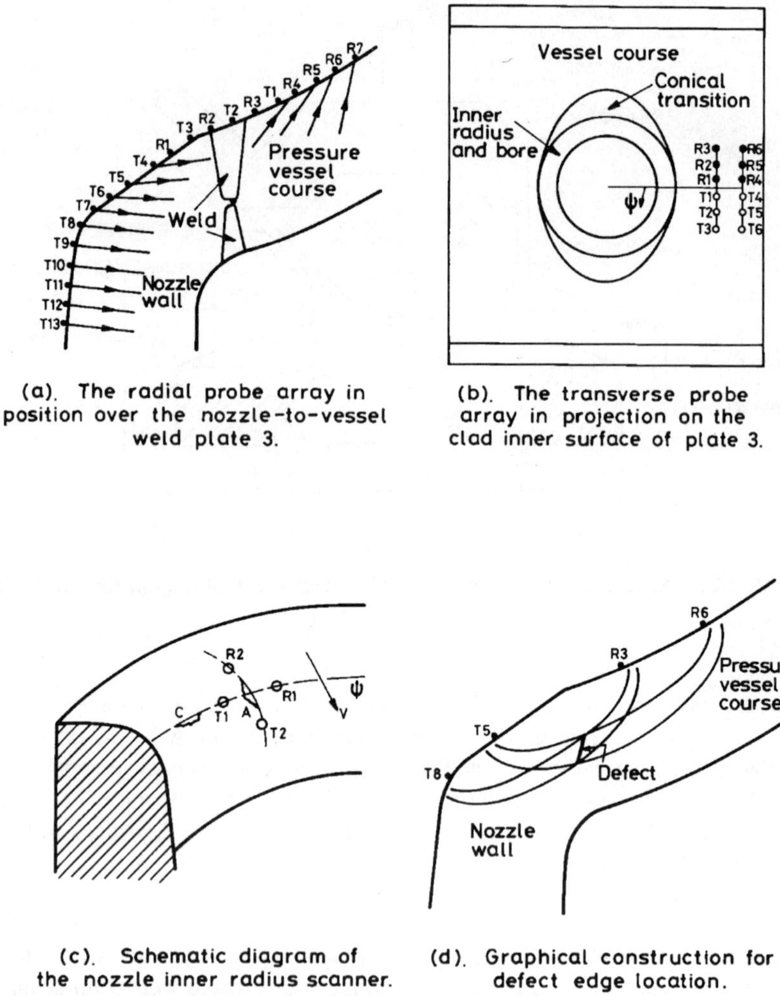


**Fig. 6.10** Coordinate system and probe deployment for inspection of the nozzle to shell weld and the nozzle inner radius (from Curtis and Stringfellow [1986]).

face with the cladding and almost parallel with the interface then defect depths could be found accurately. Detailed examples of measured crack profiles compared with those intended are given by Stringfellow and Perring [1984] who observed that, in all but three cases, the results obtained for the through-wall extent of the defects were within 2 mm of the actual values, while the remaining three cases were within 4 mm. This corresponds to an average oversizing error of 1.1 mm with a standard deviation of 1.8 mm. Apart from the two carbon cracks, which had very uncertain definitions of length, the Time-of-Flight Diffraction length measurements gave an average undersizing error of 2.4 mm with a standard deviation of 7.4 mm. This difference in accuracy between measurements of through-wall extent and defect length is expected because the through-wall extent is obtained from a time measurement whereas the defect lengths were inferred from the appearance of the signals as the probes were scanned, in effect using a dB drop method. It must be remembered that it is the through-wall extent of these defects which is of most importance in estimating the structural integrity of the component. Time-of-Flight Diffraction was shown, in this work, to be intrinsically capable of providing the degree of accuracy required for realistic safety assessments of component integrity, even in geometries as complex as the PWR nozzle inner radius, with the added complication of a layer of anisotropic austenite.

In work on PISC II Plate 3, an actual nozzle-to-vessel weld of a pressurised water reactor, the inspection with Time-of-Flight Diffraction was aimed at detecting, locating and sizing defects in the weld region. The defects were expected to be lying in circumferential planes parallel to the nozzle bore axis but inspections were designed to detect defects with any skew about a direction parallel to the nozzle bore axis. This was achieved with a design in which there were two separate probe arrays each capable of being mounted on a scanner head and rotated about the nozzle bore axis. The radial array consisted of 20 probes mounted in a plane containing the nozzle bore axis. Of these 20 probes, 13 acted as transmitters and 7 as receivers and these are shown in Figure 6.10. With this design all parts of the weld region in its plane were covered by a minimum of four transmitter-receiver pairs.

The transverse array covered an inspection plane at right angles to the plane of the radial array and was, therefore, intended to be most sensitive to defects lying in an axial plane, that is defects transverse to the weld. Two identical sub-arrays were used each with 3 transmitters and 3 receivers.

The PISC II Plate 3 contained 43 defects of which 30 were deliberately implanted planar flaws ranging in size from 3 mm diameter circle to a square of side 60 mm. Another 4 implanted defects were of a composite nature consisting of clusters of planar defects with overall dimensions of 50 – 60 mm. There were 9 unintentional defects with through-thickness heights of 2 – 4 mm. All the deliberately implanted defects were circumferential in orientation, that is parallel to the local orientation of the weld plane. The whole inner surface of the assembly was clad with about 5 mm of austenitic stainless steel [PISC, 1986c].

Scans with the radial array used 0.25° steps, corresponding to displacements along the surface of about 3 mm at the weld centreline. At each position A-scans from 38 transmitter-receiver pairs were recorded, giving at least 4 transmitter-receiver combinations contributing to defect detection and location of sub-surface defects or those near the back wall, while giving up to 20 combinations of probes at mid-wall. Pitch-catch reflection data were also recorded to assist in radial definition of defect positions. The radial coverage was from at least 695 mm out to 825 mm or more, giving inspection of at least 65 mm of the weld material and base metal either side of the weld centreline at about 760 mm radius.

Each trace was digitised at a sampling rate of 20 MHz. In order to get adequate signal-to-noise ratios, 128 traces were averaged for each probe pair and each probe position.

After analysis and reporting, five defects had been missed of which three were not more than 3 mm deep by 12 mm long. These three were not considered serious. However, two defects missed were near-surface defects, each a 10 mm diameter circle. These were just too deep to be seen by a closely spaced pair of probes such as that at 40 mm separation and they were just too shallow to be detected by a widely spaced pair such as those at 140 mm separation. It is clear that these defects would have been detected correctly with a pair of probes spaced at an intermediate value between 40 and 140 mm, say at 80 mm. The accuracy obtained for the through-thickness measurement was within ±2 mm or better for about half the defects or within about ±10% for the larger defects. Such errors were consistent with normal errors of measurement, whereas for the remaining defects, which were sized less well, the errors were due to misinterpretation of the various diffracted signals. For real reactor inspection the errors would be smaller because supplementary data on defect detection and sizing would be utilised.

The results for this inspection, together with those obtained on the PISC II flat plate (Plate 2), have been reported by Curtis and Stringfellow [1986]. They concluded that the Time-of-Flight Diffraction technique was capable of detecting and sizing defects in girth welds of pressurised water reactors with a high degree of reliability. To achieve similar accuracy and similar performance for near-surface defects in the inspection of nozzle-to-vessel welds it would be necessary for the clad inner surface of the vessel to be of higher quality than that of PISC II Plate 3.

Because the signals diffracted from the defect come essentially from the edges of the defect, the technique is less sensitive to the roughness of the defect faces than conventional pulse-echo techniques. Curtis and Stringfellow [1986] could find no difference between the diffraction responses from rough and smooth defects.

PISC II Plate 3 was also inspected by Risley Nuclear Laboratories using an automated ultrasonic technique comprising high sensitivity pulse-echo detection and predominantly Time-of-Flight Diffraction sizing. These techniques were deployed from the clad inner surface of the nozzle and made use of digital data collection, analysis, and display. With this system Risley Nuclear Laboratories detected 30 out of the 31 intended weld flaws and correctly located all 3 of the nozzle corner defects. With Time-of-Flight Diffraction sizing they achieved a mean size error of −1.3 mm and a standard deviation of 7.0 mm when their results were compared with the intended defect sizes of the 31 weld flaws [Rogerson, Poulter, Clough and Cooper, 1988]. This illustrates the way in which, for critical applications, the conventional pulse-echo techniques and the Time-of-Flight Diffraction method can provide diverse ways of size measurement, thereby enhancing confidence.

For complex geometries such as the nozzle to vessel weld of a PWR inlet nozzle, it has been found advantageous to use a mathematical model of the inspection geometry in order to display the signals in their correct relationship to the structure [Poulter, 1986]. On the PISC II nozzle, Risley used Time-of-Flight Diffraction

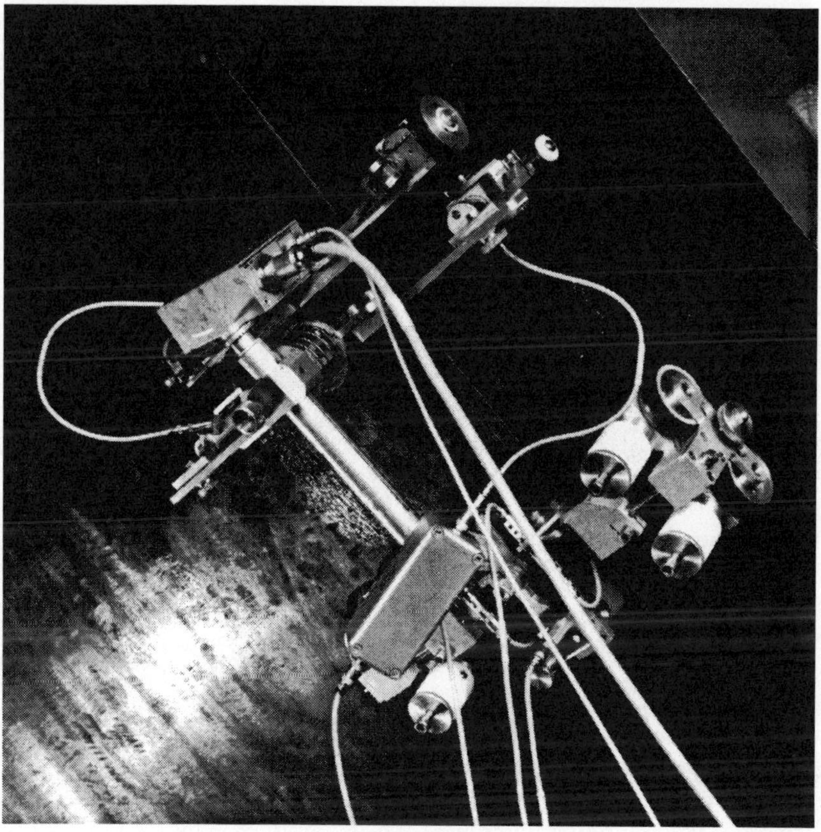

**Fig. 6.11** Close-up of the Time-of-Flight Diffraction technique crawler on the RTD plate.

sizing of the defects which they detected using pulse-echo techniques and found a mean sizing error of −0.14 mm, with a standard deviation of 3.0 mm, when comparing their results with the intended defect sizes [Poulter, 1986].

As well as scanners designed to fit standard in-service inspection masts for geometries such as the nozzles of a pressurised water reactor, there is also a requirement for inspection devices which can be easily adapted to a variety of inspection tasks. Such devices are usually, in effect, miniature vehicles which can traverse a component, carrying a probe assembly, under some form of guidance. For nozzles or pipes, the vehicle would usually be attached by straps or chains, allowing circumferential and possibly limited axial travel. Where that form of restraint is inconvenient, magnetic attachment can be used, when the component is ferritic, and the vehicle can be guided by a marked track which it follows optically. A vehicle of this type, generally referred to as a crawler is illustrated in Figure 6.11 operating on the RTD plate. This plate, so named because it was supplied by Röntgen Technische Dienst, is a part of

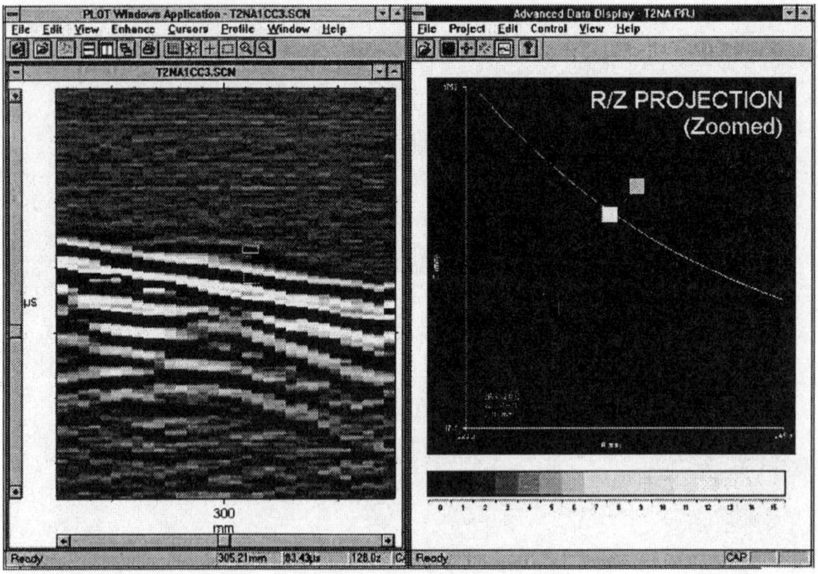


**Fig. 6.12** Images from MUSE data reconstruction, showing TOFD data in uncorrected format and selected data mapped into the component (reproduced from Daniels et al. [1996]).

a boiling-water reactor (BWR) pressure vessel shell containing a nozzle.

# 6.7 Recent developments in nozzle inspection

In the previous section, we described some of the performance demonstration exercises which took place during the period when TOFD was still in its development phase. During those exercises, tools to assist in interpretation of defect indications in the complex geometry were developed on an *ad hoc* basis. As the technique has become better established and as equipment has become more standardised, it has become possible to provide a wider range of more adaptable tools to assist in the interpretation of data.

The general principle of these tools is to enable the interpreter of the raw TOFD data to project salient features of the data onto a variety of projections of the work-piece. We shall not discuss the techniques involved in any detail but simply give two illustrative examples from published papers. The reader is referred to the cited papers for a more detailed description.

The first example, taken from Daniels et al. [1996], relates to inspection of a PWR steam generator feed-water nozzle carried as a qualification exercise for the EPRI NDE Center, Charlotte, NC, USA. Figure 6.12 shows the raw TOFD data alongside a radial-axial projection at a given azimuth. Using a system called MUSE,

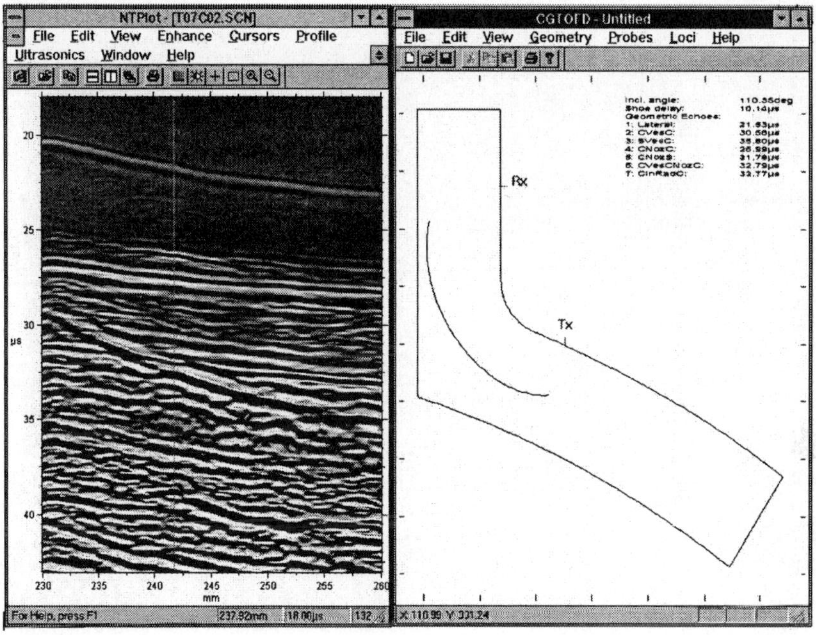


**Fig. 6.13** Data from azimuthal scan of defect showing locus constructed by CGTOFD on a projection of the nozzle (reproduced from Bloodworth [1999]).

the operator can mark features of the raw data with a cursor and the corresponding positions are simultaneously plotted on the projection.

The other example refers to the inspection of nozzle-to-pipe attachment welds in a BWR plant, carried out for the Swedish Qualification Centre [Bloodworth, 1999]. In Figure 6.13, we show data from an azimuthal scan at a fixed axial position. The operator, using the CGTOFD software package, can position a cursor on a defect signal in the TOFD data shown on the left, to define a specific time-of-flight. On the right, the corresponding locus of points of equal time-of-flight is plotted on a projection of the nozzle. These loci can be saved so that when an axial scan is performed over the location of the defect, the crossing of loci will give an unambiguous indication of the location of the defect edge, in the manner described in Section 2.3.3.

# Chapter 7

# Additional Complexities

In this chapter, we discuss some further aspects of the application of the Time-of-Flight Diffraction technique which require consideration in certain circumstances. We cover anisotropic materials, the effects of compressive stress on signals from cracks, and some subtle effects of component curvature.

Most metallic crystals show anisotropic elastic behaviour but, in fine-grained bulk samples with no preferred grain orientation, the macroscopic properties are isotropic. If, however, the grains approach in size the wavelength of the ultrasound, or are preferentially aligned, the resultant anisotropy and scattering affects ultrasonic inspection. This problem is particularly relevant to austenitic steels, both in bulk and in the form of cladding layers on ferritic steel. Section 7.1 discusses the problem of applying the Time-of-Flight Diffraction technique to such material.

Another problem arises from the differences in temperature and stress levels during service and those occurring when inspection is carried out. Examples of this are: aircraft, where in flight at 33,000 ft the temperature is −25°C and the pressure is $\sim 0.3$ bar, which contrasts with typical inspection conditions of a temperature of 20°C and a pressure of $\sim 1$ bar; nuclear reactor coolant circuits, where inspection is almost always carried out at temperatures and pressures well below their normal operating point; offshore structures, when inspection is carried out in calm weather when the wind and sea loadings are very different from those during severe weather. As a result of these changes in ambient conditions between normal service operation and those during inspection, cracks which were under tensile stress sufficient to cause growth during some conditions of service could be under compressive stress when inspected. The effect of compressive stress on the amplitude of Time-of-Flight Diffraction signals is discussed in Section 7.2.

Finally, in cylindrical geometries, the speed of the lateral wave, which is used as a timing reference, is found to vary from its value on a flat plate. It is necessary to know what this variation is, if Time-of-Flight Diffraction is to be applied confidently to curved geometries and this problem is discussed in Section 7.3.

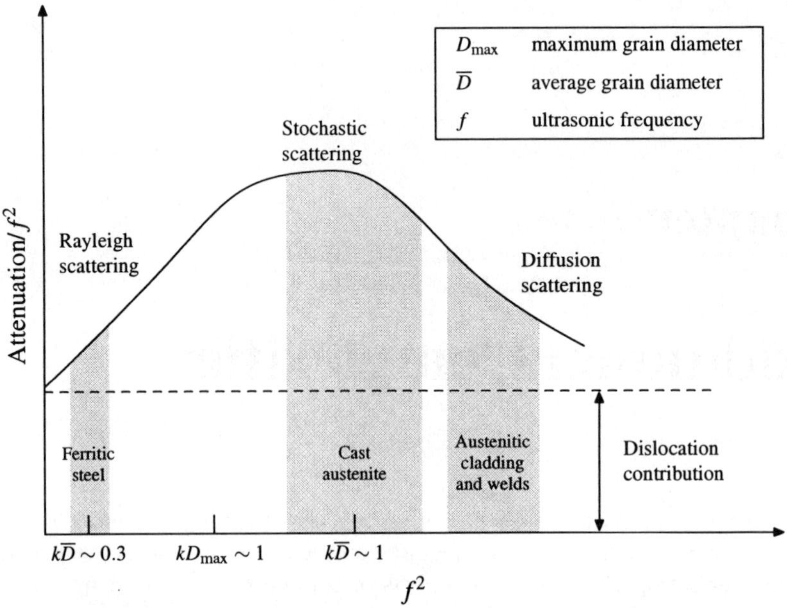


**Fig. 7.1** Frequency dependence of ultrasonic attenuation in granular media (from Reynolds and Smith [1984]).

## 7.1 Anisotropic media

In isotropic materials, each type of elastic wave travels at its characteristic speed, independent of direction. This is not so in anisotropic materials, where, for any type of wave, the velocity depends on the direction with respect to the crystal axes of the material. Clearly, for a technique such as Time-of-Flight Diffraction, which relies on the measurement of transit times, this adds an extra complication which must be allowed for if the technique is to maintain its accuracy. Studies of the propagation of ultrasound in austenitic weldments have been carried out by Silk [1979d, 1981b,c], including SH-wave propagation [Silk, 1979c] and the application of Time-of-Flight Diffraction and other ultrasonic techniques to these anisotropic structures [Silk, 1980b].

In anisotropic materials, where the axes of neighbouring grains may be differently aligned, elastic waves are scattered as they pass from grain to grain. The scattering, in effect, attenuates the signal, as well as adding a background of unwanted noise signals from the grain boundaries. The amount of attenuation depends on the relationship of the ultrasonic wavelength to the size of the grains in the material. A useful summary of these effects is shown in Figure 7.1, which is taken from Reynolds and Smith [1984].

### 7.1.1 Austenitic cladding

The pressure vessel of a pressurised water reactor consists of a thick ($\sim 250\,\text{mm}$) ferritic steel shell, covered on its inner surface by a thin ($\sim 9\,\text{mm}$) layer of austenitic steel. In ferritic steel, the grains are small and normally have no well-developed preferred orientation, so that the elastic properties are macroscopically isotropic. The austenitic cladding, however, crystallises in long columnar grains with aligned axes and, as a consequence, has elastic properties which are markedly anisotropic.

Ferritic steel crystallises with a body-centred cubic structure, whereas austenitic steel has a face-centred cubic structure. The anisotropy factor of cubic crystals is defined as the square of the ratio of the velocity of shear waves propagating along the [100] (cube edge) direction to that along the [110] (face diagonal) direction [Kittel, 1963, page 95]. This anisotropy factor A can then be expressed in terms of elastic constants in the Voigt notation, using the relationships explained in detail in Section A.8 of the Appendix, as:

$$A = \frac{2C_{44}}{(C_{11} - C_{12})} \tag{7.1}$$

For ferritic steel, the value of $A$ is about 2.4; for type 316 austenitic steel, the value is about 3.6; and for type 304 stainless steel, it is about 3.5. In this case, the austenitic steel is intrinsically more anisotropic than the ferritic steel. However, it is not the intrinsic anisotropy which governs the effective anisotropy of a granular medium but the size and orientation of the grains. Materials with grains much smaller than the wavelength of the ultrasound propagating through them appear effectively isotropic unless there is some preferred alignment of the grains. As the ratio of the ultrasonic wavelength to the grain size decreases and eventually approaches unity, the effects of anisotropy become more and more apparent. For a material with grains which are much larger than the ultrasonic wavelength, the full intrinsic crystalline anisotropy applies.

In such anisotropic materials, the speed of propagation of the different wave modes becomes a function of the direction in which they are travelling. Since, in Time-of-Flight Diffraction, the estimate of the depth of a crack extremity below the inspection surface depends on the velocity of the various waves, it is necessary to correct for the effect of variation of velocity in the cladding. It is not practicable to measure the velocities for every ray path and the detailed cladding structure is both too complicated and too imperfectly known for exact calculations to be performed. A simplified model was therefore developed and applied to the depth correction algorithm implemented in the software used for sizing defects in the Defect Detection Trials [Charlesworth and Temple, 1982].

### 7.1.2 Anisotropic cladding model

The austenitic cladding is usually applied in two layers to a total thickness up to 10mm. The first layer has a higher alloy content but suffers some dilution from diffusion into the ferritic steel and so has a final composition close to that of the second layer (AISI 308L).

The cladding is applied by strip welding. On cooling, it crystallises in columnar grains, the long axes of which are approximately normal to the isotherms during solidification. The resulting structure exhibits long grains which are nearly normal to the surface but which are tilted by up to 10°. The direction of the tilt or *layback* varies locally but is generally within 20° of the welding direction. Although the columnar grains have well aligned long axes [001], the other two principal axes do not usually show any well-developed preferred orientation. The simplest model incorporating this symmetry is a transversely isotropic medium. Such a model is discussed in more detail in the Appendix (Section A.8). The phase velocities define a slowness surface, where the slowness, $k/\omega$, is the reciprocal of the phase velocity, and the group velocity, $V_g = \partial\omega/\partial k$, corresponding to a particular wavevector $k$, is normal to the slowness surface at $k$. A section through the slowness surface for type 308 stainless steel is shown in Figure 7.2, taken from Ogilvy [1985b].

Figure 7.2 shows the three sheets of the slowness surface in the $yz$-plane. The solid line and dash-dot line represent the slowness surfaces for the two quasi-shear-wave modes in which particle motion is approximately perpendicular to the wavevector. The solid line applies to the mode which is most nearly like an SV wave, while the dash-dot line applies to the mode which is most nearly like an SH wave. The other mode, shown as a short dash line, is the P-wave-like mode in which particle motion is approximately parallel to the wavevector. This quasi-compression mode has the highest velocity and so forms the innermost sheet of the slowness surface. It never crosses or touches the other two sheets of the slowness surface.

For all three modes, the three-dimensional slowness surface for this transversely isotropic model medium is obtained by rotating the $yz$-slice shown in the figure about the $z$-axis. The two shear-like waves have the same phase velocity along the $z$-axis, that is for propagation along the axis of the transversely isotropic material, but differ in speed when propagating in the basal plane. The quasi-SV wave mode, shown by the solid line, has large variations in phase velocity with direction of propagation compared to either of the other two modes.

The group velocity, which, as we have already pointed out, is normal to the slowness surface, gives the speed and direction of energy flow. The phase velocity, which is parallel to the wavevector, governs the reflection and refraction at boundaries by generalised Snell's Law. Along the $z$-axis, or along any direction in the $xy$-plane, the phase and group velocities are in the same direction, so the energy flow is in the same direction as the wavevector. However, in other directions, such as, for instance, the one shown in Figure 7.2 at about 35° to the $-z$ direction, the normal to the quasi-SV slowness surface (depicted by the solid line), is far from parallel to the wavevector. This is the effect known as *beam skewing*, because the energy flow of the beam is skewed away from the wavevector direction. The angle between the phase-velocity and group-velocity vectors is known as the *skewing angle*. From Figure 7.2, one can see that some degree of skewing will occur with the other two wave modes but, since their slowness surfaces are more nearly spherical, the skewing angles will be smaller.

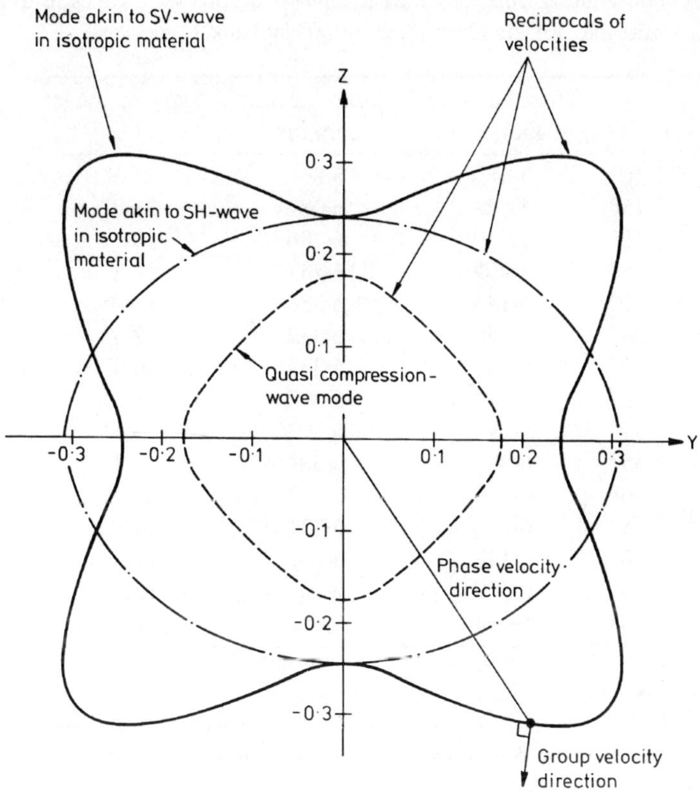


**Fig. 7.2** The intersection of the three slowness surfaces of transversely isotropic austenitic stainless steel type 308 with the (100) plane.

The quasi-SH wave mode will have the smallest skewing angles since its slowness surface is almost a sphere.

### 7.1.3 Transit times

In this section, in order to deal with the compression wave velocity in ferritic material together with phase and group velocities in the austenitic material, we use the symbols $V_f$, $V_p$ and $V_g$, instead of the symbol $C_p$ used elsewhere in the text. The velocity of the compression waves in the ferritic steel is represented by $V_f$ and is independent of direction. In the austenite, the compression waves have phase velocity $V_p(\phi)$ and associated group velocity $V_g(\phi)$. The angle $\phi$ is, in both cases, measured relative to the normal to the inspection surface and is the angle which $k$ makes with the normal. The actual direction of the group velocity is, in general, at some other angle $\theta$ to the surface normal. Values of $V_p$, $V_g$ and $|\theta - \phi|$ are tabulated

**Table 7.1** Phase and group velocities for quasi-compression waves in transversely isotropic 308 stainless steel with 0° layback.

| $\phi$ | Phase velocity mm/μs | Group Velocity mm/μs | Skewing angle |
|---|---|---|---|
| 10° | 5·453 | 5·866 | 21·6° |
| 15° | 5·642 | 6·082 | 21·9° |
| 20° | 5·830 | 6·206 | 20·1° |
| 25° | 5·999 | 6·281 | 17·2° |
| 30° | 6·143 | 6·330 | 14·0° |
| 35° | 6·256 | 6·362 | 10·5° |
| 40° | 6·336 | 6·382 | 6·9° |
| 45° | 6·382 | 6·393 | 3·3° |
| 50° | 6·393 | 6·393 | 0·6° |
| 55° | 6·370 | 6·384 | 3·7° |
| 60° | 6·316 | 6·362 | 6·9° |
| 65° | 6·233 | 6·324 | 9·7° |
| 70° | 6·127 | 6·261 | 11·9° |
| 75° | 6·009 | 6·163 | 12·8° |
| 80° | 5·893 | 6·021 | 11·8° |

in Table 7.1 for the cases where the layback is 0° and 10° (from Charlesworth and Temple [1982]). These velocities were calculated using the elastic constants listed in Table A.1.

Figure 7.3 shows the various ray paths which can occur when a clad ferritic workpiece is inspected by the TOFD method through a transversely isotropic cladding layer. The ray paths in the figure can be described as the lateral-wave path, the skip path, the critical-angle path, the defect path and the back-wall echo path; they are associated with travel times given by:

$$t_{\text{lat}} = \frac{2S}{V_g(90^\circ)} \tag{7.2}$$

$$t_{\text{skip}} = \frac{2S\sqrt{1+(h/S)^2}}{V_g(\phi)} \tag{7.3}$$

where the phase velocity direction $\phi$ is such that the group velocity direction $\theta$ satisfies the equation:

$$\theta = \arctan(S/h) \tag{7.4}$$

Also

$$t_{\text{crit}} = \frac{2h}{V_g(\phi_0)\cos\theta_0} + \frac{2(S - h\tan\theta_0)}{V_f} \tag{7.5}$$

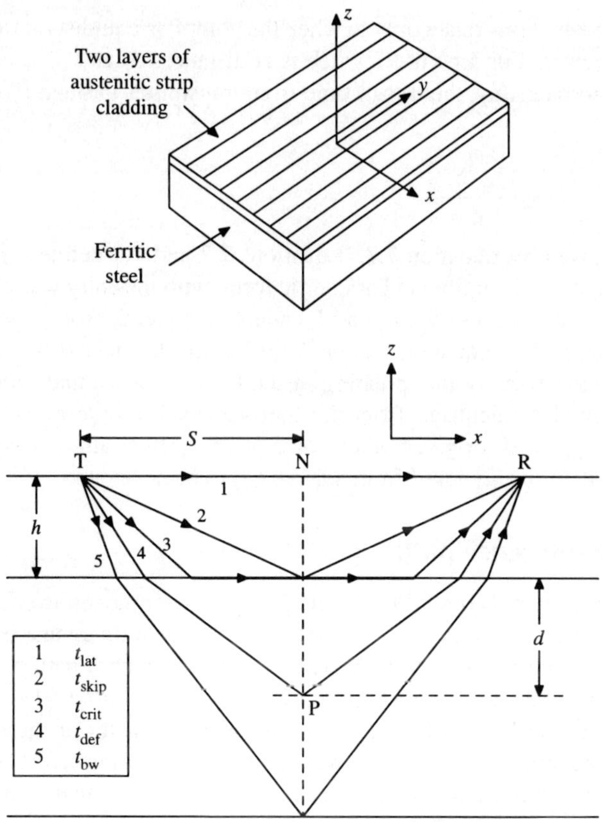


**Fig. 7.3** Ray paths into ferritic steel underneath austenitic cladding.

where $\theta_0$ is the critical group velocity angle for the interface, corresponding to the critical phase velocity angle $\phi_0$, defined by

$$\sin\phi_0 = \frac{V_p(\phi_0)}{V_f} \tag{7.6}$$

The transit time via a point P, on an upper or lower defect edge, at a depth $d$ below the interface is given by $t_{def}$, where

$$t_{def} = \frac{2h}{V_g(\phi)\cos\theta} + \frac{2(S - h\tan\theta)V_p(\phi)}{V_f^2 \sin\theta} \tag{7.7}$$

where $\theta$ and $\phi$ are related to the defect depth by

$$d = (S - h\tan\theta)\frac{\sqrt{V_p^2(\phi) - V_f^2 \sin^2\phi}}{V_f \sin\phi} \tag{7.8}$$

The above equations relate only to when the point P is equidistant from the transmitter and receiver. For a point P′ which is at distances $S_t$ and $S_r$ from transmitter and receiver, respectively, the transit time from transmitter through P′ to receiver is given by:

$$t = \frac{\left[t_{\text{def}}\left(S_t\right) + T_{\text{def}}\left(S_r\right)\right]}{2} \tag{7.9}$$

where $t_{\text{def}}$ is given by Equation 7.7. Equations 7.7 and 7.8 define the relationship between depth and transit time in parametric form, with the entry phase vector angle $\phi$ as the parameter. Because $V_p$, $V_g$ and $\theta$ cannot, in general, be expressed as simple functions of $\phi$, neither equation can be solved easily to yield $\phi$ for a given value of $t_{\text{def}}$ or $d$. However, by interpolating in the table of phase and group velocities and skewing angles calculated from the transversely isotropic model (Table 7.1), calculation of $t_{\text{def}}$ or $d$ for given values of $\phi$ is straightforward and this enables an efficient algorithm for finding $d$ from a given $t_{\text{def}}$ to be developed.

### 7.1.4 The reference path

The expressions derived above do not include any time for the ultrasonic path outside the workpiece, nor any delay in the electronics. Any such time must be determined experimentally from a reference path. The choice of reference path depends on the experimental conditions. For inspection of a region near to the clad surface, it is convenient to use either the lateral-wave path, the skip path, or the critical-angle path. A pulse travelling via the lateral-wave path always arrives before one travelling via the skip path. The critical-angle path exists only for $S \geq h\tan\theta_0$. There is a value of $S$ such that $t_{\text{lat}} = t_{\text{skip}}$, given by

$$S = h\left[\frac{1}{V_g\left(\phi_0\right)\cos\theta_0} - \frac{\tan\theta_0}{V_f}\right] \Big/ \left[\frac{1}{V_g\left(90^\circ\right)} - \frac{1}{V_f}\right] \tag{7.10}$$

For ferritic steel, $V_f$ =5.89mm/μs, which gives $t_{\text{lat}} = t_{\text{crit}}$ for $S = 6.2h$. Thus, the critical-angle path provides the best reference path for $S \geq 6.2h$. In practice, it is also usable down to $S = h\tan\theta \approx 3h$, because the amplitude received via the critical-angle path is greater than that via the lateral-wave path.

### 7.1.5 Experimental confirmation of the model

The greatest difference to transit times caused by the cladding is to paths which do not penetrate to large depths. Experiments were carried out on a specially manufactured block, 290 mm by 290 mm and 88 mm thick, made from A533B steel. One large face was covered by two layers of 308L austenitic strip cladding. A sloping saw cut was made from the clad face to a depth varying from zero at one end to 30 mm at the other, to simulate a crack of varying depth. This is depicted in Figure 7.4.

The transit time of the first arriving wave was recorded as a function of distance along the plate, parallel to the slot, the two probes being placed on opposite sides of

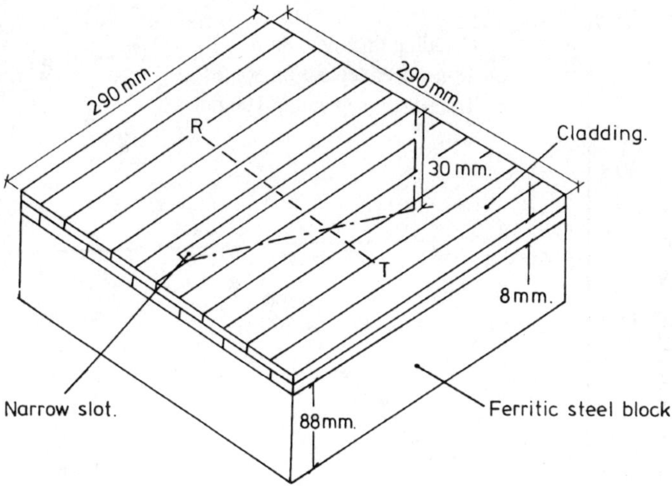


**Fig. 7.4** Experimental arrangement for comparison of predicted and actual slot depths using the Time-of-Flight Diffraction technique to size slots underneath austenitic cladding.

the slot and equidistant from it, at separations of 50 mm or 100 mm. The velocity in the ferritic material was found to be 5.894mm/μs. The ultrasonically determined slot depth below the cladding, as a function of actual slot depth is shown in Figure 7.5, where the results for a probe separation of 50 mm are shown by open circles and those for a probe separation of 100 mm are shown by solid circles.

The agreement is very good and errors do not exceed 1 mm. Systematic errors of this magnitude could have arisen from plate bowing and much of the scatter is probably the result of variations in cladding thickness.

Without the corrections for the cladding, the errors would be considerably larger. To demonstrate the size the errors could be, calculations were performed with the assumption that the cladding behaved like ferritic steel. A defect lying just under the clad-ferritic interface would then have a depth estimate in error by the thickness of the cladding layer. For defects at greater depths, the errors would decrease but would still be significant at considerable depths. The errors due to assuming the cladding to be identical to the underlying isotropic material are shown in Figure 7.6, for three probe separations, as a function of true depth.

It should be noted that this cladding model was used, with good results, for defect depth calculations in the Defect Detection Trials outlined in Section 8.4. Other methods of carrying out the depth calculations are possible and one algorithm in the Defect Detection Trials was based solely on direct application of Fermat's Principle [Curtis and Hawker, 1983; Hawker, 1983]. An alternative approach to estimating depths under cladding is to construct a calibration curve by timing signals from side-

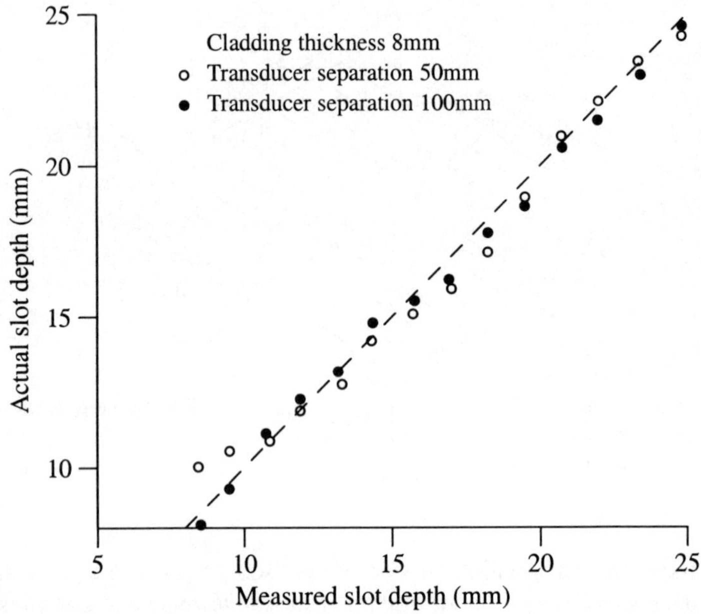


**Fig. 7.5** Experimental results for slot depth, estimated from Time-of-Flight Diffraction with depth correction, compared with actual slot depth.

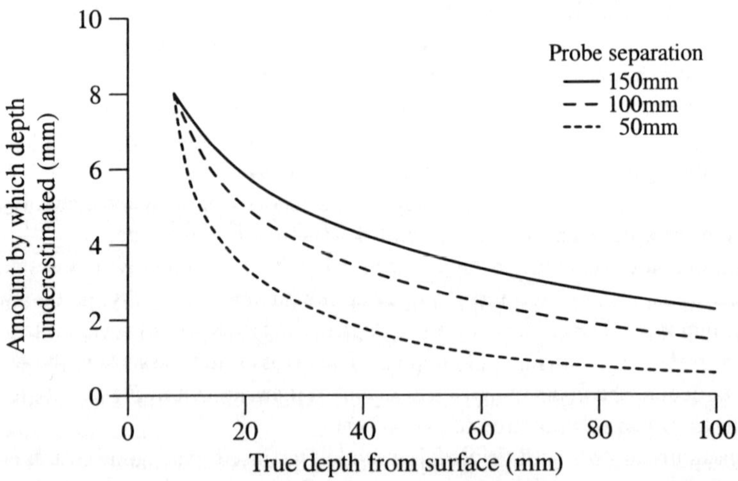


**Fig. 7.6** Errors which would arise in estimating the depth of cracks below anisotropic cladding, 8mm thick, if no correction for the cladding were made.

drilled holes in a calibration block [Murgatroyd, Seed, Willetts and Tickle, 1983]. This block must be clad by the same method and to the same thickness as the workpiece and a calibration curve will be needed for each probe separation used.

### 7.1.6 Austenitic steel

The cladding material discussed above is austenitic steel with a large grain structure. The problem was restricted to that of transmitting and receiving ultrasound through a relatively thin layer of this material, with most of the path being through isotropic ferritic material. In other applications, however, it may be necessary to inspect welds between austenitic materials, for example, in the primary circuit pipe-work of pressurised water reactors, or in the coolant vessel or internals of fast reactors. In such cases, the weld material solidifies in grains sufficiently large and locally well-aligned to show considerable anisotropy but, because the conditions producing the alignment vary as the welding proceeds, the direction of alignment varies from place to place in the weld. Conventional ultrasonic inspection of such welds with angled shear-wave probes is likely to be very unsatisfactory, because of the strong effect which the grain structure has on the propagation of the SV waves used; inspection with compression waves will be more successful [Ogilvy, 1985a,b; Silk, 1980a]. Ogilvy has shown, however, that SH waves are relatively unaffected by the structures typical of austenitic welds, which tend to have large anisotropic grains with a well defined structure determined by the direction of heat flow during welding. In equiaxed material, SH waves will suffer the same scattering and beam distortion as the other shear wave mode. In general, austenitic welds are difficult to inspect because of both beam skewing and scatter at grain boundaries. The signal arriving at the receiver probe is the combined effect of scattering at many grain boundaries and varies quasi-randomly with both transit time and probe position. This quasi-random variation with transit time makes the grain-scatter signal rather resemble thermal noise and so it is often referred to as 'acoustic noise'. It has a similar effect to thermal noise in obscuring the defect signals, but is not amenable to reduction by conventional signal averaging because, unless the probes are moved, a repeated firing will reproduce the same grain scatter signal. These signals are somewhat analogous to clutter on a radar screen and the term 'grain clutter' or simply 'clutter' is preferable to 'acoustic noise'.

Experiments carried out with compression waves to inspect welds in austenite showed that the signal-to-clutter ratio was in the region of 2. Although this is probably insufficient for reliable detection of defects, it is sufficient for accurate sizing of defects detected by other means. However, experiments carried out by Silk, Bainton, Hillier and Robertson [1986a], using SH waves, showed signal-to-clutter ratios of between 10 and 20, giving an improvement in signal detectability of between 6 and 10 dB. The only major drawback to the use of SH waves in a Time-of-Flight Diffraction approach is the difficulty of coupling this mode to the test specimen. The commonest solution to this problem is to use piezoelectric transducers with a very viscous couplant, but this reduces scanning speeds. Honey and uncured epoxy resin have been used successfully, as well as proprietary couplants. Rao and Raj [1998] have carried out a promising demonstration of the use of electromagnetic acoustic transducers (EMATs) for TOFD measurements with SH waves.

If compression waves are used to inspect austenitic welds, the B-scan images can be seriously distorted by the effects of the weld structure. This distortion is largely absent when SH waves are used. The scattering in equiaxed materials increases strongly with frequency and even the shape of the beam profile shows some frequency dependence in weld structures. Careful tailoring of the ultrasonic pulse shape and spectrum, with emphasis on low frequencies, can produce considerable improvements in signal-to-clutter ratio [Aldridge, 1987].

Although grain clutter is not reduced by conventional signal averaging, it might be expected that averaging while moving the probes by a few grain diameters should improve the signal-to-clutter ratio. However, the authors are not aware of a convincing demonstration of this effect.

When the first edition of this book went to press, ultrasonic inspection of austenitic materials was an active field of research and advances in understanding were anticipated within a short time. Several papers which clarify our understanding of diffraction in anisotropic materials have been published since then. It is disappointing to find little published evidence of improved inspection capability arising from this work.

### 7.1.7 Diffraction in anisotropic materials

Diffraction of elastic waves is more complicated in anisotropic materials than it is in isotropic materials. In Section A.4 of the Appendix, equations A.32–A.35 define the diffraction coefficients in isotropic materials such as ferritic steel. It has not been possible to derive analytical expressions such as these for the general case in an anisotropic material. Norris and Achenbach [1984] presented results for the diffraction coefficients for a crack in a transversely isotropic material. Although the grains of austenitic weld metal are typically several millimetres in diameter and never have higher symmetry than orthorhombic, a simple model based on transversely isotropic symmetry can provide quite an accurate description of the aggregate elastic properties of a volume of weld metal containing many grains, provided there is a well-developed preferred orientation of one of the principal axes of the grains.

Early attempts at calculating diffraction coefficients in complex geometries and anisotropic materials using numerical solutions to the wave equation were not wholly successful [Temple, 1993; Temple and White, 1993]. Recently, solutions for the diffraction coefficients of elastic waves in arbitrary anisotropic materials have been obtained [Lewis, Temple and Wickham, 1996a,b; Lewis et al., 1998]. These agree with those of Norris and Achenbach for transversely isotropic materials, but without some rather special experimental confirmation, of the sort supplied by Figure 3.6 for diffraction coefficients in isotropic steel, these coefficients remain as theoretical predictions. It is also difficult to devise validation for these models. Comparison with analytical results is only possible for the isotropic and transversely isotropic cases, both of which are successful. Comparison with numerical solution of the wave equation is another possibility but such approaches proved difficult to interpret

[Temple and White, 1993]. Experimental verification would require large single crystals to enable distinct measurements to be made. Growing large single crystals of austenitic steel is difficult but it might be possible to grow large single crystals of copper, which is also elastically anisotropic.

The diffraction coefficients predicted depend on the elastic constants used, and, just as in isotropic steel, the diffraction coefficients can have zeroes at particular angles of elastic wave incidence. This means that it is not entirely sensible to try and quote a figure for a typical difference between diffraction coefficients in isotropic and an anisotropic material. As the anisotropy increases there can be substantial differences between the diffraction coefficients in anisotropic material compared with those in isotropic material for a given angle of wave incidence. For backscatter, such as would be applicable to pulse-echo inspection for misaligned defects or for single probe TOFD techniques, the differences in signal amplitude are typically about 6 dB.

In practice, for real austenitic materials with large and complex grain structures, the signal amplitudes recorded will be as much a function of the paths followed from transmitter to defect and from defect to receiver as they will be of the angle of diffraction at the crack tip. This is because the path through the grains, of varying orientation, will create varying amounts of beam skew and apparent attenuation as the probes are scanned. A robust approach to design of inspections in such materials is to use computer modelling to seek particularly difficult combinations of material orientation, that is those which produce small signals, and then to design the inspection to avoid the beam angles which could lead to small signals. This was the purpose of the Ray Tracing in Anisotropic and Inhomogeneous Media program (RayTrAIM) developed by Ogilvy [1985a,b] and reviewed more recently by Harker, Ogilvy and Temple [1991].

## 7.2 Compressive stress

In any ultrasonic technique, the strength of the defect signal, and hence the likelihood of the defect being detected satisfactorily, depends on the properties of the defect. In particular, the difference in material properties between the defect and the surrounding material has an important effect, as well as other parameters, such as the orientation, shape and roughness of the defect. For crack-like defects, it is the discontinuity in stress across the faces of the crack which is the cause of scattering. This applies equally to conventional pulse-echo and tandem techniques, which, in principle, rely on specular reflection from the faces of the defect, as it does to the Time-of-Flight Diffraction technique. In the latter case, it is the signals diffracted at the extremities of a crack-like defect which lead to the detection and accurate sizing of the defect. Suppose now that there is a compressive stress applied to the crack; this will tend to push the faces together and will, if large enough, cause increased interaction between them. It is easy to imagine that this interaction will lead to a reduced discontinuity in the ultrasonic stress pattern round the defect and, hence, to less scattering and less signal amplitude available for the ultrasonic flaw detector. This is indeed what is observed in practice.

### 7.2.1 Experimental and theoretical results

The reflection of ultrasound at an interface between two media is described by a reflection coefficient which, in the case of a rough interface, such as a crack face, depends on the ultrasonic wavelength and the height of the roughness. The same reflection coefficient would be obtained from two rough surfaces at different frequencies if the ratios of ultrasonic wavelength to the height of the roughness on the two surfaces were constant. Results obtained by Wooldridge [1979] on cracks under compressive stress, and by Arakawa [1983] on rough surfaces in contact, are in agreement with the theoretical predictions of Haines [1980] for normal incidence. Arakawa studied the transmission and reflection of ultrasound at machined steel surfaces in contact under an applied load. For normal compression waves at 5 MHz, the reflected signal decreased by about 6 dB for an applied load of 200 MPa. Typical results from Wooldridge's work are similar. Wooldridge used surface roughnesses with RMS values from less than 1 μm up to about 30 μm. For an applied load of 200 MPa, the transmission coefficient for compression waves at normal incidence is 10 dB less for surfaces with about 10 μm RMS roughness than it is for surfaces with less than 1 μm RMS roughness.

The variation of ultrasonic signal amplitude from manufactured defects under compressive stress has been studied by Denby and Duncumb [1985]. Examples of defects such as lack of fusion, solidification cracking and under-clad reheat cracks were considered. It was concluded that compression to 20% of yield stress would produce no significant effect on the ultrasonic response from these manufacturing defects and this was confirmed by experimental results showing less than 1 dB change in signal compared with the unstressed state [Denby and Duncumb, 1985]. This is in contrast to the case of fatigue cracks, which would show significant reductions in signal at these stress levels.

### 7.2.2 Application to Time-of-Flight Diffraction

As well as the experimental work of Wooldridge [1979], experiments have also been carried out on BS4360-50D steel by Whapham et al. [1985a]. These latter experiments were performed with nominal 10 MHz compression wave transducers and 5 MHz shear wave transducers. The shear wave transducers used in this test produced waves with the SH polarisation, which are reflected at the crack faces without mode conversion, and are therefore qualitatively similar to compression waves at normal incidence. The experiment employed two transducers placed symmetrically, one on each side of the defect, with both transducers on the same surface of the specimen, as shown in Figure 7.7. Experiments were carried out to study how stress on the crack faces affected the diffracted Time-of-Flight signals.

The primary object of the experiment was to establish whether an applied compressive stress could remove the diffracted signal completely. The results showed that there was a reduction in signal strength but that the signal was never destroyed completely. Two configurations were tested experimentally: first, with the transducers on the side of the specimen from which the crack was grown; secondly, with

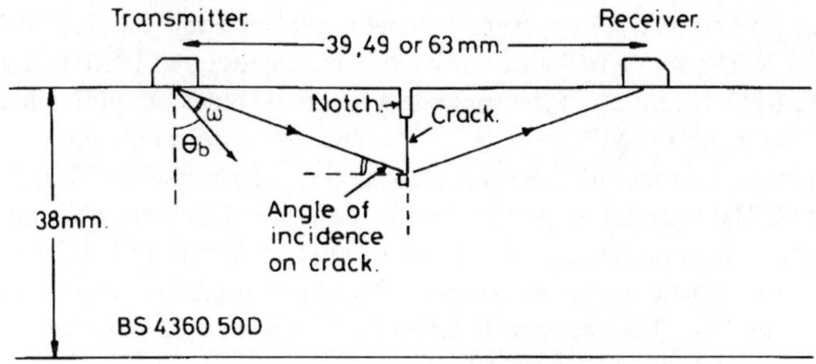


The geometry used in the experimental studies of diffracted signal strength as a function of applied compressive stress.

| Probe separation. | $\theta_b$ | $\lvert\omega\rvert$ |
|---|---|---|
| 39 mm. | 60° | 0.6° |
| 49 mm. | 70° | 4.2° |
| 63 mm. | 70° | 0.8° |

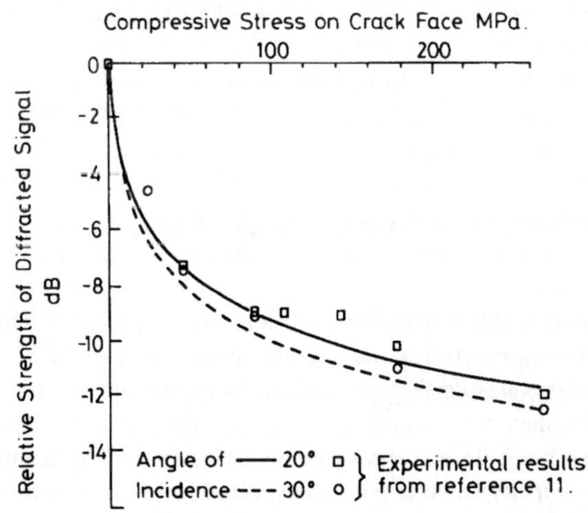


**Fig. 7.7** Experimental and theoretical results for the strength of signals diffracted by a tight fatigue crack under compressive stress. The results are for compression waves at 6 MHz and a root mean square roughness of 1.1 μm.

both transducers on the opposite face. This gives a range of incident angles on the defect face. The maximum diffracted signal was measured and results were reported relative to this for increasing compressive stress and also for applied tensile loading.

Theoretical predictions of the variation of the reflection and transmission coefficients of tight fatigue cracks at normal incidence, taken from Temple [1984b], appear in Figure 7.8. The figure includes results for frequencies up to 10 MHz, for three values of the RMS height $\sigma_c$ of the roughness and two values of applied load, 60 MPa (Figure 7.8.A) and 160 MPa (Figure 7.8.B). The reflection coefficient goes to zero at zero frequency, as it should, since a static load (i.e. zero frequency) would be entirely transmitted. The material properties used in these calculation are a Young's modulus of 210 GPa, a shear modulus of 84 GPa and a relative density of 7.9 (i.e. the material is steel); these elastic constants correspond to wavespeeds of $C_p = 5.9\,\text{mm}/\mu\text{s}$ and $C_s = 3.26\,\text{mm}/\mu\text{s}$. The material is taken to have a flow pressure of 1200 MPa as suggested by Kendall and Tabor [1971].

We obtain the following form, derived from Haines [1980], for the transmission coefficient $T$ for compression waves at normal incidence:

$$T = \frac{2}{2 + ik_p Ew/P_t} \tag{7.11}$$

where $k_p$ is the wavevector of the incident compression wave, $w$ is the perturbation displacement introduced by contact of the asperities, $E$ is Young's modulus and $P_t$ is the pressure transmitted by the interface. To a first approximation, the energy contained in the transmitted wave is lost from the energy available for diffraction. This will be particularly the case when the incident wavefront runs down the crack before reaching the tip where diffraction occurs. Thus, to the same order of approximation, we associate the diffracted compression wave signal strength with the magnitude of the signal reflected from a crack of infinite extent. Similarly, we associate the strength of the diffracted, mode-converted shear wave with the amplitude of the mode-converted reflection from an infinite crack. This is a very simple model which turns out to be a reasonable first approximation, effective in describing the actual situation.

We have plotted Whapham's results in Figure 7.7, together with our calculations for the reflection coefficient of 6 MHz compression waves incident on a crack with 1.5 μm RMS deviations from flatness on both faces. Results for angles of incidence of 20° and 30° are shown.

The actual crack profile was measured on a Surfcon 30B stylus profilometer and displays features at many wavelengths, as expected. The value obtained for the RMS roughness depends on the sample length over which it is evaluated [Whitehouse and Archard, 1970]. For example, Whitehouse and Phillips [1978] found, on a sample set of surface profiles, that the mean peak height changed by a factor of 2.5, the peak density by a factor of 4, the peak curvature by a factor of 10, and the average slope by a factor of 2, when the sample length changed from 2 μm to 24 μm. For one of the crack surface profiles used in this work, a sample length of about 2 mm gave an RMS value of about 20 μm, whereas for a sample length of about 100 μm the RMS value falls to about 7 μm.

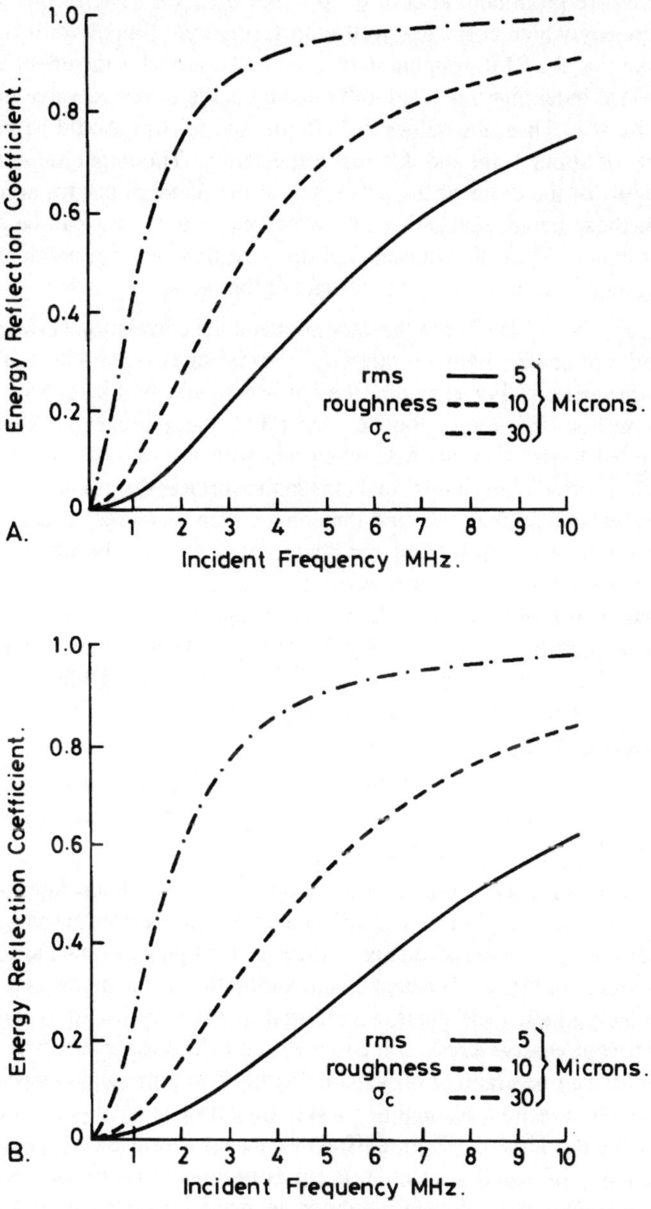


**Fig. 7.8** Predicted reflection and transmission coefficients for a tight fatigue crack as a function of frequency. A is for an applied load of 60 MPa and B for 160 MPa.

In terms of the spatial frequency of the various contributions to the overall roughness, features are prominent at both 6.2 μm and 0.75 μm. The former value has a spatial frequency which correlates well with formation of microvoids during crack growth. Note that the RMS roughness $\sigma_c$ used in the model is the effective value for a rough surface indenting into a smooth one and is the observed value on each face multiplied by $\sqrt{2}$. Thus, the values of 0.75 μm and 6.2 μm should be modelled by values of $\sigma_c$ of about 1 μm and 8.8 μm, respectively. The larger value arises from sample lengths of the order of the grain size of the material but we argue that it is precisely at those length scales that the two faces on the crack can be expected to be well correlated. Thus, length scales of this size represent waviness of the crack, rather than roughness accounting for contact of the faces.

We can see the effect of both the waviness and the correlation between the faces on the amount of contact between them by considering two periodic surfaces which have the same period. For example, the surfaces could be like egg boxes. When mountains on both faces are opposite each other, the amount of contact between them is limited to the summits but, when one surface is translated parallel to the other by half a period along a principal axis in the surface, the mountains on one face are opposite valleys on the other and the contact area increases. Clearly, the actual contact area will be determined by the degree of correlation between the faces, as well as by the microscopic roughness which is at length scales much smaller than the waviness of the two surfaces. It is then plausible that, for fatigue cracks, the contact between the two crack faces is governed by RMS roughness determined over short sample lengths, that is, at about the 1.5 μm used in the calculations depicted in Figure 7.7. This agreement between the theoretical value used and that determined experimentally is considered satisfactory.

The results also indicate that the maximum loss of signal which can be expected under loading conditions up to 70% of the load used during crack growth is about 13 dB for an RMS roughness of about 1.5 μm.

In experimental work undertaken for the offshore petroleum industry, Newton [1987] found that higher ultrasonic frequencies and beam angles gave higher signals for dry cracks under compressive stress, whereas, for tight, wet cracks, no such general trends were confirmed, because of the variability of the signals received. For pulse-echo techniques, the signals were found to decrease by 30 to 55 dB for dry cracks under compressive stress, compared with the decrease in crack tip diffraction signals from the same crack of only 10 to 20 dB. The pulse-echo inspections used specular reflection of both SV and SH waves travelling at 45°, with a frequency of 2.2 MHz, while the Time-of-Flight Diffraction inspections used compression waves with a frequency of 10 MHz. Unlike the pulse-echo measurements, the Time-of-Flight Diffraction signals showed a similar decrease for both wet and dry cracks. Newton concluded that, provided the crack tip signal can be seen, there is no significant change in sizing accuracy for either tight or filled cracks. Also, the effect of an overload, such as a 60% increase in maximum tensile load, greatly improved subsequent Time-of-Flight Diffraction signal visibility under compression. This may be due to changes in the plastic zone round the crack tip and may lead to improvements in detectability for real cracks offshore, where fatigue loading is variable.

Theoretical modelling of the signals received in pulse-echo or tandem inspections of liquid-filled defects can predict very substantial decreases in signal amplitude, especially for narrow defects [Temple, 1980, 1981a,b], with a 'worst case' value of a signal reduced by 62 dB for a 2 μm wide crack filled with rust, compared with the same defect filled with air [Temple, 1982], for inspection with 45° shear waves at 4 MHz. In purely amplitude-based techniques, such signal reductions would automatically yield incorrect defect acceptance on fracture mechanics criteria but, providing signals could still be observed with both Time-of-Flight Diffraction and probe movement techniques, the accuracy of assessment should not be significantly affected.

## 7.3 Component curvature

As we have seen in Sections 2.3 and 7.1, the Time-of-Flight Diffraction technique requires knowledge of the speed of propagation of waves over the entire signal path. In isotropic homogeneous materials, this is a well-known quantity. In anisotropic homogeneous media, the wavespeed can be adequately modelled, as seen from the results obtained on cladding, described in Section 7.1.2. Another case arises where the speed of propagation can differ from the bulk wave speed. If the component surface is curved or the defect itself is volumetric rather than crack-like, the speed with which the waves traverse the curved surfaces is not equal to the bulk wave speed. This can lead to errors in the calculation of defect depths or sizes, if it not taken into account.

Such effects could arise in inspection of a pipe, where the reference path, analogous to the lateral wave, would be a wave creeping along the curved face of the pipe; a defect signal from a cylindrical cavity would also show the effect.

The equations governing the wave motion around a cylindrical cavity are given in the Appendix, together with an indication of the derivation of the velocity of propagation (Section A.9). For the lowest compression or shear wave mode, which has the lowest attenuation, the following expression was found to describe satisfactorily the ratio of the creeping wave velocity $V'$ to the bulk compression wave velocity:

$$\frac{V'}{C_p} = \frac{1}{\left[1 + 0.928\,(k_p a)^{-2/3}\right]} \tag{7.12}$$

Replacing $k_p$ by $k_s$ and $C_p$ by $C_s$ yields the appropriate expression for the creeping shear wave.

To put these values in perspective, we note that the creeping compression wave only reaches 98% of the bulk value when $k_p a > 300$. A plot of these results is given in Figure 7.9.

Experimental tests were carried out in both steel and aluminium to confirm these predictions [Charlesworth and Temple, 1981]. These experimental results were for circular holes with radii between 0.25 mm and 3 mm at a depth of 25 mm below

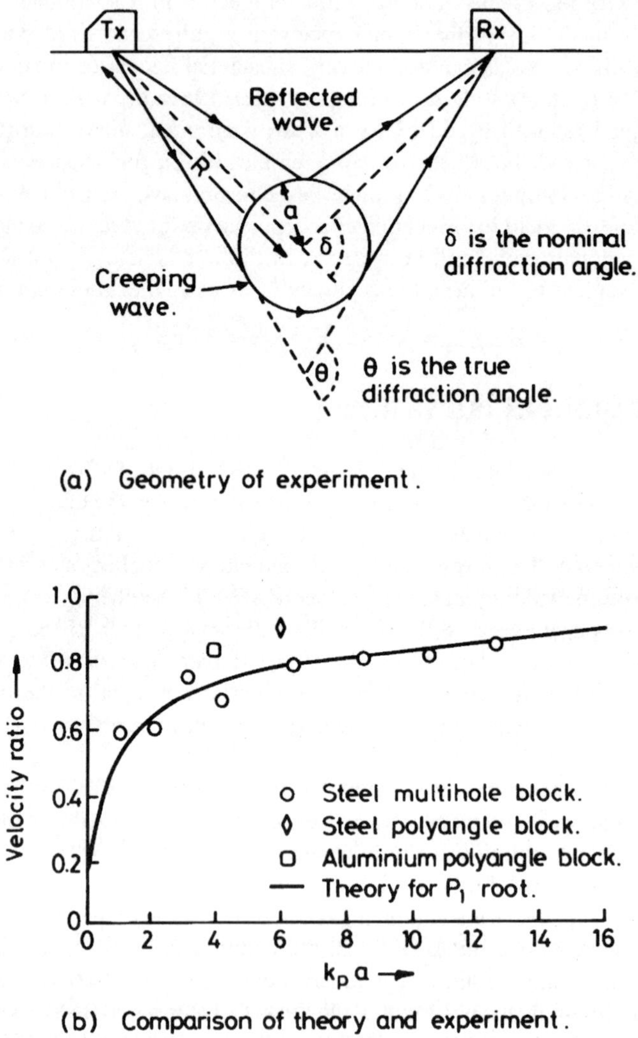


**Fig. 7.9** Creeping wave speed and attenuation as a function of the radius of curvature of the surface.

the inspection surface. The transducers operated at frequencies between 2.5 MHz and 4 MHz and the experimental results obtained were in good agreement with the theoretical predictions, as shown in Figure 7.9.

# Chapter 8

# Experimental Demonstrations of Capability

Non-destructive testing techniques, including ultrasonic inspection, are often used in safety critical applications such as the nuclear industry, submarines, offshore oil platforms, chemical plants, aircraft and gas pipelines. A characteristic of such applications is that there is often a reluctance to adopt new techniques until there has been a build up of experimental evidence of capability. The evidence which leads to successful adoption tends to start with idealised trials in the laboratory followed by an accumulation of satisfactory field experience.

Both the laboratory tests and the field experience can be embodied in a standard procedure for applying the inspection technique once it has reached a certain maturity. The Time-of-Flight Diffraction technique is now at this stage, having been encapsulated in both British and European Standards. This follows several demonstrations of capability in a wide range of large-scale test-block exercises which are reviewed in this chapter. Results from several significant test-block trials are presented in some detail to highlight the capability of Time-of-Flight Diffraction for accurate determination of the through-wall extent of cracks. The test-block exercises test technique capability, rather than reliability or repeatability in practice.

In this chapter, we confine our discussion to the principal test block exercises. A number of other, generally smaller and more specialised, exercises are covered in Chapter 9.

Capability is not sufficient in itself; reliability in practice is also required. The level of reliability required of an inspection is that which, when combined with a knowledge of the severity of defects, will lead to the desired level of structural integrity under normal operation or possible accident loading conditions. Even good techniques applied reliably will exhibit some spread of errors which have implications for the structural integrity of the component under test. This concept is reviewed with special reference to the pressure vessel of a pressurised water reactor; the approach is, however, universally applicable.

Before embarking on a discussion of the results obtained in test-block trials, we bring out some of the limitations of such tests.

## 8.1 Limitations of test-block exercises

Although there are a number of limitations to test-block exercises which we will indicate here, we should emphasise that test-block trials are useful indicators of the capability of inspection techniques to detect, size and possibly characterise defects. In order to derive the maximum benefit from a test-block exercise, careful thought must be given to the objectives and the experiments must be carefully designed to maximise the relevance of the results to the structural integrity of the component or structure which the specimens are intended to represent.

Test blocks can be expensive to produce and can usually contain only a small number of deliberately implanted defects. As a result, the number of defects studied in a trial is rarely as large as would otherwise be desirable. This was the basis of a serious criticism by Whittle and Coffey [1981] of the PISC I results [PISC, 1979]. For a review of the whole series of PISC exercises see Crutzen [1985a,b]; Crutzen, Jehenson, Nichols and Stephens [1985]. PISC was originally an acronym for Plate Inspection Steering Committee but this was superseded by Programme for the Inspection of Steel Components. Three PISC programmes have now been completed. All of them involving major international collaboration in making realistic scale test blocks, distributing them around a number of geographically disparate locations, refereeing the inspections and drawing conclusions from the results.

Because the implanting of defects in test blocks is not an exact science, the blocks must eventually undergo destructive examination to establish the precise configuration of the defects, for comparison with the results produced by the inspection teams. Since this cannot occur until all the non-destructive inspections are complete, major test-block exercises tend to take one or more years to complete.

In the next two sections we consider in more detail the difficulties mentioned above.

### 8.1.1 The number of defects

In any test, including application in real inspections in the field, there will be a certain likelihood that the defects may be missed, or, if detected, sized wrongly, thus possibly being misclassified as acceptable when they are unacceptable, or vice versa. The likelihood of correctly classifying a defect is called the *reliability*. The average reliability for a set of defects can be estimated as the proportion of defects correctly classified out of the total defect population. For example, a reliability of 0.9 (or 90%) means that, on average, 9 out of 10 defects will be correctly detected and classified. Average values are only part of the information required since it is also necessary to know the *confidence level*; i.e. how certain one can be that a result will be close to the average or above some lower threshold. Although the ideal situation would be a 100% reliability with 100% confidence, this is impossible to achieve in practice, so the aim must be to reach reliability and confidence levels as high as reasonably practicable.

Confidence levels achievable from test-block trials, in terms of the number of correct interpretations of defects, are discussed in detail in Section A.10 of the Appendix. For a test in which there are 15 defects of which 14 are correctly classified, the best estimate of the reliability is 0.93 and we can be about 83% confident that the reliability exceeds 0.80. As another example, for a test in which there are 20 defects with only 19 correct results, the best estimate of the reliability is 0.95 and we can be about 83% confident that the true reliability exceeds 0.85. In a test with 30 defects and 29 correct results then the best estimate of the reliability is 0.97 and we can be at least 82% confident that the true value exceeds 0.90. Here we are treating each defect as a separate trial. Similar results for 95% probability of detection with 95% confidence have been given elsewhere [Whittle and Coffey, 1981] as requiring 92 successes out of 93 trials.

The relatively small number of defects required to establish 90% probability of detection with about 80% confidence level is realistic and shows that test-block exercises can demonstrate that degree of reliability for a particular class of defects. However, if the organisers of a test-block trial were foolish enough to request a 99.5% reliability with 95% confidence, they would find it a very exacting task. The techniques being tested would then need to be completely successful in about 600 trials or, if only one test were failed, success would be required in 949 out of 950 trials. A very high a degree of confidence costs a great deal of time and money! Similarly, if an adequate demonstration of reliable inspection is required over many different defect classes or component geometries, then large numbers of test blocks will be required.

Another problem with test-block exercises is that, because of the desire to introduce as many defects as possible within a limited budget, the defect density in the blocks may have to be several orders of magnitude greater than would ever be found in a component in normal service. This has at least two possible effects: defects may be inserted so that they obscure each other (which would be acceptable only if it were likely to occur in practice); and the realism of scanning many metres of weld without finding a defect is lost and the inspectors may be assisted in detecting defects by their expectation of defects being present.

### 8.1.2 Comparison with destructive tests

In order to determine how successful the inspection procedures have been, it is necessary to perform a destructive examination of the test blocks. This demands an engineering capability to cut up thick-section steel plates with the tight tolerances of fractions of a millimetre necessary for comparison of the results with such a sensitive ultrasonic technique as Time-of-Flight Diffraction. In the Defect Detection Trials, the plates were cut up into small cuboids containing the defects and these were then examined using a combination of very high sensitivity ultrasonics, metallography and further sectioning.

In the destructive examination of the plates, small additional defects may be found to be associated with the intended defect. These usually result from imperfections in the welds used to implant defects. A rule must be devised in order to decide whether such associated defects should be included in the destructive results. The same rule should be followed by all the teams reporting on the ultrasonic results, especially if the comparison between ultrasonic and destructive results is to be made on the basis of simple boxes drawn round defect 'extremities'. Teams using Time-of-Flight Diffraction, in the various test-block trials to be discussed later, were not usually using the same rules as the those laid down in the destructive examination. We have, therefore, in our present assessment of the results, used the minimum volumes of the defects found during destructive examination, except where otherwise stated.

Since it is the through-wall extent of planar, crack-like defects which is generally regarded as the most significant parameter governing the likelihood of catastrophic brittle fracture, we will concentrate on this parameter in our analysis. Defect length can be an important parameter, however, during some possible accident sequences.

## 8.2 Round-robin trials

Several round-robin trials are reviewed in this chapter. They are ordered according to increasing complexity, with older trials of similar complexity appearing first. By complexity we mean the factors:

- geometry
- material
- defect type
- component access.

Thus, just as in previous chapters, we recognise that extensive flat plates of isotropic homogeneous material, such as ferritic steel, containing well defined, open, smooth (in ultrasonic terms) planar cracks will represent the simplest category. Making specimens with more complex geometries but still of ferritic steel adds complexity. Even more complexity is added by using a material which is not homogeneous and isotropic — such as austenitic steel, especially welds or forged material. Cracks which are rough, or branched, such as stress corrosion cracks (SCC) will be more difficult to detect, size and characterise than smooth planar cracks. This progression of complexity is reflected in the sequence of major round-robin trials reviewed here: Welding Institute trials (Section 8.3), UKAEA Defect Detection Trials (Section 8.4), PISC II (Section 8.5) and PISC III (Section 8.6).

In Section 8.9 these results are put into a fracture mechanics context. A comparison of TOFD and radiography is made in Section 8.7 and with amplitude based techniques in Section 8.8.

Reliability in practice demands more than a highly capable technique. This is a necessary but not sufficient condition. It is also necessary to ensure the technique is applied properly in practice. This topic will be reviewed later, in Section 10.4. Modelling studies, which may be used as a partial replacement for round-robin trials, have already been considered in Section 5.10.

## 8.3 Results obtained in the Welding Institute collaborative programme

A collaborative programme of work, to establish the sizing capabilities of several ultrasonic techniques including Time-of-Flight Diffraction, was carried out, in four phases, on behalf of the Mechanical Engineering and Machine Tools Requirements Board of the Department of Industry, by the Welding Institute, the National NDT Centre at Harwell Laboratory, United Kingdom Atomic Energy Authority, and by the NDT Applications Centre of the Central Electricity Generating Board, Northwestern Region Scientific Services Department. Phase 4 was concerned with complex geometries and has been discussed in Section 6.1. Phases 1 and 2 will be reviewed here.

Welded specimens manufactured with carefully controlled deliberately introduced defects were tested using a wide range of ultrasonic equipment. The results obtained were compared with destructive examination of the specimens and were analysed in terms of the accuracy of techniques to measure defect size and confirm defect character. The work was reported in three volumes [Welding Institute, 1979, 1982a,b].

### 8.3.1 Phase 1

The first report [Jessop, 1979] deals with the results obtained in sizing and characterising non-planar defects. In this series of tests, ten test blocks were manufactured from carbon manganese steel plate, to BS 1501 Grade 223 32B, and contained 26 defects such as slag lines, lines of porosity, slag inclusions and lack of root penetration in the weld. Time-of-Flight Diffraction was one of the ultrasonic sizing techniques applied to all ten blocks. The results obtained for vertical cross-section position error, error in length and cross-sectional area measurements are summarised in Table 8.1.

The Time-of-Flight Diffraction technique gave a mean through-wall size error of −0.32 mm with a standard deviation of 1 mm. The specimens containing these defects ranged in thickness from 37 to 95 mm. These errors compare favourably with those obtained using conventional ultrasonic techniques: with the 20 dB drop method a mean cross-section size error of −3.3 mm with an associated standard deviation of 3.2 mm was obtained, and with the maximum amplitude method a mean error of −2.1 mm and standard deviation 2.0 mm were obtained. The results quoted above for 20 dB and maximum amplitude methods were obtained with an ultrasonic frequency

**Table 8.1** Results obtained in Phase 1 of the Welding Institute tests by Time-of-Flight Diffraction sizing of non-planar defects.

| Type of measurement | Mean error | Standard deviation | Sample details |
|---|---|---|---|
| Vertical cross-section position error | 0.35 mm | 1.3 mm | 24 defects |
| Length extremities (% error) | 3% | 7.7% | 34 linear defects 40 to 121 mm long |
| Length extremities (% error) | 7.1% | 40% | 14 cluster defects 5 to 15 mm long |
| Cross-section size | −0.32 mm | 1.0 mm | 24 defects 1.5 to 7.2 mm |

of 4 MHz. At 2 MHz, the errors were smaller, giving a mean error of −0.88 mm and standard deviation of 2.3 mm by the maximum amplitude technique. Results obtained with DGS (distance gain size) sizing data were a mean equivalent reflector size of −1.7 mm and standard deviation of 1.6 mm for the linear defects and a mean error of −2.7 mm and standard deviation of 1.8 mm for the cluster defects.

From these results it was concluded that the Time-of-Flight Diffraction method *'showed better accuracy than other methods particularly for through-thickness sizing. In this instance an accuracy of +1mm could be expected'* [Jessop, 1979].

### 8.3.2 Phase 2

The second phase of this collaborative programme was carried out on similar material made into 14 specimens varying in thickness from 34 mm to 94 mm. The plates all contained a weld. Two processes, manual metal arc and submerged arc, were used in the welding and the weld preparation was chosen from one of: single V, $\frac{2}{3}/\frac{1}{3}$ double V, single U, or equal double V. Solidification cracking, lack of fusion, hydrogen cracking and a cluster of inclusions were created deliberately in the test plates. Results from Time-of-Flight Diffraction, which was used on all fourteen plates, are presented in Table 8.2 taken from Jessop et al. [1982].

The results obtained by Time-of-Flight Diffraction for accuracy of sizing of the defect through-wall cross-section were *'much superior to any of the previous tests. The slight tendency to oversize is mainly due to small defects (typically 1.5 mm to 3 mm) close to the limit of resolution. The scatter value $\sigma$ =1.8 mm is much lower than any of the previous values ($\sigma$=2.4 to 5.0 mm).'* [Jessop et al., 1982]. In Jessop's description of the results quoted above, the previous tests refer to those cited earlier in his report, namely: conventional shopfloor ultrasonic tests carried out at 2 MHz and 4 MHz; DGS sizing methods; B-scan tests; Accuscan and holography. The bald results stated above should be kept in perspective with the requirements of an in-

**Table 8.2** Results obtained in Phase 2 of the Welding Institute tests by Time-of-Flight Diffraction sizing of planar defects.

| Type of measurement | Mean error | Standard deviation | Sample details |
|---|---|---|---|
| Vertical cross-section position error | 0.56 mm | 1.8 mm | 25 defects |
| Length extremities (% error) | 5.6% | 12% | 43 defects 40 to 121 mm long |
| Cross-section size | 0.52 mm | 1.8 mm | 106 defects |

spection. Shopfloor tests with simple manual A-scans can obviously be relied on for quality control inspections with an accuracy of $-1.0 \pm 3.1$ mm, whereas fracture mechanics assessments of critical components would require the additional factor of 2 improvement in accuracy available with Time-of-Flight Diffraction, $+0.5 \pm 1.8$ mm. For shopfloor testing one can have 95% confidence that a measured value of through-wall size of a crack will lie between -7 and +5 mm of the correct value in plates up to 95 mm thick [Jessop et al., 1982]. This value should be compared with the Time-of-Flight Diffraction result, where one would have 95% confidence that the measured through-wall size lay between -3 and +4 mm of the actual value.

## 8.4 UKAEA Defect Detection Trials (DDT)

The capability of ultrasonic techniques to detect, size and characterise defects is continually evolving. A snapshot of the capability of 7 teams to detect and size representative defects in thick steel plate was provided by the results of the Defect Detection Trials organised by the United Kingdom Atomic Energy Authority (UKAEA) in 1983. Following the poor results obtained by international teams using conventional pulse-echo ultrasonic inspections in the PISC I exercise [PISC, 1979], the Defect Detection Trials were designed in 1980 with the aim of providing information for the public inquiry into the possibility of building a PWR in the United Kingdom. The trials have been described by Watkins et al. [1983b] and the results obtained summarised by Lock, Cowburn and Watkins [1983]; Watkins, Cowburn, Ervine and Latham [1983a]; Watkins, Lock, Cowburn and Ervine [1984]. Although these trials were described as 'defect detection' exercises, the results contain more information on the capability of the techniques than they do on the repeatability in practice. In particular, they can be regarded as fair experimental tests of the sizing ability of the techniques and teams, bearing in mind the cost of such test-block exercises and the small number of them that will take place.

In the Defect Detection Trials, techniques were selected on the basis of their existing use for PWR inspection or because the techniques were *'in such an advanced state of development that they could be considered as candidates for use in the first United Kingdom PWR'* [Watkins et al., 1983b]. The Time-of-Flight Diffraction technique was chosen for evaluation because of its potential for accurate measurement of the through-wall extent of a crack-like defect. The technique has the potential to evaluate accurately the most relevant parameter of the least desirable defects in pressure vessels. The Harwell Laboratory's development programme for Time-of-Flight Diffraction was reviewed at the time of the Defect Detection Trials by Gardner and Hudson [1982].

A team at Harwell designed, built and commissioned apparatus for a full-scale Time-of-Flight Diffraction inspection of welded plate and nozzle specimens typical of the geometries encountered in the reactor pressure vessel of a pressurised water reactor. Viewed retrospectively, this strategic decision to restrict the Harwell investigations solely to Time-of-Flight, which was subsequently carried over into the PISC II trials, was of crucial importance for the position of Harwell in the nuclear non-destructive testing field [Collingwood, 1987]. This artificial restriction to a single technique led to significant developments in data analysis and interpretation as well as defining the capability of the technique.

In the Defect Detection Trials, there were four specimens, of which three were flat plates (Plates 1, 2 and 3) and one (referred to as Plate 4, although not actually of plate geometry) simulated the geometry of a pressurised water reactor (PWR) nozzle inner radius. The specimens used were of full thickness and of reactor quality, clad as though each was actually part of a PWR vessel. Plate 1 contained 29 deliberately introduced flaws and Plate 2 contained 16. The defects in these plates were of planar, crack-like type distributed throughout the entire weld volume of the 250 mm thick steel plates. Plate 3 contained 26 deliberately introduced flaws in the region near the austenitic cladding, while Plate 4 contained 20 flaws near the inner radius and extending into the nozzle bore and to the vessel face. Thus there was a total of 91 flaws, a number which must be viewed in the context of the discussion of confidence limits which appears in Section 8.1.1.

The defects introduced into the blocks cover a range of sizes which are thought to contribute most to possible vessel failure under certain accident conditions in the range 10 to 55 mm through-wall extent. The restriction to defect sizes less than 55 mm does not mean that a single very large defect would not be highly likely to lead to vessel failure but high standards of workmanship and inspection ensure that such a defect is very unlikely to be produced and even more unlikely to go undetected before the vessel is put into service. Hence, such defects contribute little to the total failure probability. Very small defects will occur more commonly and may not be detected by inspection but the presence of a single such defect is highly unlikely to lead to failure. Hence, these defects, again, contribute little to the total failure probability. The bulk of the probability arises from defects of intermediate size, with intermediate probabilities of occurrence and of detection, and intermediate likelihood of individually leading to failure [Cameron, 1984; Cameron and Temple, 1984; Marshall, 1982]. This is the basis of the restriction to the 10 to 55 mm through-wall size range examined in the Defect Detection Trials.

### 8.4.1 Caveats concerning the Defect Detection Trials

We note that the German teams performed their inspections to a cash cost and were therefore limited in the time available for inspection and interpretation. Some of the German ALOK work was reviewed by Barbian et al. [1984b]. In the case of some of the French work, we note that the inspection equipment, which is actually used for in-service inspection, is not designed to cope with the number of defect indications per cubic metre that existed in the DDT plates. Good results, based on pulse-echo detection methods and sizing measurements involving transit times of signals (but not Time-of-Flight Diffraction), were reported by Bowker, Coffey, Hanstock, Owen and Wrigley [1983]. We have already noted, in Section 4.1.2.2, that the Harwell Time-of-Flight equipment was not designed to detect very small defects near the clad interface. Another potential criticism of the Defect Detection Trials was that the defect types were not sufficiently representative of real defects. While this may be true of Plate 1, in which the defects were rather well defined planar inserts, the defects in the other three plates comprised a mixture of machined defects, fatigue crack inserts and deliberately induced weld cracking, and hence more clearly modelled the types of defects which could occur in real pressure vessel welds.

### 8.4.2 A comment on automated inspections and Time-of-Flight Diffraction

Most of the inspections in the Defect Detection Trials used automated equipment for scanning the plates and recording the indications. The repeatability in practice of results from such equipment is governed largely by the setting-up procedures and the degree of built-in self checking. Automated equipment will produce more consistent results than manual inspections but, if the equipment is incorrectly set up or operated, or develops a fault during operation, the results may be consistently wrong. Incorrect setting up or operation can be avoided by the use of carefully designed procedures but fault monitoring may require modifications to equipment design.

In the Time-of-Flight Diffraction technique, the presence of the lateral wave provides assurance that the signal acquisition equipment is working satisfactorily. When the lateral wave is absent because it has been interrupted by a surface-breaking defect, there will usually be a diffraction signal from the internal edge of the defect (unless it is a through-wall defect). Thus, while it is not straightforward to make the equipment totally self-checking, monitoring of lateral wave amplitude can be used to alert the operator to possible malfunction. A closer inspection of the signals will then reveal whether the alarm was raised by a true malfunction or by the presence of a surface-breaking defect.

In the commonly-occurring case of flat plate geometry, the back-wall echo can also be monitored and it will be very rare for both lateral wave and back-wall echo to be absent while the equipment is still functioning.

In the Time-of-Flight Diffraction inspections in the Defect Detection Trials, coupling of the ultrasound was by water immersion, so no coupling monitor was required. However, the technique can be, and frequently has been, applied with contact probes. The technique described above using the lateral wave and the back-wall echo also provides a means for monitoring the coupling efficiency.

### 8.4.3 Sizing capability

The measured defect size will usually have an error associated with it. In order to use the measured value in an assessment of the acceptability of the defect some relationship between the measured and true values needs to be established. If a calibration experiment has been carried out, in which several defects were sized using ultrasonic measurements before the test pieces were examined destructively, we can calculate the mean and standard deviation of the sizing error for defects in each class. If, further, we know the distribution of these errors then we can put confidence limits on the 'actual' value as inferred from the measured size. For example we might assume that the errors in sizing are normally distributed (but they appear not to be, see Section 8.4.8).

### 8.4.4 Summary of results from the Defect Detection Trials

In the Defect Detection Trials, the detection of defects was very good, especially for those defects which would have been classed as *referable*, meaning that they would have been marked out for detailed analysis and possibly repair or rejection of the component containing them. All the teams detected all the defects in the inspection of Plates 1 and 2 from the clad side [Watkins et al., 1983a,b, 1984]. The results from the clad side are especially important since current in-service inspection of many PWR vessels has to be carried out from inside, that is, from the clad side. It had previously been thought that the anisotropic nature of the cladding could hinder the detection and sizing of defects, though it is worthy of note that the Central Electricity Generating Board team obtained results of comparable accuracy for Plates 1 and 2 using the conventional methods to be used for the Sizewell 'B' station. The results of the defect detection exercise show that it is possible to take account of the cladding in such a way that defects can be detected and accurately sized through it (see also Section 7.1). The detection of defects in Plates 3 and 4 was also good, with all teams detecting all the defects in Plate 3 from the clad side and in Plate 4 all the defects were detected using automated equipment [Watkins et al., 1984]. One defect, which, although detected, was not reported in Plate 4, may be considered as an example of human error.

More detail of other team's results can be found in Barbian et al. [1984b]; Bowker et al. [1983]; Grohs et al. [1983]; Murgatroyd et al. [1983]; Poulter, Rogerson, Willetts and Dyke [1982]; Wüstenberg, Erhard, Montag and Schenk [1982]. A review and analysis of the capability of the different techniques appear in Murgatroyd and Firth [1985] and a summary and conclusions on the outcome of this exercise and the preliminary conclusions on PISC II exercise were provided by Nichols [1985]. Only

**Table 8.3** Results for defect through-wall size as measured with Time-of-Flight Diffraction by Harwell in DDT Plates 1 and 2 and compared with the minimum defect volumes determined destructively.

| Plate | Side | Correlation with destructive tests | Mean error | Standard deviation |
|---|---|---|---|---|
| 1 | clad | 0.984 | −1·4 | 2.5 |
| 1 | unclad | 0.988 | −1·3 | 2.0 |
| 2 | clad | 0.896 | 1·6 | 8.6 |
| 2 | unclad | 0.932 | 2·1 | 6.9 |
| 1 &2 | clad | 0.925 | −0·4 | 5.5 |
| 1 & 2 | unclad | 0.943 | 0·0 | 4.7 |

two teams, Harwell and Risley, inspected all four plates. For these two teams, at least, the evidence of the Defect Detection Trials is that, excluding human error, the reliability of automated inspection of thick steel sections of PWR geometry is governed by the capability of accurate sizing of the defect through-wall extent coupled with the repeatability of application in practice. Both teams used Time-of-Flight Diffraction to achieve their accurate sizing of the through-wall extent of defects.

The integrity of the PWR vessel was the main concern of the Defect Detection Trials and so we must be aware of the consequences of the results for vessel integrity. Detection of a defect is not the only important part of inspection; once detected, the defect must be sized as accurately as possible in order to test whether it is acceptable or should be repaired. The Defect Detection Trials were important tests of detection and sizing.

### 8.4.5 Results obtained for through-wall size

The results for the inspection of Plates 1 and 2 are presented in Figure 8.1. This is a scatter plot of the ultrasonically determined through-wall dimension of the defects compared with that found destructively and shows the results from all teams using a variety of ultrasonic inspection techniques from both sides of the plates. The results from the clad face are shown as solid circles, while those from the unclad face are shown as open circles.

The information from the Harwell Time-of-Flight Diffraction results alone is shown in Figure 8.2. The reduced scatter evident in Figure 8.2 brings out very clearly the high sizing accuracy achieved by the Time-of-Flight Diffraction technique.

### 8.4.6 Errors in TOFD through-wall sizing for Plates 1 and 2

The errors in the Harwell team's TOFD through-wall sizing results on in Plates 1 and 2 are set out in Table 8.3.

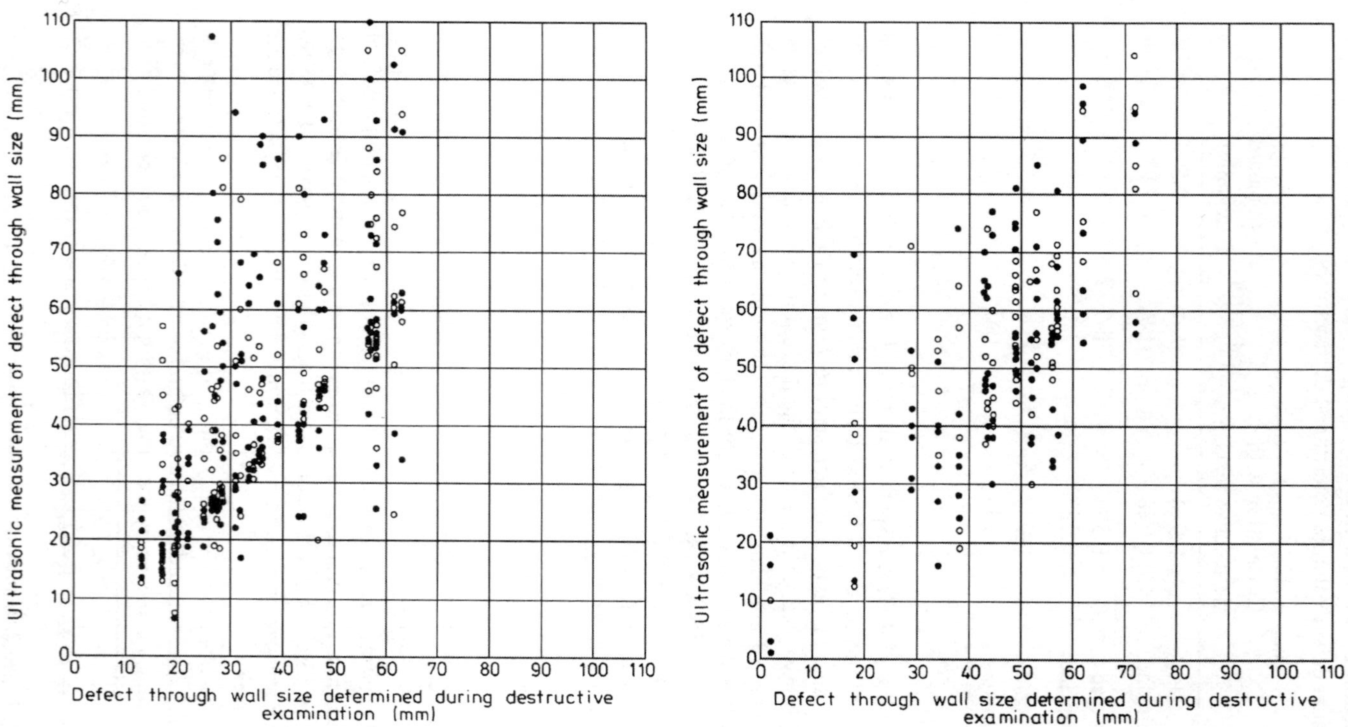


(a) DDT Plate 1

(b) DDT Plate 2

**Fig. 8.1** Scatter plot of results for defect through-wall size determined by all teams inspecting Plates 1 and 2 of the UKAEA Defect Detection Trials. Solid and open circles denote inspections from the clad and unclad sides of the plates respectively.

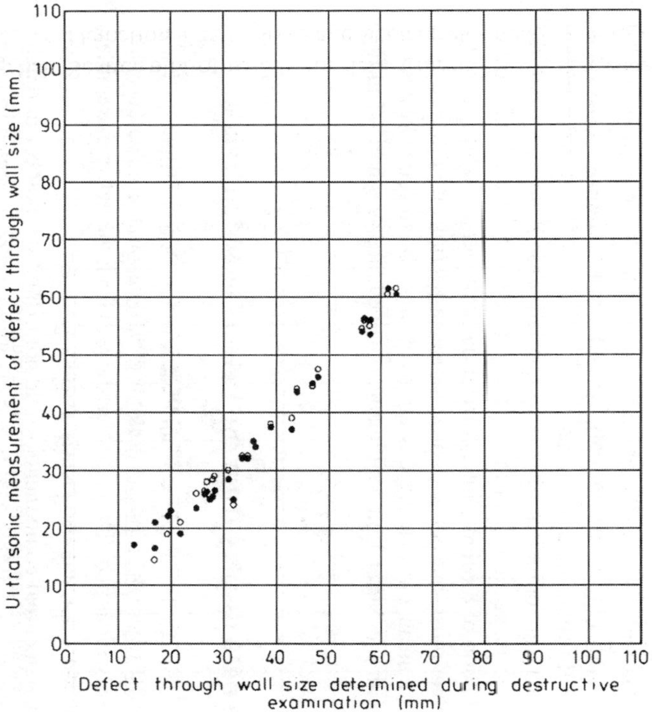


(a) DDT Plate 1

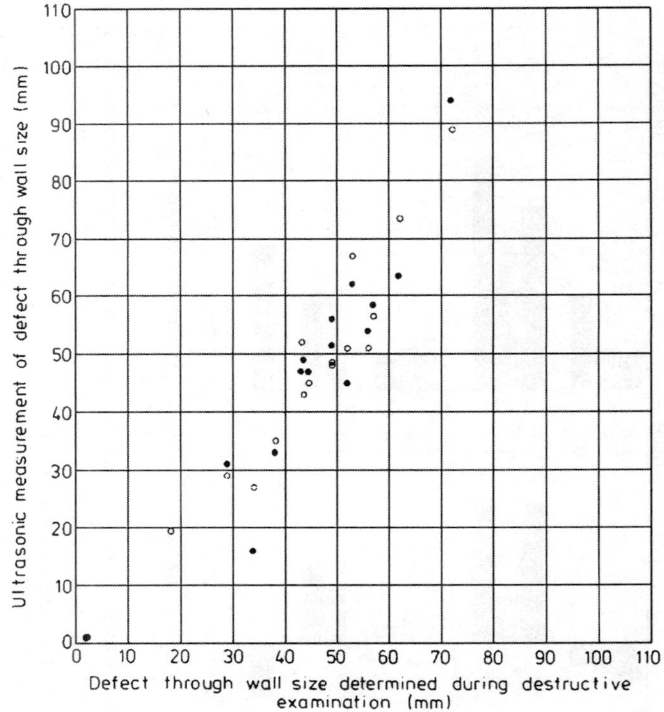


(b) DDT Plate 2

**Fig. 8.2** Scatter plot of results by obtained by Harwell with ultrasonic Time-of-Flight Diffraction on Plates 1 and 2 of the Defect Detection Trials organised by the UKAEA. Solid and open circles denote inspections from the clad and unclad sides of the plates respectively.

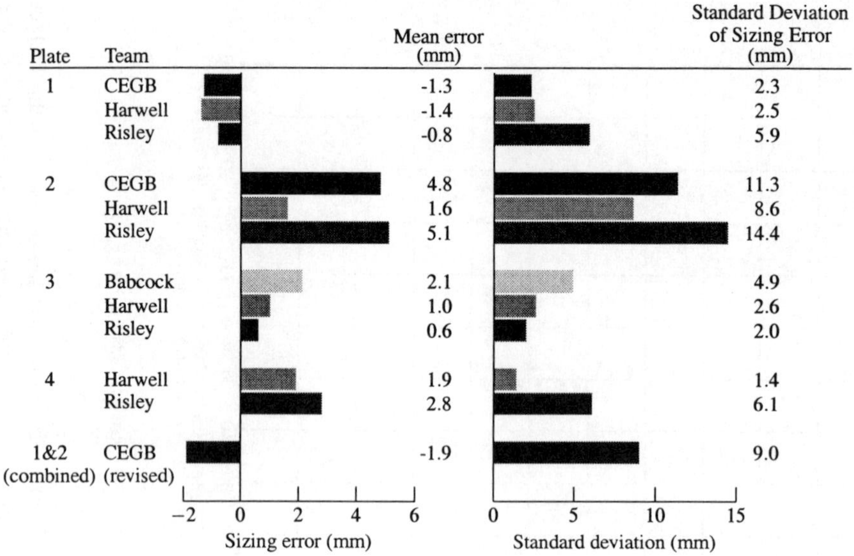


**Fig. 8.3** Mean and standard deviation of through-wall sizing measurements with inspection from the clad side of the plates. Results obtained by the U.K. teams in the Defect Detection Trials.

Even the worst Harwell Time-of-Flight Diffraction results, those from the unclad side of Plate 2, achieved a mean error of only 2.1 mm. For the clad-side inspections of Plate 1 the Harwell results are a mean error of −1.4 mm with standard deviation 2.5 mm and a correlation coefficient of 0.984. Similarly, for Plate 2, we find the Harwell result for the inspection from the clad side to be a mean error of 1.6 mm and a standard deviation of 8.6 mm with a correlation coefficient of 0.90. These results were better than most, but not all, conventional inspections used in the same test-block trials. The mean and standard deviations obtained by the three best teams overall, together with the correlation coefficients obtained, are summarised in Figure 8.3.

## 8.4.7 Typical data display from the Defect Detection Trials

An example of the data display obtained from Plate 1 of the Defect Detection Trials is shown in Figure 8.4 where the tops and bottoms of various numbered defects have been clearly and easily identified. The characteristic arcs from the defect extremities, as discussed in Section 2.3.4, are also clearly visible.

Although, in practice, real components would not exhibit the number of defects shown in this picture, signals of this quality and clarity would be expected from any fine grained equiaxed material with low inclusion content.

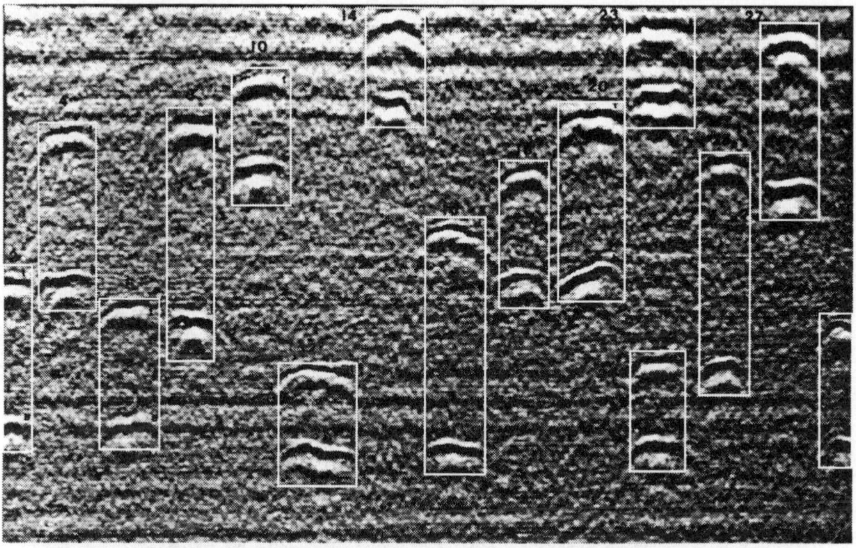

**Fig. 8.4** Time-of-Flight Diffraction signals observed on Plate 1 of the Defect Detection Trials. Related tops and bottoms of defects are linked by a white rectangle. Note that these rectangles are *not* intended to represent the extent of the defects [after Curtis and Hawker, 1983].

## 8.4.8 Characterisation of defects

The defects in Plate 1 were fabricated by welding patches into recesses in the weld preparation prior to the main welding process. The defects thus simulated lack of side wall fusion with clearly defined boundaries and gave rise to little controversy during comparison of the inspection results with the destructive test results. Plate 2 contained a wider selection of more complex defects aimed at simulating natural defects more closely. These included implanted fatigue crack coupons, cracks of unknown morphologies produced by carbon and copper contamination and some slag lines. Some of the cracks were of fragmented or branched type and raised some problems when comparisons of the inspection results with destructive test data were carried out on the basis of boxes drawn round defects.

To illustrate this point, we show, in Figures 8.5 and 8.6 respectively, the raw Time-of-Flight Diffraction data obtained from defect 15 in Plate 2 together with the report of the defect which was made during the defect detection trials [Curtis and Hawker, 1983].

A highly fragmented defect is apparent and the difficulty of drawing a simple box round the defect is obvious. Other examples of such fragmented defects in Plate 2, the Time-of-Flight Diffraction signals obtained from them, and the reports made of them at the time, can be found in Curtis and Hawker [1983]. To some extent, the correlation achieved between ultrasonic measurements and those obtained destruc-

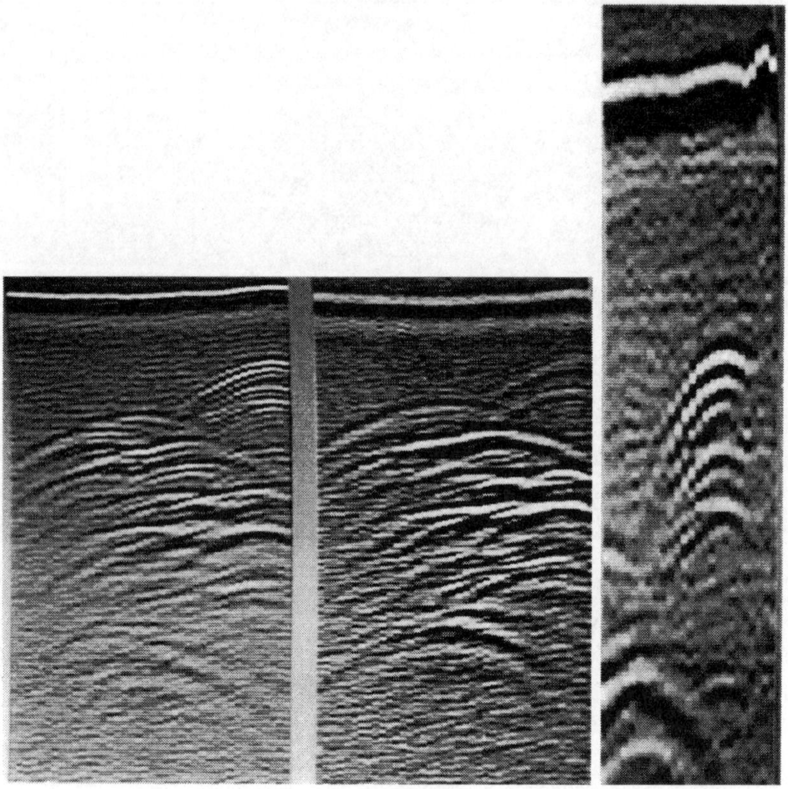

T5–R5 T5–R6 T4–R5

Defect and satellites Satellites

**Fig. 8.5** Raw ultrasonic data obtained from the clad-side inspection of defect number 15 in Plate 2 of the Defect Detection Trials.

tively will be a measure of the box drawing ability of the team as well as its intrinsic ultrasonic capability. The emphasis should then be placed on characterisation of the defects which have been found and sized. An interesting observation is that the correlation coefficients tend to improve, if the ultrasonic data are compared with the results of an extended destructive examination which included small welding defects associated with the coupon implants. The comparison between the results from this extended destructive examination and those obtained from the minimum volumes highlights the problem of drawing boxes around defects. These decisions should be based on unambiguous rules which are the same for the ultrasonic inspections as for the destructive examination. It is not known whether each team would reach the same conclusions on fragmented defects or defects with satellite indications each time the same defect signals were examined.

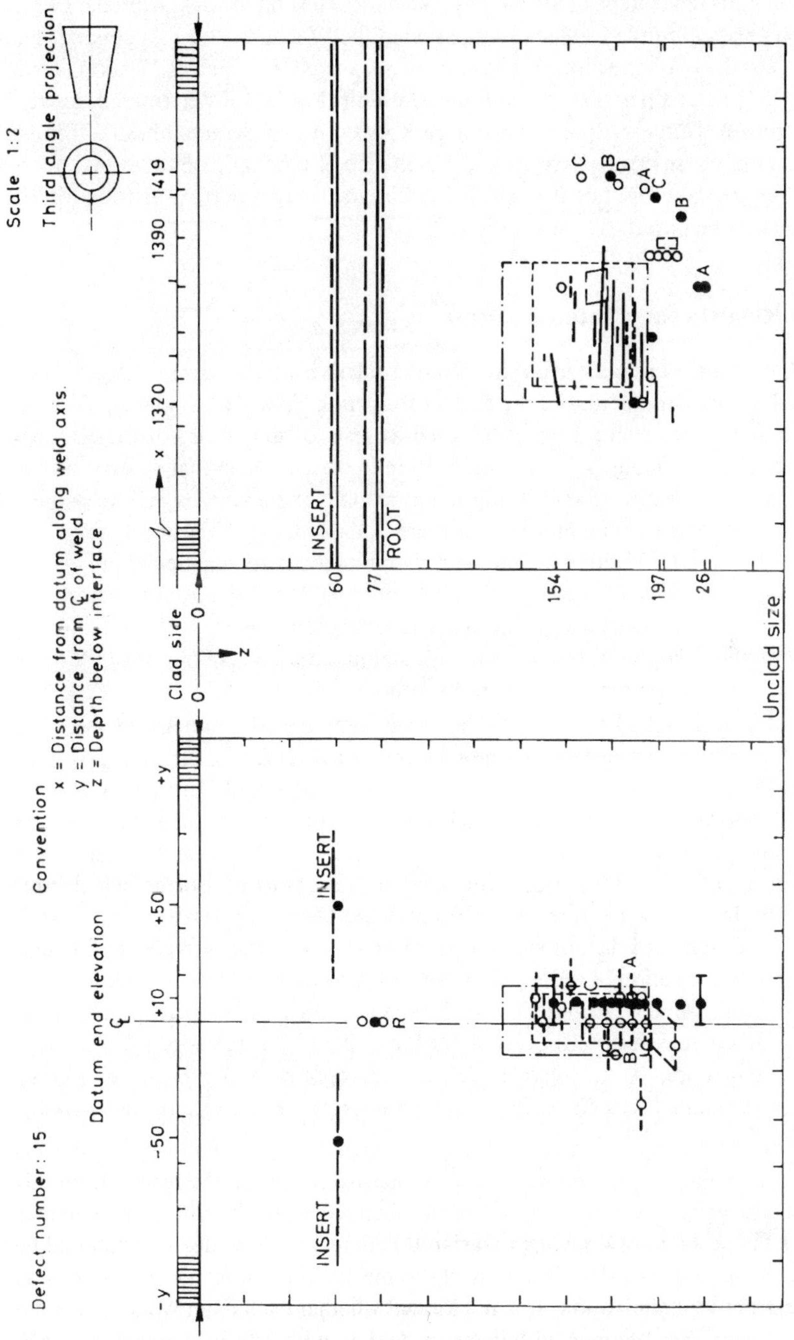


**Fig. 8.6** Report made by ultrasonic inspector characterising defect number 15 of Plate 2 of the Defect Detection Trials.

The scatter plots of Figure 8.1 suggest that the results may not be normally distributed and this tends to be confirmed by a statistical test on the data from the Defect Detection Trials. Temple [1984c, 1985] applied the W-statistic (see Appendix, Section A.11) to the published information on the measured defect sizes [Watkins et al., 1983a, 1984] as compared with the minimum defect volumes determined destructively [Crutzen, Bürgers, Violin, Di Piazza, Cowburn and Sargent, 1983]. Temple concluded that these errors have only a 2% chance of coming from a normal distribution. We are therefore not strictly justified in assuming a normal distribution but should seek more descriptive statistics.

### 8.4.9 Results for Plates 3 and 4

Two reactor nozzle cut-outs made from representative SA508 class 2 forging steel were used in the manufacture of the Defect Detection Trial Plates 3 and 4. The defects introduced into Plate 3 were designed as tests of the ability of the teams to detect and size sub-cladding cracks. In addition to the 26 intentional defects in Plate 3, three others were discovered during the ultrasonic examinations and subsequent destructive sectioning of the blocks. For Plate 3, the Harwell Laboratory team used the Time-of-Flight Diffraction technique for simultaneous search, detection and sizing, as a demonstration of the limitations of applying Time-of-Flight Diffraction in the unfavourable near-surface geometry. The team from Risley Nuclear Laboratories used Time-of-Flight Diffraction only for sizing, after detection of the defects by a 70° twin crystal compression-wave pulse-echo technique.

Plate 4 was designed to simulate the more complicated geometry of the PWR nozzle inner radius. The surface was prepared to a final value of 3 μm average roughness. On Plate 4, Harwell used a coarse raster Time-of-Flight Diffraction scan for detection, followed by more detailed sizing scans, while Risley used methods similar to those they used on Plate 3. A mean error in Plate 3 of 1.0 mm was achieved by Harwell and 0.6 mm by Risley with standard deviations of 2.6 mm and 2.0 mm respectively. In Plate 4 the mean errors found were 1.9 mm by Harwell and 2.8 mm by Risley with standard deviations of 1.4 mm and 6.1 mm respectively. Full details of the Harwell inspection of these plates can be found in the papers by Charlesworth and Hawker [1984] and Stringfellow and Perring [1984]. Note that the above results are based on the destructive results for Plates 3 and 4 as reported by Lock et al. [1983] and not simply on the intended defect sizes reported by Watkins et al. [1984]. Except for very small defects, there is a general tendency to oversize the cracks in both Plates 3 and 4.

## 8.5 The PISC II programme

The Programme for the Inspection of Steel Components (PISC II) carried out between 1981 and 1986 [PISC, 1986d] constituted a more detailed evaluation of the best performance obtainable with modern ultrasonic techniques under optimal conditions. The international programme grew from PISC I which was aimed at establishing the capability of ASME Code Section XI ultrasonic procedure.

The PISC I programme which ran between 1976 and 1980 was designed to investigate the appropriateness of the 1974 ASME Code, Section XI, ultrasonic inspection procedure for detecting, sizing and sentencing flaws in nuclear reactor pressure vessel components. The round-robin trial involved three plates, each 200 mm thick and containing a number of artificially induced flaws, being shipped to ten countries in turn where a number of teams applied ASME XI techniques or a selected set of alternative ultrasonic inspection techniques. The results were reported in 1980 to the CSNI Working Group on Safety Aspects of Steel Components in Nuclear Installations. The Working Group noted the urgent need for further work to develop the alternative techniques which were seen as being able to cover the weaknesses of the then conventional ultrasonic inspection techniques. The results obtained in PISC I were highly variable between teams. A number of teams, working to the 1974 ASME XI procedure undersized large cracks perpendicular to the plate surfaces (the critical direction from a fracture mechanics point of view). When these experimental flaws sizes were plotted on an ASME accept/reject diagram, they always appeared closer to acceptable than the true flaw sizes. Conversely a number of teams oversized small flaws. In contrast, the alternative procedures did significantly better at both detection and sizing [Crutzen, 1988].

The inspections in PISC II took place more recently than those in the Defect Detection Trials, although effort available to participate was more limited and the results were not obtained on the full range of specimens. Time-of-Flight Diffraction was used by one team in PISC II as a stand-alone detection and sizing tool and by another team for sizing only. Both teams achieved better than average sizing results. The results on the nozzle geometries have been discussed in Section 6.6; here we note the results obtained on Plate 2, in which the mean through-wall size error obtained by Harwell with Time-of-Flight Diffraction was 6 mm with an associated standard deviation of 13 mm. On the nozzle plate (Plate 3) the mean error was 8 mm (oversizing) with an associated standard deviation of 13 mm. Risley Nuclear Laboratories achieved a mean sizing accuracy of −1.3 mm (undersizing) with an associated standard deviation of 7.0 mm on the nozzle Plate 3 using Time-of-Flight Diffraction [Rogerson et al., 1988]. These results for Plate 3 are particularly noteworthy, since they demonstrate that good results can be obtained in difficult geometries.

Plate 1 was not attempted, since it contained so many parent metal defects that large areas of the plate would have been described as a single defect if the indications had been combined together according to standard proximity rules such as those in ASME-XI.

On the whole, the defects in PISC II were not as carefully manufactured as those in the Defect Detection Trials, since several defects were badly introduced and their envelopes resulted in very large defects, or the defects were surrounded by satellites which modified the detection rate of the defects [PISC, 1986a,b].

The PISC II round-robin trials were developed to demonstrate the effectiveness of in-service inspection and to cover defects in the size range 20 to 70 mm through wall extent which had not been covered in PISC I. In the spirit of testing in-service inspections, teams had to write procedures for their inspections and then follow these during the trials. The scheme for evaluating the results of the trial was worked out in detail in advance. The plates used in PISC I had been of relatively old types of steel manufactured to older acceptance standards so techniques were developed for implanting artificial defects into plate of the cleaner material typical of more modern production. A summary of the plates and the defects in them is given in Table 8.4 [from Nichols and Crutzen, 1988a].

In summarising the results from many teams from several countries, and several different procedures, Nichols and Crutzen conclude that *'TOFD alone is found in this work capable of doing most of the job and it is clear that a combination of techniques involving TOFD must reach high performances'* [Nichols and Crutzen, 1988b]. The teams using TOFD were careful to point out that they did not claim the technique was capable of detecting defects very near to, or penetrating, the cladding layer.

In trials such as PISC, it would be prohibitively expensive to provide enough defects to be able to put tight confidence bounds on the results. In principle, if all the defects in PISC II were taken to represent a single class of defects, there are enough defects to establish a lower bound of 99% reliability with 95% confidence (see Section 8.1.1 in this chapter and Section A.10 of the Appendix). In practice the defects cannot all be classed as similar. However, while the numbers of defects in each class were not sufficient for really high confidence in the inspection performance to be established, there were enough to indicate a good mean level of reliability.

## 8.6 The PISC III Programme

Nuclear reactor pressure vessels and primary circuit pipes are often made from materials which are not homogeneous and isotropic and neither are the geometries of nozzles simple. These additional complications, treated individually in Chapter 6 of this book, might lead to ineffective non-destructive inspection if the techniques employed were designed incorrectly. It was, therefore, logical to extend the testing of ultrasonic inspection techniques to materials more similar to those found in real reactors; with more realistic, though still artificially inserted flaws; in geometries more akin to those in actual reactors. This aim was fulfilled by the PISC III series of experimental round-robin trials completed in 1993, with destructive evaluation and assessment of the results afterwards.

The materials used, austenitic stainless steels, are characterised by a tendency for weld metal or cast material to solidify with a grain size of several millimetres and for the grains to show a degree of crystallographic alignment, governed by the direction of heat flow during solidification. These grains are comparable with, or larger than, the wavelength of ultrasound which would otherwise be the best to use for inspections. Because of this large grain size, relative to the ultrasonic wavelength used, the material exhibits anisotropy, with different wavespeeds in different directions. Because the crystal axes of neighbouring grains are not exactly aligned, the ultra-

**Table 8.4** The test plates used in the PISC II programme and the defects they contained.

| Plate | Country of manufacture | Type of specimen | Welding process | Plate material | Plate dimensions (mm) | Nozzle material | Nozzle dimensions (mm) | Total weight ($10^3$N) | No. of defects | Type of defect |
|---|---|---|---|---|---|---|---|---|---|---|
| 1 | Germany | Flat longitudinal weld in clad plate | Submerged arc under lower bound conditions | 20MnMoNi | 1050 × 1040× 248 | | | 21.5 | 20 | Fabrication defects |
| 2 | United Kingdom | Flat longitudinal weld in clad plate | Automatic submerged arc | ASME SA533B Class 1 | 1525 × 1525× 250 | | | 45 | 27 | Service induced defects |
| 3 | Italy & CEC | Curved with clad nozzle | Automatic submerged arc | ASME SA533B Class 1 | 2300 × 2600× 250 | ASME SA508 Class 2 | PWR nozzle OD 1370 ID 709 weld c/line ∅ = 1530 | 156 | 40<br>3 | Service induced & welding defects<br>Inner radius cracks |
| 9 | Japan | Flat with nozzle, clad | Automatic submerged arc | ASME SA533B Class 1 | 1950 × 1950× 200 | ASME SA508 Class 2 | BWR nozzle OD 535 ID 292 weld c/line ∅ = 890 | 65 | 17<br>3 | Subsurface flaws including cold cracks and lack of fusion<br>Fatigue cracks at nozzle inner radius of depth 15, 25 & 25 mm. One of the 25 mm cracks was repaired |

**Table 8.5** Results obtained by the Risley Nuclear Laboratory (UKAEA) on PISC II Plate 3 using high sensitivity pulse-echo detection with TOFD and SAFT sizing. The figures represent mean error and standard deviation in mm.

| | Through-wall ($z$) Defect location and size | Across-weld ($x$) Defect thickness | Along-weld ($y$) Defect length |
|---|---|---|---|
| Sizing | $-1.3 \pm 7.0$ | $-0.6 \pm 9.2$ | $-0.6 \pm 15.5$ |
| Location | $2.1 \pm 7.1$ | $2.4 \pm 6.6$ | $0.4 \pm 11.5$ |

**Table 8.6** Results obtained by the Harwell Laboratory (UKAEA) on PISC II Plate 2 using TOFD detection and sizing. The figures represent mean error and standard deviation in mm.

| | Through-wall ($z$) Defect location and size | Across-weld ($x$) Defect thickness | Along-weld ($y$) Defect length |
|---|---|---|---|
| Sizing | $1.0 \pm 13.0$ | N/A | $14.0 \pm 22.0$ |
| Location | $3.0 \pm 9.0$ | $2.0 \pm 3.0$ | $-3.0 \pm 5.0$ |

sonic properties vary from place to place, making the material inhomogeneous. The effect on the ultrasonic inspection can be likened to looking through frosted glass into a distorting mirror and trying to make accurate estimates of the size of a dimly discerned object.

PISC III defined eight areas of study (*actions*), with different material types, geometries and scale of specimen. Only two of the actions were relevant to the subject of this book. They were:

**Action 3** Nozzles and dissimilar metal welds. "*A round-robin test of four safe-end welds representing some of the most difficult technical aspects of in-service inspection*" [Crutzen, 1994]. The specimens were a Japanese-Italian BWR assembly with a nozzle and safe-end; an American BWR assembly with two nozzles and safe-ends; and a Spanish PWR safe-end. These were inspected in 13 countries and we present some conclusions relevant to TOFD.

**Action 4** Austenitic steel testing. This involved different configurations of austenitic material. There were wrought-to-wrought joins, wrought-to-cast joins, and cast-to-cast joins. Each has a distinctive grain structure and differing degrees of inspection difficulty. We present results from this study.

## 8.6.1 PISC III Action 3 — Nozzles and dissimilar metal welds

Three specimens representative of reactor BWR and PWR pressure vessel safe-end welds, PWR steam generator and surge line dissimilar metal welds, were used in this round-robin trial of in-service inspection techniques.

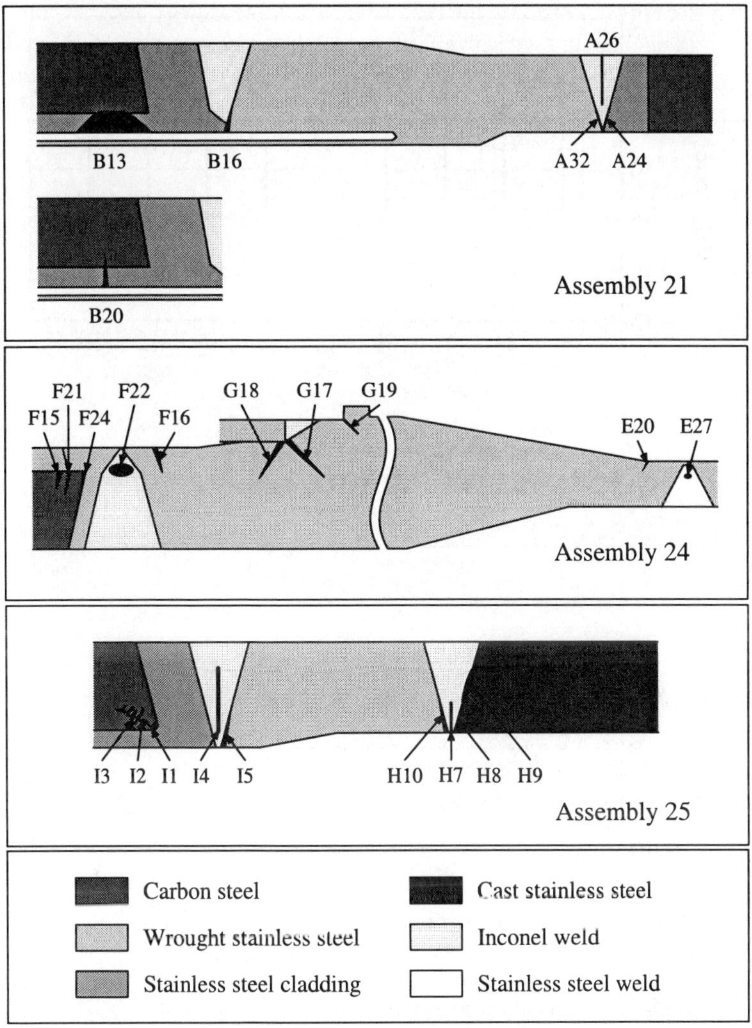


**Fig. 8.7** Flaw distribution in the assemblies used in PISC III, Action 3 (Redrawn from Dombret [1994]).

A single UK team was resourced from AEA Technology, Nuclear Electric, Babcock Energy, Rolls Royce and Associates and OIS. The team was led by Nuclear Electric and the assemblies were examined in Nuclear Electric's Wythenshawe laboratory. Pulse-echo inspection using an RTD Primscan scanner, the MIPS/GUIDE software and commercially available compression wave probes. Sizing made use of the pulse-echo results and Time-of-Flight Diffraction measurements made with a Zipscan instrument. Good detection performance was achieved except for two large defects, one in Assembly 21 and one in Assembly 25, which were not detected. Prior

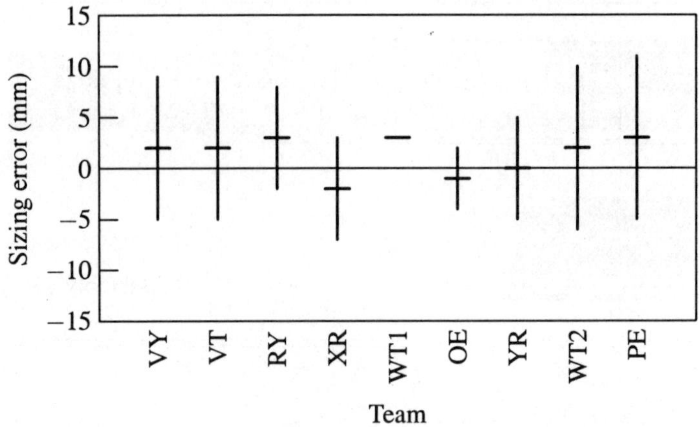


**Fig. 8.8** Sizing errors for defects in PISC III assembly 21.

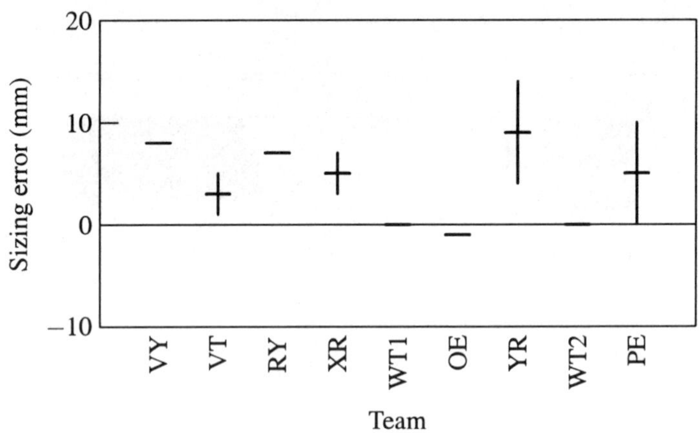


**Fig. 8.9** Sizing errors for defects in PISC III assembly 22.

to the tests, the team had considered the weld designs and modelled the inspection using RayTrAIM [Harker et al., 1991] with a structure based on what information could be gleaned from the drawings and on assumptions about the structure to be expected from the horizontal-vertical welding position. When the structures were finally revealed they turned out to be radically different from what had been assumed and the failure to detect some defects was thereby explained. This experience served to emphasise the wisdom of following the normal UK practice which requires qualification welds to be made so that the macrostructure of welds of each characteristic type can be studied prior to ultrasonic inspection.

Figure 8.7 shows the distribution of defects in Assemblies 21, 24 and 25. Results for mean sizing error and associated standard deviation are given for each team and

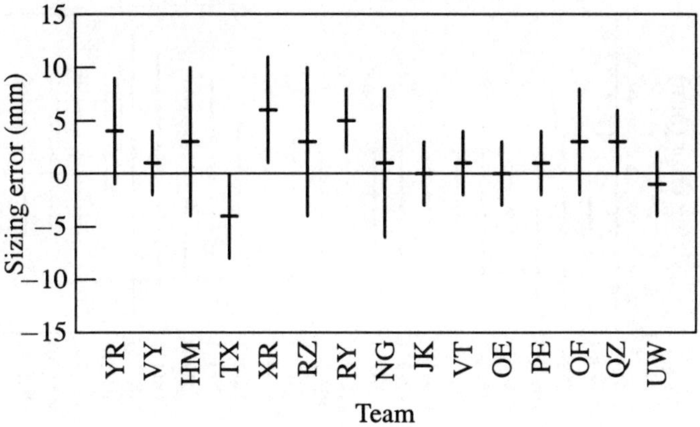


**Fig. 8.10** Sizing errors for defects in PISC III assembly 24.

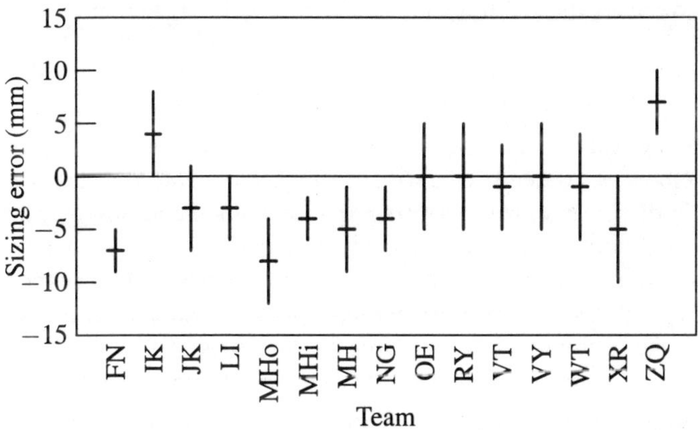


**Fig. 8.11** Sizing errors for defects in PISC III assembly 25.

assembly in Figures 8.8, 8.9, 8.10 and 8.11.

The combined UK team using TOFD sizing is team VT. These represent inspection of 25 flaws intentionally introduced into the assemblies. Of these 25 flaws, 3 were located in the thermal sleeve area of Assembly 24; 13 in the dissimilar metal welds and 9 in the homogeneous welds [Dombret, 1994].

### 8.6.2 PISC III Action 4 — Austenitic welds

Action 4 comprised three separate trials. One was a series of six wrought-to-wrought stainless steel assemblies numbered 31 to 36, containing a range of flaws such as intergranular stress corrosion cracking, fatigue cracks and electric-discharge-machined slots. A second trial used the wrought-to-cast assembly number 51. This assembly

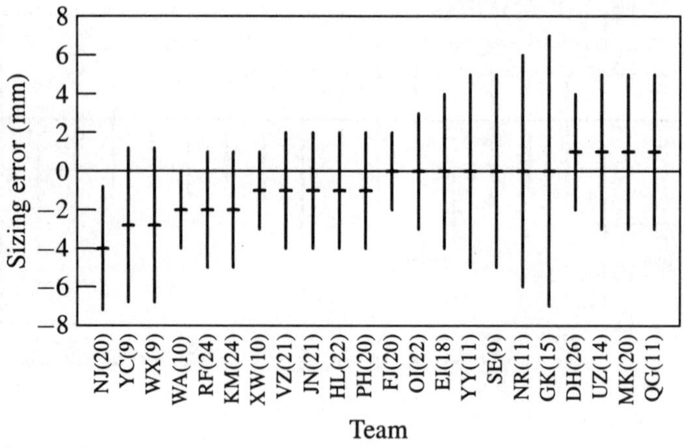


**Fig. 8.12** Mean sizing errors and standard deviations for the participating teams for the wrought-to-wrought assemblies of PISC III Action 4.

was a large wrought stainless steel pipe section with a centrifugally cast section welded on one end. At the other end a short section of centrifugally cast stainless steel pipe elbow was welded to the wrought pipe. The whole assembly was about 3 m long, 1 m in diameter, weighed 5750 kg and caused some handling difficulties. The third trial used cast-to-cast assemblies 41, 42 and 43. One of these pipe assemblies was welded into a support with good access and contained two seam welds. The other two assemblies were made by cutting a pipe into sections, growing or implanting flaws in the sections and then welding all the pieces back together again into two cylinders with extensions on the ends to provide necessary inspection run-outs.

PISC Report 33 [Lemaître and Kobl, 1995a] covers the ultrasonic inspection results of the wrought-to-wrought assemblies numbers 31, 32, 33, 34, 35 and 36. Six wrought-to-wrought assemblies were inspected by 23 teams from 10 different countries. In total 26 flaws were introduced. These comprised 12 intergranular stress corrosion cracks, 4 fatigue cracks, 7 surface breaking and 2 embedded notches, and 1 lack of weld-root penetration. Amongst the conclusions drawn it was noted that (sic) "*The key of success to performing a good depth sizing of surface-breaking cracks is the capability to detect crack tip diffractions. Amplitude drop methods are not suited to size the depth of surface breaking cracks*" and "*An ASME type performance demonstration test was simulated. It was confirmed that the detection and the false call performance were satisfactory but that the sizing performance was poor. Of the 11 teams considered for the simulation 10 were successful for detection, 9 for false calls, 3 for depth sizing and none for length sizing. The three teams that were successful for depth sizing all made use of crack tip diffraction. Two of them also used mode conversion.*" The mean sizing error and standard deviation are shown in Figure 8.12. The numbers in brackets are the number of defects used in determining the mean and standard deviation of sizing error for that team. The UK team using

**Table 8.7** Number of false calls on the wrought-to-wrought assemblies for each team participating in PISC III Action 4; the figure in parentheses is the number of false calls classed as rejectable flaws.

| Team | Weld | Heat affected zone HAZ | Weld plus HAZ | Counter-bore | Base material | Total | False rejects |
|---|---|---|---|---|---|---|---|
| DH | 0 | 3(1) | 1(0) | 0 | 0 | 4 | 1 |
| EI | 1(0) | 0 | 1(1) | 0 | 0 | 2 | 1 |
| FJ | 0 | 0 | 0 | 0 | 0 | 0 | 0 |
| GK | 0 | 0 | 0 | 25(9) | 0 | 25 | 9 |
| HL | 6(4) | 4(0) | 2(1) | 0 | 1(0) | 13 | 5 |
| JN | 0 | 0 | 0 | 0 | 0 | 0 | 0 |
| KM | 0 | 6(1) | 0 | 1(1) | 2[1](0) | 9 | 2 |
| LP | 1(0) | 5(2) | 0 | 0 | 0 | 6 | 2 |
| MK | 1(1) | 0 | 0 | 0 | 0 | 1 | 1 |
| NJ | 0 | 3(0) | 0 | 1(0) | 2(0) | 6 | 0 |
| NR | 0 | 1(0) | 0 | 0 | 0 | 1 | 0 |
| PH | 0 | 0 | 1(1) | 0 | 0 | 1 | 1 |
| OI | 0 | 4(3) | 11(11) | 5(5) | 1(1) | 21 | 20 |
| QG | 0 | 0 | 0 | 0 | 0 | 0 | 0 |
| RF | 0 | 1(0) | 1(1) | 1(0) | 3(1) | 6 | 2 |
| SE | 2(2) | 1(0) | 0 | 0 | 0 | 3 | 2 |
| UZ | 0 | 3(1) | 0 | 0 | 0 | 3 | 1 |
| VZ | 0 | 1(0) | 0 | | 0 | 1 | 0 |
| WA | 0 | 0 | 0 | 0 | 0 | 0 | 0 |
| WX | 0 | 4(3) | 0 | 0 | 1(1) | 5 | 4 |
| XW | 0 | 0 | 0 | 0 | 0 | 0 | 0 |
| YC | 1(0) | 4(0) | 0 | 8(0) | 0 | 13 | 0 |
| YY | 0 | 6(6) | 1(1) | 0 | 0 | 7 | 7 |

1. False calls due to seam weld

TOFD sizing is team FJ. This team was formed from personnel and techniques supplied by AEA Technology, Nuclear Electric, Babcock Energy and Rolls Royce and Associates.

In difficult inspection tasks such as these, it is possible to increase detection rate by increasing sensitivity. This leads to more false calls which, if classed as rejectable flaws would lead to expensive grinding out and reworking of material. The false call rates reported in PISC III Report 33 [Lemaître and Kobl, 1995a] are reproduced in Table 8.7.

PISC Report 34 gives the results of the cast-to-cast trial. In the UK it was not possible to resource a team to carry out inspections on the cast-to-cast material.

PISC Report 35 [Lemaître and Kobl, 1995b] gives details of the results of ultrasonic inspections from the wrought-to-cast weld on assembly 51 and from the weld between the wrought and centrifugally cast material in assembly 43. Assembly 43

**Table 8.8** False calls on the wrought-to-cast assemblies for each team participating in PISC III Action 4; the figure in parentheses is the number of false calls classed as rejectable flaws.

| Team | WCC43[1] | CCW51[2] | WSC51[3] | Total | False rejects |
|---|---|---|---|---|---|
| AT | 0(0) | 0(0) | 1(1) | 1 | 1 |
| DH | N/I[4] | 0(0) | 1(0) | 1 | 0 |
| EI | 2(0) | 1(0) | 0(0) | 3 | 0 |
| FJ | N/I | 0(0) | 1(0) | 1 | 0 |
| NM | 0(0) | 2(2) | N/I | 2 | 2 |
| PH | 0(0) | 0(0) | 0(0) | 0 | 0 |
| UZ | N/I | 0(0) | N/I | 0 | 0 |
| YC | 34(23) | N/I | N/I | 34 | 23 |
| YY | 2(0) | N/I | N/I | 2 | 0 |
| ZD2 | N/I | 1(0) | 3(0) | 4 | 0 |

1. Wrought to centrifugally cast weld in assembly 43
2. Centrifugally cast to wrought weld in assembly 51
3. Wrought to statically cast weld in assembly 51
4. N/I signifies not inspected

also contained another weld, between two sections of centrifugally cast material. A single team from the UK carried out the inspections reported and was a combination of personnel and techniques supplied by AEA Technology and Nuclear Electric (now British Energy).

The false call rates of the different teams are shown in Table 8.8. Some of the conclusions drawn in the report on inspection of wrought-to-cast stainless steels are (sic):

- *The best detection results were obtained with twin crystal compression wave probes working at* 1 MHz *with an angle of incidence of 45° or 60°.*
- *The use of focusing probes did not improve substantially the detection performance. However, the focusing probe technique seems promising for depth sizing.*
- *The detection performance of the shear wave probes was in general lower than that of the compression wave probes.*
- *Depth sizing proved to be difficult in these assemblies. Therefore, more effort should be devoted to develop probes that exploit crack tip diffraction. In this respect the focusing probes seem promising.*

Mean sizing errors and associated standard deviations are shown in Figure 8.13. The UK team is FJ.

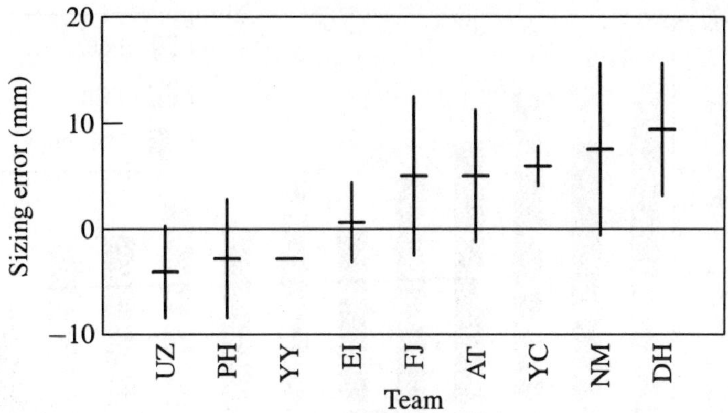


**Fig. 8.13** Mean sizing errors and associated standard deviations for the wrought-to-cast welds in PISC III Action 4.

## 8.7 Comparison of TOFD with radiographic inspection

The Netherlands Institute of Welding (NIL) organised a test-block trial in round-robin fashion with a series of artificial workpieces ranging in thickness from 6mm-15mm. This round-robin trial and the results have been reported by Stelwagen [1995]. Some 21 workpieces, containing a total of 244 artificial, but very realistic, defects were inspected by eleven methods. The defects included lack of fusion, lack of weld penetration, slag, cracks and gas inclusions. The aim of the trials was to compare mechanised ultrasonic methods with more traditional NDT approaches so inspection methods ranged from mechanised ultrasonic scanning, to manual ultrasonic tests and included radiography. In all, eleven approaches were used, each adhering rigidly to a predefined written inspection procedure. Of these eleven methods, a total of seven were for mechanised ultrasonic inspection: three using TOFD and four using pulse-echo. Completing the set were manual ultrasonic inspection and three distinct radiographic techniques. One of the outcomes of this round-robin exercise was a clear demonstration of the benefit of using combined pulse-echo and TOFD giving excellent defect detection and defect sizing. This is shown in Figure 8.14 which plots a performance factor. Both missed defects and false calls were used to define the performance factor. As a result of this trial, MicroPlus, the world leader in commercially available TOFD equipment, now offers a unit which collects both pulse-echo and TOFD data simultaneously in a single pass. This approach has been used by AEA Technology for NDT of a pipeline during pipe-laying operations in Brazil, in preference to radiography, saving time without losing quality of NDT information and so saving the pipe-laying company money.

The significance of the NIL study for the establishment of standards appropriate to the TOFD technique is discussed in Section 10.2.

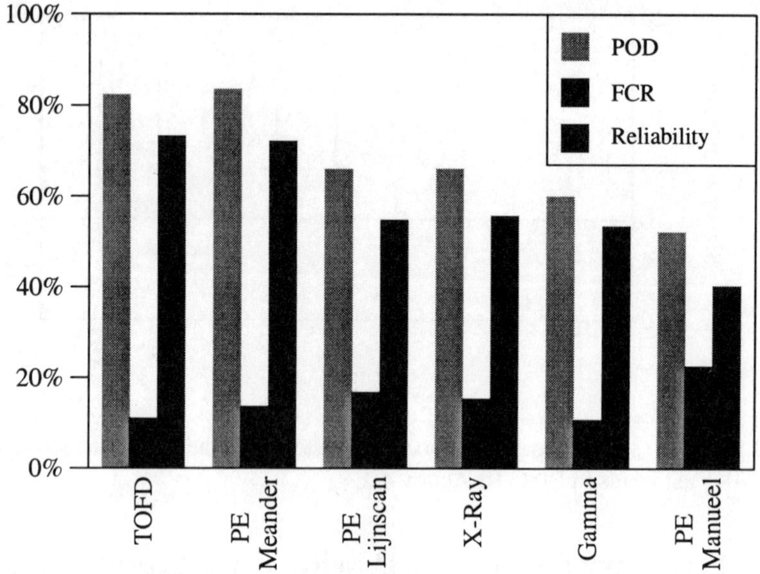


**Fig. 8.14** Comparison of TOFD with other NDT techniques, organised by the Netherlands Institute of Welding [Stelwagen, 1995]. POD is probability of detection, FCR is false call rate and Reliability is the probability of correct classification.

## 8.8 Sizing accuracy of TOFD compared with amplitude based techniques

Ammirato and Willetts [1989] record the results of a round-robin test of sizing accuracy by a variety of amplitude based techniques and by TOFD. Two measures of accuracy are required. First there is the average error attained by a particular technique over the set of artificial defects. Second there is a measure of how variable the results are, again for a particular technique, over the set of artificial defects. The measure of this is the standard deviation of the results about the mean. A perfect technique would have zero mean error and would also have zero standard deviation. Good techniques will therefore have small values for these two measures. Ammirato and Willetts [1989] give the results illustrated in Figure 8.15.

To understand the significance of such numbers we need first to know what the defect set used was. In this case, intentional flaws had been introduced into the test pieces to represent three classes of cracks of particular interest to the nuclear power generation industry. These were cracks under the cladding; defects embedded in welds; and defects in nozzle-to-shell welds. For these realistic defects, appropriate to a clad, thick-walled, pressure vessel, we see that TOFD would be the preferred technique with the other diffracted signal method, backward scattering tip diffraction

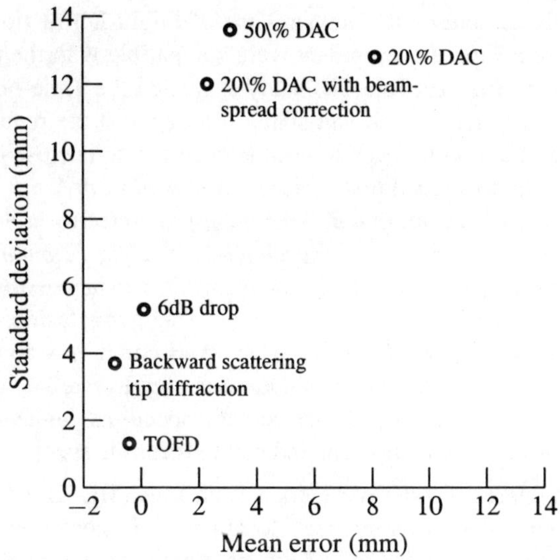


**Fig. 8.15** Comparison of the accuracy of TOFD and amplitude-based ultrasonic techniques [after Ammirato and Willetts, 1989].

a second choice, followed by the 6 dB drop method.

The fact that standard deviations for the various sizing methods have been quoted could be taken to imply that the sizing errors are random and distributed according to the Normal distribution. This would imply that errors could be reduced by repeated measurements, so that, for instance, the 6 dB drop method could equal the accuracy of TOFD if repeated 20 times. This is probably far from the truth, since a large part of the spread in sizing results is likely to be related to the range of defect types and geometries employed in the trial. The use of the standard deviation is a convenient way of indicating the spread of measurements, rather than a precise statement about the distribution of results.

## 8.9 Implications for structural integrity

The defects of most concern in typical engineering structures are those which could lead to failure. This usually means planar, crack-like defects orientated perpendicular to the principal stresses. Fracture mechanics criteria of one form or another can be used to give precise definitions of a critical defect size for a given material strength and loading. These criteria can be chosen from linear elastic fracture mechanics or can include elastic-plastic analysis and will not be discussed in any more detail here. One common set of rules for assessing defect significance, based on linear elastic fracture mechanics, is Section XI of the Boiler and Pressure Vessel Code of the American Society of Mechanical Engineers [ASME, 1974,1977,1983]. Silk carried out a study to determine whether Time-of-Flight Diffraction data obtained with the then current Zipscan equipment were compatible with the requirements of the ASME-XI code [Silk, 1987b]. The study evaluated the Time-of-Flight Diffraction technique, in its basic search and sizing role, against the requirements of the ASME-XI code and a modified version of the code which is close to the European industrial norm. Silk concluded that *'Operation in conformity with ASME-XI is expected to be possible for all internal defects and for all defects which lie deeper than 30% of the specimen thickness in steel specimens exceeding 12 mm in thickness. Operation in conformity with the modified code is expected to be possible for all defects in steel specimens exceeding 10 mm in thickness.'* These conclusions applied only to the basic use of Time-of-Flight Diffraction, as it was commonly applied in the field with Zipscan equipment. When the technique was used to size known defects, or in specialised uses such as nuclear pressure vessel inspections, higher precision could be achieved by tailoring the equipment and methods for the specific task.

As well as engineering codes of practice, such as ASME-XI, which concern the acceptability of defects of different sizes, locations and orientations, other ways of assessing defect significance and the relationship between the reliability and precision of non-destructive testing techniques and structural integrity have been developed. Marshall [1982] and Lucia and Volta [1983] used probabilistic analyses to determine the size range, aspect ratio and location of the flaws which have the greatest influence on integrity of the pressure vessel of a PWR during possible accident sequences. As we have already seen in Section 8.4, the greatest contribution to the vessel failure rate is expected from cracks in a limited size range, which depends both on the chance that cracks in that size range will be present and the chance that the material properties in the region of the crack will be such that the crack is of a critical size for some possible transient stress. The cracks contributing most to the predicted failure rate, under conditions appropriate to large loss-of-coolant accidents (LOCAs) or steam line breaks, are those planar, crack-like flaws orientated perpendicular to the principal stresses (i.e. lying in planes perpendicular to the pressure retaining surfaces) and with a through-wall extent of between 10 and 50 mm [Cameron, 1984]. The most important locations of the cracks are the nozzle-to-shell weld, nozzle corners and the belt-line welds, and these are, therefore, the geometries appropriate for test-block exercises. For conservatism in predictions of the failure rate of vessels, it is usually assumed that the cracks are all surface breaking or at least would be classed as surface-breaking cracks according to proximity rules such as given by ASME [1974,1977,1983]. If the assumption that the cracks are all near the surface is not valid then the estimated failure rates of vessels decrease by at least three orders of magnitude [Lucia and Volta, 1983].

The hazard presented by the failure of a component should determine the reliability required of that component. If the component is required to survive various possible excess transient stresses, for example, then non-destructive testing may well be used to identify flawed components before any catastrophic failure occurs.

A defect is classified as *unacceptable* if it poses a threat to the integrity of the structure and *acceptable* if it does not. Basing his assessment on probabilistic fracture mechanics applied to analysis of the expected failure rate of PWR pressure vessels, Marshall [1982] suggested a target to be achieved for the reliability of classifying defects according to their through-wall extent. The through-wall extent is, of course, precisely what the Time-of-Flight Diffraction technique measures, whereas, for other inspection techniques, it may only be derivable indirectly. Marshall's target was a 50% chance of detecting and correctly classifying a defect of 6 mm through-wall extent coupled with a 95% chance of detecting and correctly classifying a defect of through-wall extent 25 mm. This is now believed to be a conservative estimate of the reliability of ultrasonic techniques but nevertheless yields a failure rate of $10^{-7}$ per vessel year for a PWR pressure vessel. In general, probabilistic fracture-mechanics assessments have assumed that a single parameter of the defect, through-wall size, governs the likelihood of vessel failure. However, this parameter is not what is measured most readily by most ultrasonic inspections except by Time-of-Flight Diffraction.

Even if the chance of failing to correctly classify a defect were as low as $10^{-4}$ independent of defect through-wall extent, then the failure rate of the pressure vessel would only decrease to a little below $10^{-8}$ per vessel year. Thus there is a limit to the advantage that can be gained by increasing the inherent capability of inspection techniques. There are many assumptions in these analyses which are beyond the scope of our present brief discussion. For more detail the reader is referred to Marshall [1982] and Cameron [1984]. Section A.12 of the Appendix discusses these points in a little more detail.

The important point is that targets outlined above define a scale for how reliable inspection should be for the pressure vessel of a pressurised water reactor. As we have shown, Time-of-Flight Diffraction can achieve much greater accuracy and reliability than this target. The fact that such performance is also possible with well designed conventional pulse-echo methods gives confidence that diverse techniques are available in situations where the highest performance is demanded.

# Chapter 9

# Applications of Time-of-Flight Diffraction

As we have demonstrated in earlier chapters, the Time-of-Flight Diffraction technique is a powerful and accurate tool; it is now routinely used to size defects in a large range of components both as a complement to detection by more conventional methods and in stand-alone applications where both detection and sizing are carried out by Time-of-Flight Diffraction.

It is in the nature of routine applications that they rarely give rise to published papers. Much of the work cited in this chapter on applications could more accurately be described as studies of capability, undertaken before embarking on routine deployment of the technique. Some of the applications have been referred to in earlier chapters but are presented here again to make this survey as comprehensive as possible. The content of the cited papers is described only briefly and the reader is referred to the original references for greater detail.

Wedgwood [1995] reviews the advantages and disadvantages of TOFD vis-à-vis other ultrasonic inspection methods, citing better reliability as one of the major reasons for choosing TOFD. He describes some applications of TOFD to offshore and nuclear plant but does not attempt a comprehensive list of all applications to date. In the following sections we present applications grouped into specific areas.

## 9.1 Water-cooled nuclear pressure vessels and nozzles

Rolls-Royce and Associates Limited has been involved in the design, procurement and operation of pressurised water reactors (PWRs) since 1959 [Anon., 1987]. Up to mid-1987, they had carried out 30 pre-service and in-service inspections, and had more than twenty PWRs to inspect regularly with more under construction, giving them, at that time, more experience than any other UK company in inspecting this type of reactor. Since TOFD became well established, they have adopted it as one of their main inspection techniques.

Browne [1988] describes in-service inspection of primary circuit nozzle and pipe welds in a German nuclear power station, citing reliability and accuracy as the reason for choosing the TOFD technique.

Lilley [1989] describe the detection and sizing of under-clad cracks in a ferritic component clad with austenite, using the TOFD technique from the unclad ferritic surface, so that the crack signals appear near the back-wall echo.

Pitcher [1989] used TOFD to inspect a circumferential weld in the primary circuit of a pressurised water reactor. The detailed procedure was validated with the appropriate regulatory authority. An advantage cited is the rapidity with which data can be collected, allowing analysis and processing to be carried out off-line. Processing techniques used included time-to-depth linearisation to simplify interpretation and synthetic aperture focusing (SAFT) to improve resolution and signal-to-noise ratio.

Pers-Anderson [1991] describes the detection and repair of a crack in a feed-water nozzle of a boiling water reactor (BWR) in Sweden. It is not clear from the paper how the defect was first detected but it was monitored in service by both TOFD and an eddy-current technique. When it became clear that the crack was surface-breaking, it was repaired during the next scheduled outage. Crack samples taken during the repair were consistent with the ultrasonic results.

Daniels et al. [1996] describe the use of TOFD for sizing cracks in the feed-water nozzles of PWR steam generators. System, procedure and personnel performance were tested in blind trials at the EPRI NDE Center, Charlotte, NC, and the first "live" use of the system was successfully completed at a nuclear power plant in the USA. The paper describes the sophisticated analysis tools provided to help the operators interpret the data and gives details of the performance achieved in the blind trials. A screenshot of one of the data analysis tools is reproduced in Figure 6.12.

Bloodworth [1999] describes the development of procedures for detection and sizing of defects in the nozzle to pipe attachment welds of a Swedish BWR. Both the nozzle and the pipe are ferritic steel with austenitic cladding on the inner surface. The accuracy required for through-thickness sizing of the defects was $\pm 2.3$ mm, which is very demanding. A TOFD procedure was developed for this purpose and achieved the required accuracy when tested on a qualification specimen with documented defects. Data collection and analysis personnel subsequently passed qualification tests on blind-trial specimens. At the time of writing no non-TOFD procedure had achieved the required accuracy. A screenshot of an analysis tool used in this work is reproduced in Figure 6.13.

## 9.2 Gas-cooled nuclear pressure vessels

An article in Nuclear Engineering International [Anon., 1992] reviews ultrasonic inspection methods for the inspection of pressure vessels used in the gas-cooled Magnox reactors which are now operating beyond their design life. Use of the TOFD technique to produce real-time D-scan images has enabled a clear view of the defects in their true relative positions and size to be produced and this capability has been central to the granting of plant life extension.

Pennick [1993] gives a detailed description of the deployment of TOFD inspection equipment on the pressure vessels of the Calder Hall and Chapelcross Magnox reactors. The steel vessels contained one surface breaking defect, less than 2 mm deep, and three buried defects, all less than 25 mm long, with through-wall sizes of 2.4, 4.0 and 6.8 mm. These results were compared with previous inspection findings and with calculated limiting crack sizes. Destructive examination of the defects was not possible, as the vessels were still in service.

## 9.3 Other nuclear components

Broere, Hagedoorn and Lodder [1991] describe the Nerason instrument for the ultrasonic inspection of the internal bores of steam-generator tubing. TOFD is one of the techniques which can be deployed with this instrument.

Threaded studs and fasteners are used to retain the top dome on a PWR pressure vessel. Load cycling in service can sometimes gives rise to fatigue cracks, usually developing from the thread root. Gartside and Hurst [1994] have developed a system for TOFD inspection of the studs on the Sizewell 'B' PWR vessel, deploying the ultrasonic probes from the 'heater hole' in the bore of the stud.

## 9.4 Non-nuclear pressure vessels

Anliker and Cilauro [1988] used TOFD to detect, size and profile cracks on the surface of a hot (200°C) pressure vessel used in the pulp and paper industry.

In a trial made on a thick-walled pressure vessel taken from the petrochemical refining industry, Yokote, Ishizuka, Tahara, Bagdasarian, Gougler and Stellina [1994] compared TOFD with the 6 dB drop method for crack sizing. The vessels, used as hydroprocessing reactors, were made from $2\frac{1}{4}$Cr-1Mo steel clad in the inside surface with successive layers of 310 and 308 austenitic steel and were about 150 mm thick. They had been exposed to 26 years service at high temperature and high hydrogen levels.

The performance of the ultrasonic techniques was demonstrated on test blocks, prior to testing the vessels. The five vessel cracks tested had previously been detected using radiography and ultrasonic pulse-echo inspection. Three of them were sectioned after the NDT tests and real crack depths obtained from the macrographs. The results are shown in Table 9.1. Both pulse-echo and TOFD appear to have performed well but TOFD is described as having excellent accuracy. Radiography was not satisfactory.

## 9.5 Turbine and generator components

Browne [1988] cites the use of TOFD in the sizing of cracks in turbine discs. Lilley and Pitcher [1989] describes the detection and sizing of cracks in turbine rotor shafts.

**Table 9.1** Results of crack sizing trials on thick-walled pressure vessels from the petrochemical refining industry [after Yokote et al., 1994].

| Inspection technique | —— Block 5 —— | | | Block 6 | Block 15 |
|---|---|---|---|---|---|
| 6 dB drop | 16·5 | 14·5 | 4·0 | 21·0 | 14·0 |
| TOFD | 16·0 | 10·0 | 5·9 | | 11·0 |
| Sectioning | 15·0 | 9·0 | | 18·0 | |

They claim that axial cracks in the bore and radial cracks at the outer surface are readily detected and sized using probes on the bore surface and quotes a through-wall sizing accuracy of $\pm 0.1$ mm. They also report that individual beach marks of a growing fatigue crack can be distinguished in a TOFD D-scan image, provided the signals are separated in time from neighbouring ones by at least $1\frac{1}{2}$ wave periods.

Ashwin [1989] has also applied TOFD to retaining rings and turbine discs and claims improved sizing accuracy compared with pulse echo techniques as well as readier recognition of defect signals.

Dube and Helleringer [1989] studied stress corrosion cracking (SCC) and fatigue cracking in low pressure turbine rotors used in nuclear power plant. Using a computerised TOFD system they were able to obtain rapid and repeatable results and size cracks on site.

In a study of samples taken from a low pressure steam turbine rotor, good agreement was also found between TOFD inspection data and destructive examination. A sizing accuracy of better than 1.5 mm for defects of actual height between 2.5 mm and 15 mm, with a consistent 0.75 mm undersizing [Helleringer and Salin, 1990].

Day [1992] used an automated TOFD system to inspect retaining rings from a generator at a geothermal power plant in New Zealand. These rings were made from different types of steel: carbon steel, austenitic steel and a martensitic steel. Each type of steel is associated with different defect types and locations and so different inspection procedures are appropriate. Flaws in ferritic and martensitic material could be accurately sized using TOFD and the advantage of such a capability was demonstrated by monitoring a known flaw in a martensitic end ring. Stress corrosion cracking (SCC) at the back wall in end rings made from austenitic steel could not be reliably detected with conventional ultrasonics. However, using TOFD, it was possible to use the phase differences between the signals to distinguish crack-tip signals from reflections from the back wall, or from changes of form which occur with shrink fitting of the rings.

Nottingham and MacDonald [1988, 1989, 1990] were also concerned with intergranular SCC in retaining rings. Once again the advantage of being able to prolong the life of a flawed component by deploying an accurate crack sizing technique such as TOFD was demonstrated. They found TOFD to be advantageous in discriminating cracks from geometric reflectors and concluded that *'TOFD was the only method investigated which could be used to estimate the depth of a crack with confidence'*. MacDonald [1990] described this work at greater length and reported that SAFT processing of the TOFD data improved the spatial resolution. At that time, he thought that SAFT processing was too slow to be of practical use; however, computer processing speeds have increased by a very large factor since then, so this criticism would no longer apply.

## 9.6 Offshore structures

Bainton et al. [1975] published an early review of the inspection requirements of fixed offshore platforms and the possible techniques which could be used. At that time TOFD was in its infancy but was recognised as having potential for application in this area.

Gardner and Bosselaar [1984] reported the results of applying the TOFD technique to the sizing of defects in samples relevant to offshore structures. The samples used were a butt weld between flat plates, a 90° T-butt weld and a section of tubular node. Sizing accuracy of $\pm 1$ mm was achieved for defects more than 5 mm below the inspection surface.

This work led to a successful series of trials of a prototype underwater sizing apparatus in a diver training tank [Hawker et al., 1985; Newton et al., 1986]. The UKAEA subsequently patented equipment for applying TOFD to underwater structures [UKAEA, 1988]. Newton [1987] assessed how inspection performance might be affected by compressive stresses causing crack transparency and, more recently, Newton [1990] reviewed the programs carried out by the Harwell Laboratory for the offshore industry, including the use of TOFD to size defects in subsea node welds.

Osborne [1989] reported successful trials of the TOFD method for monitoring weld root condition of underwater pipe welds. Browne [1990a] described the application of TOFD to detection of corrosion, weld defects and chemically induced cracks in pipelines used to transport oil in the North Sea. Browne and Verkooijen [1991] proposed the wider use of TOFD for quality control during construction of pipelines for undersea use. Lilley and Osborne [1991] compared the use of TOFD with other ultrasonic and radiographic techniques for inspection of tubular components for the oil and gas industry and suggested that TOFD should become the standard technique.

Winchester [1989] described a remotely operated underwater inspection vehicle deploying a number of inspection techniques, including TOFD.

Wall, Haywood, Slesenger, Gunderson and Chilton [1990] reported a design study for a remotely operated vehicle for inspection of deep water tendons and risers with limited internal access. The intention was to use TOFD for accurate sizing after detection by other means.

AEA Sonomatic's application of TOFD to weld inspection was recently reviewed [Anon., 1996] and the Nautilus subsea manipulator described. This tool, which can apply TOFD as well as other inspection techniques, can be used for inspection of risers, caissons, closure welds, access windows, spiral welds, pipework and bends.

## 9.7 General weld inspection and plant monitoring

A novel application of the technique incorporates the use of lasers to generate and receive ultrasound [Scruby, Dewhurst, Hutchins and Palmer, 1981, 1982] to inspect hot steel billets for defects prior to rolling.

Browne [1990b] argues that the TOFD technique should not be confined only to very demanding NDT applications but can be deployed as a very effective and rapid means of defect detection, with meaningful reporting on very many weld inspection tasks at lower cost that is possible using more traditional methods.

Verkooijen [1995] reports that the use of the TOFD technique as an alternative to radiography during the construction of a refinery in Rotterdam has resulted in major cost savings and increased confidence in the end-product.

Takeuchi, Morimoto, Hamana, Taniguchi and Hiraga [1996] report techniques used for inspection of water pipes and constructional members in power stations and other plant. The TOFD technique has been adopted for increased accuracy.

## 9.8 Monitoring defect growth

Cecco and Broomfield [1984] measured the profiles of fatigue cracks in compact tension fracture specimens using the TOFD technique. Mudge [1980] describes the use of the technique for measurement of fatigue pre-crack depth in fracture toughness specimens. Sigmond and Lien [1980] used it to make in-situ measurement of fatigue crack growth in single notch bend specimens.

Silk, Hillier, Hammond and Jones [1986b] showed that TOFD was a suitable technique for monitoring defect growth in a hydrocracker reactor pressure vessel at British Petroleum's Grangemouth refinery. During plant shutdowns a cracked region of the reactor was monitored with four scans taken over the period 1982 to 1985. The precision with which defect growth can be monitored depends on the equipment used, the precision with which scans can be repeated from year to year, and the migration of growing cracks from one scan line to another with position and over time. This last restriction imposes a limit of about 0.7 mm on the absolute measurement of defect through-wall extent, but does not impair the performance as far as detecting changes in defect size. The estimated accuracies of 0.5 mm were believed to have been achieved and detectable crack growth was demonstrated.

As engineering practice turns more towards design based on likelihood of fracture failure, assessed from an understanding of fracture mechanics, and on the ability of NDT to estimate remaining ligaments and crack sizes, techniques such as Time-of-Flight Diffraction will become increasingly important.

If the precision of the technique can reach 0.1 mm or below, the monitoring of the early stages of fatigue crack growth will be possible. Such an increase in precision will also be beneficial in the inspection of thin materials or for the near-surface regions of thick components. This need has already led to developments in higher frequencies and compact-pulse transducers so as to improve timing accuracy. Work has been carried out on pulse compression [Silk, 1987].

Dawson, Clough and Silk [1989] developed an automated ultrasonic system to measure the rate of growth of thermal fatigue cracks in stainless steel cylinders of 6 mm wall thickness, using the TOFD technique.

Silk [1989a] and Silk, Whapham and Hobbs [1989] discuss ways of extending the life of components by accurate monitoring of the size of known flaws. They suggest that alternating current potential drop (ACPD) and TOFD can achieve the required accuracy of 0.25 mm.

Terpstra, Pasma and van Woerkom [1989] describe the use of TOFD to monitor weld defects in a vessel which had already been in operation for 25 years. Previously detected cracks were scanned regularly along two sections of weld, one of 700 mm length and 30 mm wall thickness, the other over 300 mm length in a wall thickness of 22 mm were scanned regularly to monitor previously detected cracks. As a result of the high sizing accuracy and reproducibility within 0.75 mm obtainable with TOFD, it could be demonstrated that the defects were stable and the vessel could remain in service. Even better repeatability might have been obtained if the crack had been less irregular in shape and with a more reliable way of ensuring that the probe placing was the same for successive scans.

In another study of flaw monitoring by Silk and Hobbs [1990], the depth of machined slots was increased in stages and inspections were carried out with a procedure which had been constructed to minimise errors in a monitoring situation. Two cases were studied. In the first the transducers were left fixed in place whilst the slots were extended. This demonstrated that notch extension could be measured to better than 0.1 mm. In the second test, however, the probes were deliberately removed and replaced at each stage. An RMS extension error of about 0.15 mm was found with a maximum error of 0.2 mm. Silk and Hobbs concluded that TOFD is a practical way of monitoring crack growth, provided care is taken to minimise other sources of error.

Bergmann and Bergner [1994] have developed a crack growth monitoring device based on the TOFD technique. It is especially suitable for application to small samples such as Charpy-type bend specimens, for use in fracture-mechanics testing.

## 9.9 Inspection of steel bridges

One particularly impressive application is to sizing of defects in steel bridges [Mudge and Duncumb, 1985]. Many of the steel bridges in existence have already seen a long service life and there is a widespread desire for more quantitative information about their integrity. Since the turn of the century welded components have been increasingly used and the stiffened plate or box section construction now common involves long lengths of weld.

The British Standard applicable to bridge inspection (BS 5400) now places greater reliance than it formerly did on the capabilities of non-destructive testing to detect and evaluate weld discontinuities from a structural integrity viewpoint. In the United States, the provisions of the American Welding Society Structural Welding Code AWS D1.1 are widely used to determine the acceptability of welds. However, Mudge and Duncumb showed that, using these ultrasonic procedures, which are basically pulse-echo amplitude measurements, a high proportion of cracks with a size equal to 7.5% of the wall thickness were very likely to be accepted and there was a 30% chance of accepting even larger flaws. These larger flaws, incorrectly judged acceptable, were all planar in nature. In comparison, on specimens representative of those found in major tension flanges on steel bridge structures, Mudge and Duncumb were able to achieve a mean accuracy of 0.2 mm with a standard deviation of 1.0 mm for the through-wall size of 21 planar defects in samples 10 to 95 mm thick with Time-of-Flight Diffraction sizing. The 20 dB drop technique applied to the same set of defects yielded a mean accuracy of only −4.8 mm with a standard deviation of 3.1 mm. Mudge and Duncumb concluded that *'The very small sizes of significant defects for higher fatigue classes in bridges preclude the use of probe movement ultrasonic sizing techniques to evaluate them. Simple amplitude comparison techniques have also been shown to be inadequate ... Time-of-Flight ultrasonic testing does have the potential to size small flaws ...* '

There has been one report [Anon., 1998b] of the deployment of TOFD for inspection of bridge components but it is disappointing that the work of Mudge and Duncumb has not been followed up more widely.

## 9.10 Other applications of TOFD

As a search and sizing tool, the technique is now used as a routine service by the National NDT Centre (AEA Technology), by the Welding Institute, by Atomic Energy of Canada at Chalk River, by operators offshore in the North Sea and elsewhere, and also in France [de Vadder and Dosso, 1984].

Rusbridge and Roberts [1982] reported on the ultrasonic examination of artificial defects in diffusion bonded steel samples using Time-of-Flight Diffraction to detect and size these very difficult defects satisfactorily.

Published Russian work has demonstrated the advantages of Time-of-Flight Diffraction, both for cracks and for assessing the depth of the case-hardening on mill rolls for cold rolling of steels [Vopilkin, 1985].

## 9.11 Future potential

In the first edition of this book, we speculated on future applications of TOFD. We foresaw an increased application to cracking in thin-wall tubing, to monitoring of defect growth and to inspection in high-operating-cost areas such the North Sea. The papers already cited in this chapter show that TOFD has made inroads into each of those areas. We also expected that it would be more extensively used for austenitic steel and other large-grained materials with 'difficult' ultrasonic properties. In this we were encouraged by an expectation of imminent advances in understanding of how to optimise ultrasonic inspection of these materials, particularly through such techniques as digital signal processing. We have to confess that we have not found any published evidence that major advances have occurred. Research effort into these materials was largely funded by the nuclear industry at that time and the absence of progress probably reflects the fact that nuclear power plant development has effectively ceased.

Given the probability that many applications have gone unrecorded outside the organisation which carried them out, the picture is encouraging and affirms that TOFD is now accepted as as standard ultrasonic technique. There is room for some concern about the position of NDT in general however, as a result of the increasing dominance of financial as opposed to technical expertise in the boardrooms of large engineering-based organisations.

A compelling example is provided by the recent disruption to travel in the United Kingdom caused by gauge-corner cracking in railway track [Coster, 2000]. After a fatal derailment on a curve at Hatfield, apparently caused by rail failure, an emergency programme of track inspection over the whole network revealed that gauge-corner cracking was widespread [Anon., 2001c]. Severe speed restrictions were applied during the time it took to replace about 450 miles of track. The track at the site of the accident was known to have been in poor condition for a considerable period and was due to be replaced the following month [Anon., 2000] but manual ultrasonic tests had failed to show the progressive deterioration in its condition. The manual ultrasonic technique applied had poor detection capability for cracks away from the centre of the rail, had not been corrected for the rail cant and had performed badly because of the poor condition of the rail surface [Anon., 2001a].

For some time prior to this accident, the Office of the Rail Regulator had been concerned about an apparent increase in the incidence of broken rails and, jointly with the Health and Safety Executive, had commissioned a report from Transportation Technology Center Inc. [Sawley and Rieff, 2000]. The report, published two weeks after the Hatfield accident, raised a number of concerns about the track maintenance policies of Railtrack, the network owner, but only those concerning non-destructive testing will be mentioned here.

For a long period up to 1995, track inspection had been carried out by the Ultrasonic Test Unit (UTU), a train fitted with ultrasonic and eddy-current inspection equipment, supplemented by manual ultrasonic inspection of areas where indications had been found. The UTU could operate at speeds up to 40 mph but detection of defects still relied on manual analysis of chart recorder output. Use of the UTU was abandoned in 1995, on the grounds that it produced too many false calls, and complete reliance was placed on manual inspection techniques reported in the press to have had poor detection capability [Anon., 2001a]. The UTU is now to be recommissioned and improved.

Railtrack is a large organisation which, given the nature of its business, might be expected to have an active research effort in NDT. There is little evidence, however, of any attempt to develop improved inspection methods, or even to keep up with the latest technology [Sawley and Rieff, 2000]. A more forward looking policy would have been to update the techniques and equipment of the UTU to solve the false call problem and allow more rapid and efficient deployment. If NDT techniques with good crack depth capability and good reproducibility had been employed, the rate of deterioration could have been monitored and faulty track replaced in a timely fashion. In that context new techniques like TOFD could have been considered for deployment. It is reported that research into gauge-corner cracking is to be greatly increased but it is not known whether this includes investigation of improved NDT techniques [Anon., 2001b].

The rail inspection problem is comparable in economic importance with the PWR inspection problem which was such a spur to the development of the TOFD technique. It is to be hoped that similar resources will be made available to bring about a radical improvement in rail inspection.

# Chapter 10

# Application of Codes and Standards to TOFD Inspection

The aim of any ultrasonic inspection must be to determine whether the inspected component is fit for its purpose. A component that is fit for its purpose will be one which has a very high probability of continuing to perform its function for its designed life, i.e. a very low probability of failure in service. However, the precise probability required will depend on the consequences of failure. Clearly, if the failure of a component could lead to many deaths, it must be many orders of magnitude less likely to fail than one which would merely cause a short maintenance outage.

The ultrasonic inspection is designed to detect, size and possibly characterise defects in the component. The next stage of assessment is to classify those defects as acceptable or unacceptable. Whether a defect is acceptable or not depends on the component in which it is found and the stresses to which it will be subjected. Defects which are sufficient to cause the component to fail under applied loads which might occur in practice will be classed as unacceptable. In order to ensure that the assessment process is properly carried out, procedures are laid down in codes and standards.

## 10.1 Types of standard

The terms code and standard are often used somewhat loosely as if they were interchangeable. We should like to restrict the term *code* to a definition of the types and sizes of defects which are acceptable or rejectable in specified components in specified service. The term *standard* would describe a definition of how components should be inspected in order to verify code compliance. However, many documents do not fall clearly into either of these categories, since they attempt to specify acceptable inspection results rather than acceptable defects.

Most modern codes, and certainly those for safety critical components, base acceptance criteria on a fracture mechanics approach to failure of the component under a variety of normal and abnormal loads. There are other types of code which try to assess the quality of the fabrication process, according to 'good workmanship' criteria. These codes typically restrict the numbers of defects of particular size ranges which are allowed in a structure, or a weld. Obviously, large defects should be equally unacceptable in these codes as they are in those based on fracture mechanics. However, it is common for the good workmanship criteria to take account of defects that would be too small to be of structural concern simply because they are being used as a quality control measure. Codes based on good workmanship criteria are often called acceptance standards.

If codes are written in terms of the number, size, position and nature of defects, they do not, in principle, impose any restriction on the method by which the information was obtained and can be applied to a new technique without difficulty. Unfortunately, many existing codes have been written with a particular inspection technique in mind and are couched in terms of the response of the inspection instrument, such as signal levels, rather than defect sizes. This approach has the laudable aim of eliminating errors and subjectivity in translating instrument responses to defect sizes but can be criticised on two grounds. First, it can give an unjustified impression that a single instrument response, such as a signal amplitude, is always a totally reliable indicator of defect significance, and secondly, it can hamper the introduction of new techniques because the existing codes will not be directly applicable.

## 10.2 Development of standards for TOFD

Browne [1997a,b] makes the point that the majority of standards in use today were created decades ago when ultrasonic testing techniques were different. This has undoubtedly handicapped the acceptance of TOFD which is still sparsely represented in codes and standards. The American Petroleum Institute is reviewing it. The German DIN organisation accepts it by default for inspection of nuclear reactor pressure vessels. TOFD has now been demonstrated, on a thick section (350 mm) qualification block, to meet the requirements of ASME Code Case 2235, *Use of ultrasonic examination in lieu of radiography, Section VIII, Divisions 1 and* 2 which became effective in 1996 [Anon., 1999]. The British Ministry of Defence (Navy) has accepted TOFD as a prescribed method of weld inspection in critical components, covering detection, sizing and characterisation. The effective cost of slow uptake of an improved inspection technique could be very high in terms of lost production and unnecessary repair.

There is little point in pressing for British and European standards for use of TOFD in control of fabrication quality, if major fabrication codes effectively exclude its use [Browne, 1997b]. However, in-service inspection codes are more often specified in terms of defect sizes and here there is more scope for TOFD. Acceptance criteria are the subject of a recent paper by Dijkstra, de Raad and Bourna [1997]. The authors observe that the current good workmanship criteria embodied in most NDT standards measure the performance of the welder rather than evaluating weld integrity and argue that existing acceptance criteria are limited to this because this is the best that can be done. If it were possible to balance testing the welder's performance against a fracture mechanics assessment, without introducing undue conservatism, this would be more nearly ideal. It could be achieved by combining modified acceptance criteria with a more informative NDT technique, one which is capable of detecting small defects and measuring the through-wall size of planar defects.

In the TOFD technique, the amplitude of the signal does not bear any direct relationship to the defect through-wall size. Most of the current standards are, therefore, to a greater or less extent, inappropriate, because they are based on amplitude-based techniques which were the only sort available at the time of their inception. We can ask, however, whether the sizing capability of TOFD satisfies the requirements of existing codes. Silk [1989b] has discussed this in detail, as we summarise below.

Engineers use codes as a way of assessing defects. The American Society of Mechanical Engineers (ASME) produces codes for designing and testing many components, especially pressure components. This work arose originally in the 19th century from an effort to reduce the large number of deaths then occurring from steam boiler explosions. ASME, like other engineering bodies, produces codes concerned with assessing whether defects found in structures can be tolerated by the structure with the expected loads. In particular, ASME XI rules provide a comprehensive set of criteria for the most serious, planar, defects in nuclear reactor pressure vessels. These rules or other similar ones will be adopted increasingly in different industrial sectors as ultrasonic inspection becomes tied more closely to insurance and asset life management of all manner of structures. ASME XI Appendix 8, which applies to pressure vessels and piping, allows the use of any inspection technique which can meet the specified performance requirements and so is no barrier to the adoption of TOFD.

Silk [1989b] examined ASME XI and similar rules from other industries to determine the implications of these for the TOFD technique in non-nuclear applications. The rules in question are those for defect significance and not those for defect detection which are inappropriate for TOFD because they are couched in terms of pulse-echo amplitudes. The ASME XI defect significance rules may be too stringent when applied to structures other than the nuclear reactor pressure vessel for several reasons. The material used may well be different, with different strengths and fracture properties; the inspection intervals will be different; or single failures may be less important.

Silk found that TOFD applied in its simplest form (a single probe pair at fixed separation) and with the precision available in 1989, would easily meet all the requirements of ASME XI, provided the defects of concern were not in the top 30% of the full material thickness and were in steel specimens at least 12 mm thick. One can deduce from this that, with an appropriate set of probe separations, the requirements could be met for all defects more than 5 mm from the inspection surface. Nor is 5 mm the absolute lower limit as much of the previous material in this book should show. It is true, however, that *detecting* very shallow defects in a large workpiece might be more rapidly and efficiently carried out with a combination of techniques, because a TOFD probe pair of small separation has a small volume coverage from any given position.

Having determined that TOFD sizing satisfies existing code requirements, we can ask how reliable is it when used to both detect and size defects. Much of this book is devoted to just this topic. Here we draw on some recent work which may eventually lead to a revolution in international codes and standards.

A good inspection technique will detect defects with a high degree of probability. The *probability of detection* (POD) should be close to 1 and the closer the better. For all techniques there will be some parameters which need to be set, such as amplifier gain, frequency etc., and the POD will be to some extent dependent on those settings. A parameter value chosen to give the largest POD may, however, lead to the observance of signals which look as if they arise from defects but are actually spurious, arising from noise, grain boundaries, reflections from small harmless inclusions, or other extraneous features. This leads to a finite probability of falsely reporting a significant defect, i.e. the *false call rate* (FCR) will be greater than 0. To optimise the technique, we need a measure of reliability which takes both POD and FCR into account. The product POD$\times$(1-FCR) is a convenient measure of reliability, since it is equal to 1 when all defects are found and there are no false calls and falls below 1 when either defects are missed or false defects are reported.

In a project by the Netherlands Institute of Welding, the reliability of TOFD was compared with radiography on steel sections between 6 mm and 15 mm thick. TOFD was found to be about 25% more reliable than X-radiography and 45% more reliable than conventional manual ultrasonic inspection [Verkooijen, 1995]. The results from this test have already been referred to in an earlier chapter (Section 8.7 and Figure 8.14). As a result of this trial, AEA Sonomatic used TOFD on a large scale as an alternative to radiography during the construction of a refinery in the Rotterdam area. The result was a major cost saving and increased confidence in the end-product.

Following this success, a project was launched in the Netherlands to formalise inclusion of TOFD in acceptance standards for welds in their Rules for Pressurised Equipment (RTOD) and in European Standards. Dijkstra et al. [1997] refer to this project, *The development of acceptance criteria for the TOFD Inspection Method*, carried out by the Netherlands Society for Non-Destructive Testing and Inspection Techniques (KINT), coordinated by the Project Bureau of the Netherlands Institute of Welding. Zeelenberg [1998] has also contributed to the development of acceptance standards for TOFD applicable in the Netherlands.

The advantage of using TOFD and pulse-echo inspections together to achieve a high probability of defect detection with a low false call rate, can be seen from Figure 8.14. Since this work was carried out there have been moves towards using combined TOFD and pulse-echo ultrasonic inspections to replace radiography in pipeline construction. AEA Technology has carried out work for Allseas in Brazil in which this combination was used for pipeline construction with much reduced inspection costs [Anon., 1998a].

# 10.3 Current standards specific to TOFD

## 10.3.1 British Standard BS7706:1993

In this standard [British Standards Institution, 1993], the simple theory of the TOFD technique is described, followed by criteria for the choice of ultrasonic probes and the setting-up procedure to be applied. Discussion of the errors that can occur and their typical effect on accuracy is included. The standard is at pains to point out that, since the technique does not rely on a direct correlation between defect size and the amplitude of the signal received, artificial reflectors should be used only for: verifying the angular distribution of energy within a specimen; as a means of reproducing inspection sensitivities; or to demonstrate inspection resolution. Advice is given on gain settings to be used with electric-discharge-machined slits or side-drilled holes. The standard also considers the interpretation of the signals obtained. Five categories of flaws are recognised, of which four are distinct:

- Planar flaws such as cracks, lack of fusion;
- Volumetric flaws such as lack of penetration, larger slag lines;
- Thread-like flaws, those with significant length but small (less than about 3 mm) through-wall extent;
- Point flaws such as pores, small pieces of slag;
- Uncategorised flaws

The reasons for possible false indications of the various types of flaws are discussed together with some of the special techniques included in this book. The document in cludes several annexes, dealing with reporting of results, characterisation of defects, examples of typical D-scans and recommendations for operator training.

## 10.3.2 European Standard ENV 583-6

The European Committee for Standardisation (CEN) oversees the creating of standards applicable in the member nations. CEN has representation from the national standards bodies of Austria, Belgium, Denmark, Finland, France, Germany, Greece, Iceland, Ireland, Italy, Luxembourg, Netherlands, Norway, Portugal, Spain, Sweden, Switzerland and the United Kingdom.

CEN Standard EN 583 is entitled *Non-destructive testing. Ultrasonic examination.* It consists of six parts, the first five of which, EN 583-1 to EN 583-5, deal with conventional ultrasonic techniques. The draft sixth part, ENV 583-6 is entitled *Time-of-Flight Diffraction technique as a method for defect detection and sizing.* This draft standard, [European Committee for Standardisation, 1996] was put to a formal vote in January, 1997. It was accepted by several countries in Europe but not by the UK, since a number of comments were submitted which the UK authorities will want to take into account in implementing the standard. At the time of writing,

**Table 10.1** CEN recommendations for choice of compression-wave probe in steel plate up to 70mm thick [European Committee for Standardisation, 1996].

| Wall thickness (mm) | Centre frequency (MHz) | Crystal size (mm) | Nominal probe angle |
|---|---|---|---|
| <10 | 10 – 15 | 2 – 6 | 50°– 70° |
| 30 – < 70 | 2 – 5 | 6 – 12 | 45°– 60° |

**Table 10.2** CEN recommendations for choice of compression-wave probe in steel plate from 70 to 300mm thick [European Committee for Standardisation, 1996].

| Depth region from insspection surface (mm) | Centre frequency (MHz) | Crystal size (mm) | Nominal probe angle |
|---|---|---|---|
| 0 – 30 | 5 – 10 | 2 – 6 | 50°– 70° |
| 30 – 100 | 2 – 5 | 6 – 12 | 45°– 60° |
| 100 – 300 | 1 – 3 | 10 – 25 | 45°– 60° |

some NDT practitioners in other European countries are known to have reservations about this standard.

ENV 583-6 covers: the principles of the technique; the qualification of the operating personnel (to EN 473 Qualification and Certification of NDT Personnel — General Principles); the choice of ultrasonic probe diameter, frequency and angle, as function of defect depth, as shown in Tables 10.1 and 10.2; and a discussion of precision and resolution in line with the discussions in this book.

## 10.4 Inspection qualification

For any NDT technique to be reliable, it is necessary for the technique to have been designed with the defects of concern in mind; to be then applied according to a tried and tested procedure by competent operators or by tested automatic systems. This process of design, documentation and testing is known as inspection qualification, although the term *performance demonstration* was used in the U.S.A., when the process was first introduced. Inspection qualification has recently been reviewed by Waites and Whittle [1998]. The aim of this process is to justify that the ultrasonic inspection technique will meet the requirements of fracture mechanics when applied in the industrial context. Waites and Whittle make the point that such proof is required in two cases: for safety critical components in any industry; and when a technique is sufficiently new that experience may be limited in the industry and codes and standards may not yet exist. There are five component parts to the performance demonstration and evaluation:

- Certification of personnel to agreed standards.
- Written procedures for the inspection, be it manual or automated.
- Theoretical justification of the technique, including calculations and modelling to demonstrate capability.
- Test-block trials employing defects of the type which, if found in the industrial context would be of concern. This includes service induced defects as well as fabrication flaws. Often this will require some way of comparing the actual defect with that reported and this may mean destructive final examination of test blocks.
- Audit of an inspection company's results, possibly repeating 5 – 10% of the measurements in the field.

In the USA, mandatory appendices were added to the 1989 ASME XI code [ASME, 1989], which underpins ultrasonic inspection of pressure vessels. These mandatory appendices specify how a performance demonstration and evaluation should be carried out. Waites and Whittle observed that this approach, and some of the underlying statistical assumptions, run counter to European methods. In response to this, the utilities operating nuclear power plant have set up the European Network for Inspection Qualification (ENIQ). The Joint Research Centre of Petten is the Operating Agent and the Reference Laboratory of the Network.

ENIQ has developed a framework and principles for performance demonstration [European Network for Inspection Qualification, 1997]. The principles are:

- Qualification is obtained by a mixture of practical trials and theoretical justification.
- Procedures and equipment can be qualified using open trials in which those applying the procedure have knowledge of the defects in the test pieces;
- Any specific test pieces used to test personnel should be done blind, that is, the personnel should have no knowledge of the defects except information that would be available before a normal on-site inspection.

There is more to qualification than success in a blind trial. Another important part is a written technical justification. This is a document pulling together all previous results of capability and evaluation exercises; making use of experience gained from on-site inspections; and putting forward results from applicable and validated theoretical models and other physics-based reasoning. Because full-scale test pieces with realistic defects are very expensive, providing a sufficient number of defects to establish acceptable confidence levels in this form is not economically viable. Defects in small test block can be provided much more cheaply. Physical reasoning and theoretical understanding may be used to extrapolate from these small test blocks to the full-scale situation and a relatively small number of full-scale tests can then be used to establish confidence in these extrapolations.

## 10.5 Qualification of TOFD

Time-of-Flight Diffraction was the only technique to qualify in one such qualification test for steam generator feed-water nozzle inspection run by the Electric Power Research Institute (EPRI) in the USA [Daniels et al., 1996]. This in-service inspection was designed for use on PWR steam generator feedwater nozzles but would be generally applicable to any heavy section nozzle inspection.

The inspection was carried out from the outside surface. Inspection of pressure-vessel nozzles is technically more satisfactory from the internal surface but that requires removal of the vessel cap and dismantling of some internal equipment, so the expense can only be justified at a time when such dismantling is required for other reasons. Inspection from the outside surface requires only removal of external insulation.

The system developed includes:

- an ASME compatible inspection procedure, specifying computer designed scanning for optimum performance;
- a versatile, semi-automated scanner;
- MicroPlus as the automated data collection system;
- personal computer based inspection modelling and data analysis software developed by AEA Technology and called MUSE (see Figure 6.12).

This system was designed to be sensitive to defects, on the inner surface of the nozzle, of 1.27 mm through-thickness extent or more. These defects can be located anywhere from the safe end weld on the pipe side of the nozzle to the vessel side of the nozzle blend. Defect misorientations of up to $\pm 10^\circ$ were allowed for in the design. The defects were detected by the pulse-echo technique and then sized by Time-of-Flight Diffraction.

Trials carried out during development demonstrated 100% detection capability and an RMS sizing error of 1.02 mm. In the qualification trial at EPRI, Charlotte, North Carolina, the system performance achieved was 100% detection and a sizing error of only 0.76 mm RMS.

## 10.6 Coda

This book has described at length each of the pieces of the framework for establishment of TOFD as a fully proven NDT technique. Since its invention nearly 30 years ago, the technique has consistently demonstrated its capability and versatility, and more than anything else, its accuracy for measurement of the dimension usually most relevant to component failure. The range of applications has increased steadily and as the new millennium begins, it is poised to make a continuing contribution to the safety of all manner of structures and to the economic benefits which can accrue from appropriate ultrasonic inspection.

# Appendix

## A.1 Helmholtz potentials

Any vector representing a physical quantity, such as the particle displacement $\vec{u}$, can be split into two parts

$$\vec{u} = \nabla\phi + \nabla \times \vec{\psi} \tag{A.1}$$

where $\phi$ and $\vec{\psi}$ are *potentials*. Since there are four quantities in $\phi$ and $\vec{\psi}$ and only three in $\vec{u}$, we have some freedom in choosing $\vec{\psi}$; this is called a choice of gauge and the most useful choice is

$$\nabla \cdot \vec{\psi} = 0 \tag{A.2}$$

The potentials $\phi$ and $\vec{\psi}$ are called *Helmholtz* potentials and are often easier to work with than the displacement $\vec{u}$. The potentials $\phi$ and $\vec{\psi}$ satisfy *wave equations*

$$\nabla^2\phi - \frac{1}{C_p^2}\frac{\partial^2\phi}{\partial t^2} \tag{A.3}$$

$$\nabla^2\vec{\psi} = \frac{1}{C_s^2}\frac{\partial^2\vec{\psi}}{\partial t^2} \tag{A.4}$$

where $t$ is the time and $C_p$ and $C_s$ are the speeds of the compression and shear waves respectively.

## A.2 Other wave motions in isotropic media

The Rayleigh wave propagates along the surface at a speed which is distinct from the speed of the waves in the body of the material. This speed, denoted by $C_r$, is given by the solution of the equation [Graff, 1975]

$$x^3 - 8x^2 + \left(24 - 16\frac{C_s^2}{C_p^2}\right)x - 16\left(1 - \frac{C_s^2}{C_p^2}\right) = 0 \tag{A.5}$$

where $x = \left(\frac{C_r}{C_s}\right)^2$, or approximately by the result [Achenbach, 1973]

$$C_r = \frac{C_s\,(0.862 + 1.14\,\nu)}{1+\nu} \quad \text{where } \nu \text{ is Poisson's ratio} \tag{A.6}$$

which gives a value of $C_r \sim 0.92C_s$ in steel.

## A.3 Geometrical theory of diffraction

The central idea of this theory is that a field quantity $u$ travels along rays. The ray paths are determined by an extension of Fermat's Principle as follows: a ray connecting two points and singly diffracted from a vertex $V$ is a curve the length of which is stationary among all curves connecting these two points and passing through $V$ [Keller, 1957]. In the case of an elastic wave, the field quantity $u$ could be an elastic displacement, or its potential. $u$ has an amplitude $A\,(s)$ at some distance $s$ along the ray and a phase $k\Psi\,(s)$, so that

$$u = A\,(s)\,e^{ik\Psi(s)} \tag{A.7}$$

The amplitude $A$ is a vector or a scalar and is not restricted to being real. The difference in phase between two points on a ray is assumed to be equal to $k$ times the distance between them, so that

$$\Psi\,(s) = \Psi_0 + s \tag{A.8}$$

The amplitude variation along the ray can be obtained in a simple way from the assumption of conservation of energy and can be formally derived, at least for the leading term, in an expansion of powers of $(ka)^{-1}$, without this assumption [Karal and Keller, 1959]. The flux of energy is taken to be the same at every cross-section of a narrow tube of rays, so that the quantity $A^2 d\sigma/C$ is conserved, where $d\sigma$ is the cross-sectional area of the tube and $C$ is the speed of propagation. Consideration of two cross sections along a narrow tube yields

$$\frac{A^2 d\sigma}{C} = \frac{A_0^2\,d\sigma_0}{C} \tag{A.9}$$

Hence, $A = A_0\,(d\sigma_0/d\sigma)^{\frac{1}{2}}$. If $\rho_1$ and $\rho_2$ are the principle radii of curvature of the wavefront normal to the ray at point $P_0$, then the radii at $P$, a distance $s$ along the ray, are $\rho_1 + s$ and $\rho_2 + s$, giving [Keller, 1957]

$$\frac{d\sigma_0}{d\sigma} = \frac{\rho_1\rho_2}{(\rho_1 + s)\,(\rho_2 + s)} \tag{A.10}$$

and hence

$$A = A_0\left[\frac{\rho_1\rho_2}{(\rho_1 + s)\,(\rho_2 + s)}\right]^{\frac{1}{2}} \tag{A.11}$$

and finally that

$$u = A_0 \left[ \frac{\rho_1 \rho_2}{(\rho_1 + s)(\rho_2 + s)} \right]^{\frac{1}{2}} e^{ik(s+\Psi_0)} \tag{A.12}$$

with the interesting consequence that, for large distances $s$, the amplitude of the field decreases as $s^{-1}$, as in a spherical wave. This is true provided both $\rho_1$ and $\rho_2$ are finite. If one radius of curvature is infinite, the field falls off as $\sqrt{s}$, as in a cylindrical wave. When both radii of curvature are infinite, the amplitude does not decrease with distance and is like a plane wave.

When the ray is diffracted somewhere along its path, the amplitude is further modified and this is taken into account by including a diffraction coefficient $D$ in the equation for the amplitude. Since the diffraction effect is localised in the region of the discontinuity, $D$ can depend only on the local conditions, such as: the angles which the incident and diffracted rays make with some direction characteristic of the local cause of diffraction, such as the edge of a planar crack; the nature of the incident wave field; and the frequency of the excitation. Solutions to canonical problems can be used to determine these diffraction coefficients. The canonical problem for smooth planar cracks is diffraction by a semi-infinite plane. Results for this problem are given in Section A.4.

### A.3.1 Diffraction by curved edges

In Equation A.12, the amplitude along a ray is given in terms of the amplitude at some reference point on the ray. It is convenient to choose the reference point to be on the crack edge, which is itself a caustic of the diffracted rays. This implies that one of the two principal radii of curvature of the wavefront, $\rho_1$ or $\rho_2$, vanishes. Denoting the remaining radius of curvature by $\rho$, the amplitude becomes [Keller, 1957]

$$u = A_0 \left[ \frac{\rho \lambda_i}{(\rho + s) s} \right]^{\frac{1}{2}} e^{ik_i(s+\Psi_0)} \tag{A.13}$$

where $\lambda_i$ and $k_i$ represents the wavelength and wavevector of the diffracted wave (compression or shear) and the factor $\lambda_i^{\frac{1}{2}}$ renders the constant $A_0$ dimensionless [Chapman and Coffey, 1982]. The radius of curvature $\rho$ is now the distance from the edge to the remaining caustic of diffraction and is given by [Keller, 1957]

$$\rho = \frac{-\eta \sin^2 \beta}{\eta \frac{d\beta}{ds} + \cos \delta} \tag{A.14}$$

where $\beta(s)$ is the cone of diffracted rays, given in terms of the arc length $s$ along the edge, $\delta$ is the angle between the diffracted ray and the normal to the edge and $\eta$ is the radius of curvature of the diffracting edge.

For a scan which passes directly over the centre of an elliptical crack, and where the normal to the crack surface lies in the vertical plane containing the scan line (that is, for a crack which is not skewed), the radius of curvature of the edge is

$$\eta = \frac{E_b^2}{E_a} \tag{A.15}$$

where $E_a$ and $E_b$ are the semi-axes of the ellipse, with $E_a$ in the through-wall direction. In this geometry, the distance $\rho$ to the caustic is given by [Chapman and Coffey, 1982]

$$\frac{1}{\rho} = \frac{1}{r_1} - \frac{1}{\eta}(\cos\beta + \cos\theta) \tag{A.16}$$

where $r_1$ is the distance from the point of diffraction to the centre of the transmitter. The angles $\beta$ and $\theta$ are, respectively, the angles of the incident and diffracted rays, measured anticlockwise from the face of the crack.

### A.3.2 Incident potential

In the far field of the transmitter, the incident potential on the beam axis is

$$\psi_{inc} = \frac{A_{\text{probe}}}{\lambda_i r_1} e^{ik_i r_1} \tag{A.17}$$

where $A_{\text{probe}}$ is the area of the probe, and $k_i$ and $\lambda_i$ denote the compression or shear wavevector and wavelength respectively, depending on the type of probe. If the diffraction point is not on the beam axis, this amplitude is modified by the transducer beam profile. The transducer beam profile used is given by the familiar Bessel function form

$$2J_1(x)/x \tag{A.18}$$

where

$$x = \frac{2\pi f a \sin\Omega}{C_\alpha} \tag{A.19}$$

Here $f$ is the frequency, $a$ the radius of the assumed piston source, $C_\alpha$ the speed of the elastic wave, with $\alpha$ denoting either compression or shear waves, and $\Omega$ the angle relative to the beam centreline. With this model, which behaves well in the far field of the probe, there are sidelobes associated with the Bessel function. The points of diffraction may not be on the central maximum of the amplitude functions of either transmitter or receiver, so the angles away from the beam maximum, denoted $\Omega_1$ and $\Omega_2$ (see Figure A.1), are defined respectively as

$$\Omega_1 = \left| \arctan\left\{ \frac{X_t}{h - Y_t} - \theta \right\} \right| \tag{A.20}$$

where $\theta$ is the beam angle, $h$ is the plate thickness and the coordinates of the defect top are $X_t$, $Y_t$, measured from the bottom of the plate (as in Figure 3.3). For Time-of-Flight Diffraction with the receiver separated from the transmitter by a distance of $X_{TR}$, or for pulse-echo inspections of cracks, the extremity of the crack might not lie on the beam axis of the receiver. The angle $\Omega_2$ is given by

$$\Omega_2 = \left| \arctan \left\{ \frac{X_{TR} - X_t}{h - Y_t} - \theta \right\} \right| \tag{A.21}$$

The amplitude which arrives at the receiver is then also subject to the directional sensitivity of the receiving transducer which is taken to be the same as that for the transmitting transducer. Including the geometry of the curved crack edge, the final expression for the signal diffracted from the crack is given by [Chapman and Coffey, 1982]

$$\psi_{rec} = \tag{A.22}$$

$$\left[ \frac{4A_{probe}^2 J_1(x_1) J_1(x_2)}{\lambda_s^2 r_1 x_1 r_2 x_2} e^{ik_s(r_1+r_2)} \right] D(\theta,\beta) \left[ \frac{\lambda_s^3 \eta r_1 r_2}{\eta(r_1+r_2) - r_1 r_2 (\cos\beta + \cos\theta)} \right]^{\frac{1}{2}}$$

and $x_1$ and $x_2$ are given by Equation A.19 above.

### A.3.3 Calibration reflector

For Time-of-Flight geometries, and for the calculations used here, the signals are measured relative to those from a flat-bottomed hole situated symmetrically between the transmitter and the receiver, with the flat surface of the reflector horizontal so that the maximum signal is transferred by the calibration reflector to the receiver [Temple, 1984a]. To complete our description of the model used, we outline how the amplitude from the calibration reflector is calculated. The ratio of scattered to incident potentials is given by

$$\frac{\psi_{scat}}{\psi_{inc}} = -iRA_{\text{cal}} \cos\beta \frac{e^{ikr}}{r} \tag{A.23}$$

where $\beta$ is here the angle of incidence on the calibration reflector, measured from the normal, and $R$ is a reflection coefficient for plane waves. The calibration reflector is at range $r$ from the transmitter and is of area $A_{\text{cal}}$. For compression waves, as normally used in Time-of-Flight Diffraction, the reflection coefficient $R$ is given by [Graff, 1975]

$$R = \frac{\sin 2\beta \sin 2\theta_s - q^2 \cos^2 2\theta_s}{\sin 2\beta \sin 2\theta_s + q^2 \cos^2 2\theta_s} \tag{A.24}$$

where $q = C_p/C_s$, $C_p$ and $C_s$ being the speeds of compression and shear waves respectively, and $\theta_s$ is given by Snell's Law as

$$\theta_s = \arcsin \left[ \frac{C_s}{C_p} \sin\beta \right] \tag{A.25}$$

For shear waves at oblique incidence on the flat-bottomed hole, the reflection coefficient R would be [Graff, 1975]

$$R = \frac{\sin 2\beta \sin 2\theta_p - q^2 \cos^2 2\beta}{\sin 2\beta \sin 2\theta_p + q^2 \cos^2 2\beta} \tag{A.26}$$

where $\theta_p$ is given by

$$\theta_p = \arcsin\left[\frac{C_p}{C_s}\sin\beta\right] \tag{A.27}$$

provided $\theta_p$ is real; otherwise $R = 1$ for shear waves at angles of incidence greater than the critical angle, i.e. at angles greater than about 33° in steel.

The potential diffracted by the crack, given by Equation A.22, is then divided by the potential defined by Equation A.23 for the flat-bottomed hole and this ratio is converted to the decibel scale to give a result quoted in dB.

To convert the signal amplitudes from those relative to a flat-bottomed hole calibration reflector to those measured relative to a side-drilled hole reflector, we use the relationship that the signal strengths differ by a factor of [Bowker et al., 1985]

$$20\log_{10}\left[\frac{2\pi a_{\text{fbh}}^2}{\lambda\sqrt{r a_{\text{sdh}}}}\right] \tag{A.28}$$

where $a_{\text{fbh}}$ and $a_{\text{sdh}}$ are the radii of the flat-bottomed and side-drilled holes, respectively, both at range $r$ from the transmitter. The wavelength of the ultrasound is $\lambda$. The above expression gives a value which is added to the signal levels relative to a flat-bottomed hole in order to give signal levels relative to those from a side-drilled hole. Note that as $\sqrt{r}$ is greater than $a_{\text{fbh}}$ or $a_{\text{sdh}}$, the correction is actually negative, so that the signals measured relative to a side-drilled hole are smaller than those measured relative to a flat-bottomed hole. Typical values of this difference in these calculations are about 10 dB. Results are given in Temple [1987] for signal amplitudes from some typical defects taken from the PISC II parametric studies [see Oliver, 1984, for the background to PISC II].

## A.4 Diffraction of plane elastic waves by straight crack edges of infinite extent

The results of the mathematical analysis of diffraction of elastic waves are important for the successful implementation of Time-of-Flight Diffraction and are briefly stated here. These results were first produced by Maue [1953] and were developed by Coffey and Chapman [1983] as the basis of a model of pulse-echo and tandem inspection of misoriented smooth flat cracks. The theoretical approaches of Maue and Coffey and Chapman were compared and reported by Ogilvy and Temple [1983] who also derived results appropriate to the development of the Time-of-Flight Diffraction technique.

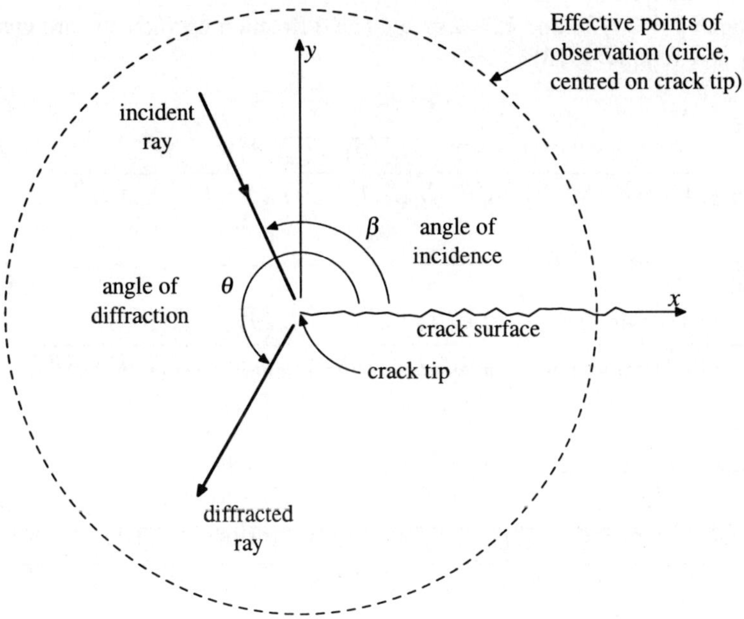


**Fig. A.1** Definition of angles used in describing diffraction by a straight crack edge of infinite extent.

Consider Figure A.1, in which the diffraction geometry is defined for a buried crack. For a plane wave incident at angle $\beta$ and an observer located at an angle $\theta$, the Helmholtz potentials of the diffracted field, denoted by $\phi_d$ and $\psi_d$, are given by

$$\begin{pmatrix} \phi_d \\ \psi_d \end{pmatrix} = \begin{pmatrix} F_{p,p} & G_{p,s} \\ G_{s,p} & F_{s,s} \end{pmatrix} \begin{pmatrix} \phi_i \\ \psi_i \end{pmatrix} \tag{A.29}$$

where $\phi_i$, $\psi_i$ are the incident Helmholtz potentials and the $F_{d,i}$ and $G_{d,i}$ are the scattering amplitudes, or diffraction coefficients, from and incident wave of type $i$ to a diffracted wave of type $d$. The diffracted potentials propagate away from the scatterer according to

$$\phi_d \rightarrow \phi_d \left( \frac{\lambda_p}{r} \right) e^{ik_p r} \tag{A.30}$$

and

$$\psi_d \rightarrow \psi_d \left( \frac{\lambda_s}{r} \right) e^{ik_s r} \tag{A.31}$$

where $r$ is the distance from the crack edge and $\lambda_p$, $\lambda_s$ are the wavelengths of the compression and shear waves and are related to their respective wave vectors $k_p$,

$k_s$ through $k_p = 2\pi/\lambda_p$ and $k_s = 2\pi/\lambda_s$. The diffraction coefficients are given by [Ogilvy and Temple, 1983]

$$F_{s,s} = e^{i\pi/4} \times \tag{A.32}$$
$$\frac{k_s^3 \sin\beta/2\left(k_s S + T\sqrt{Q_{ps}(\theta)}\sqrt{Q_{ps}(\beta)}\right)}{2\pi\left(k_s^2 - k_p^2\right)(\cos\theta + \cos\beta)\, Q_{rs}(\theta)\, Q_{rs}(\beta)\, K^{+}(-k_s\cos\theta)\, K^{+}(-k_s\cos\beta)}$$

$$F_{p,p} = e^{i\pi/4} \times \tag{A.33}$$
$$\frac{\sin\beta/2\left(\sin(\theta/2)\, R(\theta)\, R(\beta) + k_p^3 T\sqrt{Q_{sp}(\theta)}\sqrt{Q_{sp}(\beta)}\right)}{2\pi\left(k_s^2 - k_p^2\right)(\cos\theta + \cos\beta)\, Q_{rp}(\theta)\, Q_{rp}(\beta)\, K^{+}(-k_p\cos\theta)\, K^{+}(-k_p\cos\beta)}$$

$$G_{p,s} = e^{i\pi/4}\sqrt{\frac{k_s}{k_p}} \times \tag{A.34}$$
$$\frac{k_s^2 \sin\beta/2\left(-k_p^2\sqrt{2k_s}\, U\sqrt{Q_{sp}(\theta)} + 2\sqrt{2k_p}\, V\, R(\theta)\sqrt{Q_{ps}(\beta)}\right)}{4\pi\left(k_s^2 - k_p^2\right)(k_p\cos\theta + k_s\cos\beta)\, Q_{rp}(\theta)\, Q_{rs}(\beta)\, K^{+}(-k_p\cos\theta)\, K^{+}(-k_s\cos\beta)}$$

$$G_{s,p} = e^{i\pi/4}\sqrt{\frac{k_p}{k_s}} \times \tag{A.35}$$
$$\frac{k_s^2 \sin\beta/2\left(\sqrt{2k_p}\, R(\beta)\sin 2\theta\sqrt{Q_{ps}(\theta)} - 2k_p^2\sqrt{2k_s}\, T\sqrt{Q_{sp}(\beta)}\right)}{4\pi\left(k_s^2 - k_p^2\right)(k_p\cos\theta + k_s\cos\beta)\, Q_{rp}(\theta)\, Q_{rs}(\beta)\, K^{+}(-k_p\cos\theta)\, K^{+}(-k_s\cos\beta)}$$

where $k_r$ is the wavevector of Rayleigh waves in the medium at the frequency of interest. The function $K^{\pm}$ is given by the expression

$$K^{\pm}(\alpha) = \exp\left\{\frac{-1}{\pi}\int_{k_p}^{k_s} \arctan\left[\frac{4x^2\sqrt{(x^2 - k_p^2)}\sqrt{(k_s^2 - x^2)}}{(2x^2 - k_s^2)^2}\right]\frac{dx}{x \pm \alpha}\right\} \tag{A.36}$$

The other functions used are $Q_{xy}(\alpha) = k_x - k_y\cos\alpha$ and $R(\alpha) = 2k_p^2\cos^2\alpha - k_s^2$ and the substitutions $S = \cos 2\beta\cos 2\theta\sin\theta/2$, $T = 2\cos\beta/2\cos\beta\sin 2\theta$, $U = \cos 2\beta\sin 2\theta$ and $V = 2\cos\beta/2\cos\beta\sin\theta/2$ have been made.

Equations A.32 – A.35 tell us the phase of the diffracted signal as well as its amplitude. For all the equations, there is an $\exp(i\pi/4)$ factor which is typical of diffraction problems. Then there are the complicated angular factors. For the usual TOFD configuration using compression waves, it is Equation A.33 which is applicable. Since $k_s > k_p$ always, the square root factors are always real, so the phase of the diffracted signal will be $\pi/4$ or $5\pi/4$ depending on the sign of the complete angular factor. These are the phases extracted experimentally by Ravenscroft et al. [1991] (see also Achenbach et al. [1982]).

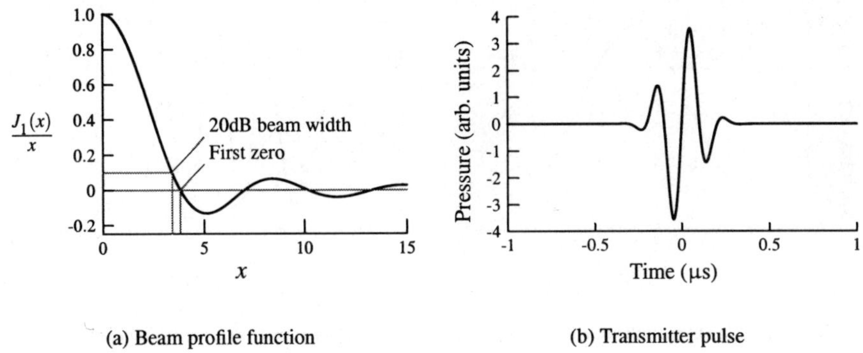


**Fig. A.2** The beam profile function and the model transmitter pulse.

# A.5 Pulse shape from a piston source

In this section we study how the pulse shape from a circular disk transducer behaving as an ideal piston source varies with angle from the beam axis.

First we consider how the amplitude of the ultrasound would vary with angle from the beam axis, if the transducer were vibrating continuously at a fixed frequency. If we wanted the absolute amplitude at some arbitrary point away from the transducer, we would need to calculate the contribution from each small element of the transducer face and integrate over the whole disk. However, we are only interested in relative values, so we can take advantage of the well known result for Fraunhofer diffraction from an aperture. Although this ignores the variation in range and inclination across the transducer face, these factors turn out to be of minor importance in the final result and would not affect our conclusions.

The amplitude $\Phi$ of the beam at angle $\Omega$ to the axis, at frequency $f$, is proportional to

$$\Phi(\Omega, f) = 2\frac{J_1(x)}{x} \qquad \text{where} \quad x = \frac{2\pi f a \sin\Omega}{C} \tag{A.37}$$

Here $a$ is the radius of the piston source, $C$ is the velocity of propagation and $J_1$ is the first-order Bessel function of the first kind. The resultant profile is shown in Figure A.2(a).

The first zero of $J_1(x)/x$ is at 3.381 and it has fallen to 0.1 of its on-axis value at $x = 3.08$. At this point $\sin\Omega \cong \lambda/2a$, the standard expression for the half-width of a transducer beam. For a centre frequency of 5 MHz, a velocity of 5.9 mm/μs and a probe radius of 4 mm, the first zero is at an angle $\Omega_{zero} = 0.181$ rad ($\sim 10.4°$) from the beam axis.

Next, we need to define a realistic shape for the on-axis pulse, which we do by assuming that the vibration of the transducer face can be modelled as a sine wave at the resonant frequency, modified by an amplitude envelope of Gaussian form. The

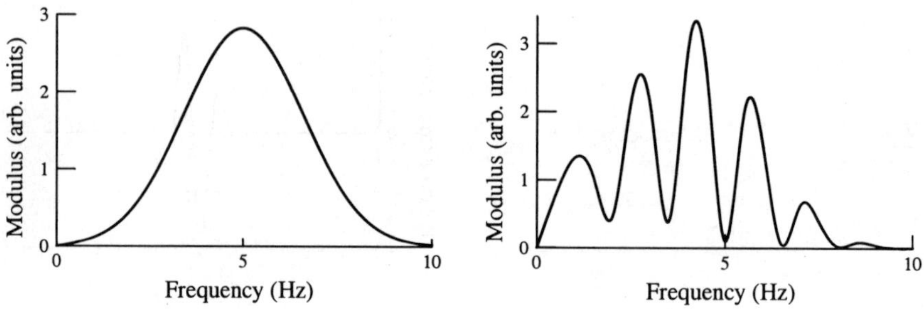


(a) On the beam axis

(b) At angle Ω from the beam axis

**Fig. A.3** The frequency spectra of the on-axis and off-axis pulses.

pulse amplitude function $p(t)$ is then given by

$$p(t) = \frac{\sin 2\pi f t}{\sigma\sqrt{2\pi}} \exp\left(-\frac{(t-\mu)^2}{2\sigma^2}\right) \tag{A.38}$$

If we choose $\mu = 0$ and $\sigma = 0.1$, we obtain the pulse shape shown in Figure A.2(b).

In order to obtain the pulse shape at some arbitrary angle $\Omega$ from the beam axis, we must first calculate the frequency spectrum of the on-axis pulse (Figure A.3(a)). We then multiply every frequency component in this spectrum by the corresponding amplitude $\Phi\{\Omega, f\}$. This produces a spectrum looking like Figure A.3(b), which is calculated for $\Omega = 0.5$, as would apply to the lateral wave in a TOFD inspection, when 60° probes are being used. The main feature is the appearance of notches in the spectrum but there is also a shift to lower frequency. To get the pulse shape, the spectrum must be transformed back into the time domain, giving the results shown in Figure A.4(a).

The appearance of two pulses, leading and trailing the zero time position is physically explained by the fact that, because the wavelets from different parts of the transducer face arrive at the measurement point with different phases, they almost all cancel and the only remaining contributions are the edge waves, those which come from the points on the transducer face which are nearest and furthest from the measurement point.

What we have calculated so far is what would be seen by a point detector immersed in the inspection medium. However, in all practical cases, the pulse is detected by another probe. We shall assume that the receiver probe is identical with the transmitter probe and is in a symmetrical position, as is commonly the case with TOFD inspection. In that case, we can simply multiply the pulse spectrum again by the identical beam spread function to take account of the second transducer and transform into the time domain as before, arriving at a pulse shape like that if Figure A.4(b).

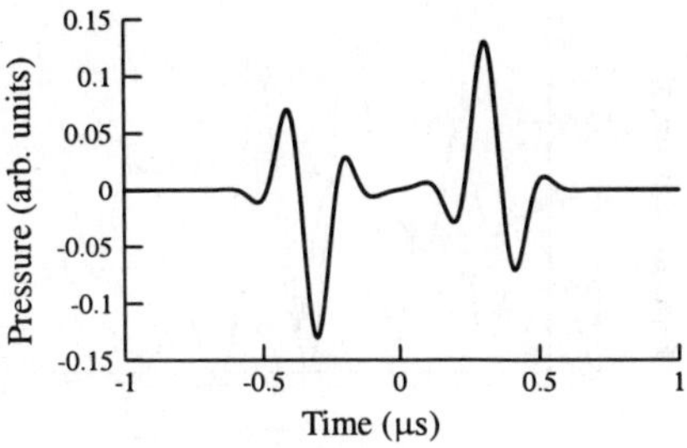


(a) Off-axis internal pulse shape

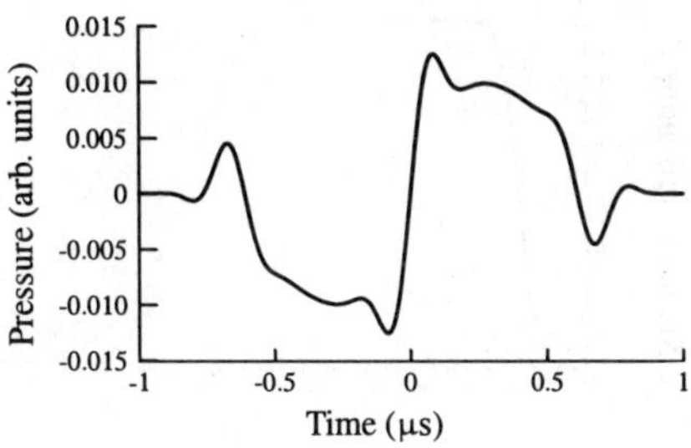


(b) Off-axis pulse shape at receiver

**Fig. A.4** The pulse shape within the inspection medium and the shape of the pulse detected by the receiver transducer.

The shape obtained is rather sensitive to the precise assumptions about the original pulse. In this case we have used a rather short pulse (small $\sigma$) with a broad spectrum and hence considerable energy at the low frequency at which the leading and trailing edge waves are in phase. Had we used a longer pulse (greater $\sigma$), there would have been less low frequency energy and the pulse shape would have looked more like a central pulse with leading and trailing pulses of half amplitude.

In practice the pulse shape shown in Figure A.4(b) will rarely be seen, because we have not yet taken into account the frequency response of the receiver amplifier. Thus far, there has been an implicit assumption that the amplifier has a completely flat response but, in practice it is more likely to be something like Figure A.5(a). Here, the roll-off at low frequency is the important feature, whereas the high frequency roll-off has very little effect. When this function is used to envelope the pulse spectrum, the time domain pulse shape looks like Figure A.5(b), more like the pulse shape we should have obtained had we started with a longer on-axis pulse.

This characteristic shape, with a central pulse and leading and trailing pulses of about half the amplitude, is easy to reconcile with the edge-wave picture invoked earlier. For the typical TOFD probe pair, the transmitter probe will act like two sources at the points nearest and furthest from the receiver probe, while the receiver probe will act like two detectors at the points nearest and farthest from the transmitter probe. Hence, for any point in the workpiece, there will be four possible paths along which detected signals could have travelled. In the case of either the lateral wave or a diffraction point lying in the plane of symmetry between the probes, two of the paths will have identical range and the other two will differ from these by equal amounts in opposite directions. Since ranges and angles differ very little between the paths one would expect the four signals to have roughly equal amplitudes, leading to the pulse arrangement we have already seen. Once the diffraction point is moved away from the symmetry plane, there will almost always be four pulses.

In practice, it often seems to be the case that the leading and trailing pulses are

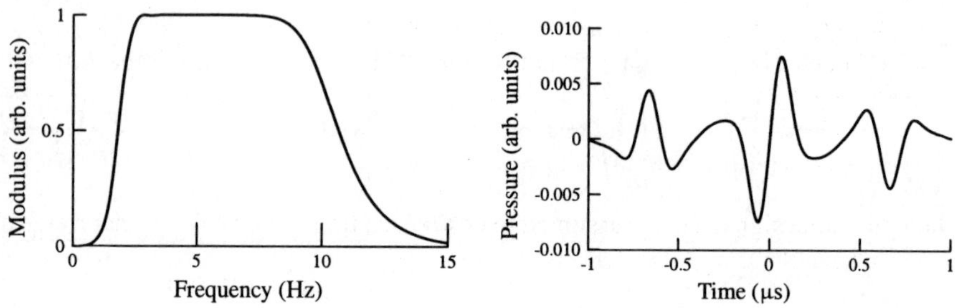


(a) Receiver frequency response

(b) Modified received pulse shape

**Fig. A.5** A typical receiver frequency response and the resultant shape of the received off-axis pulse.

much less than half the amplitude of the central pulse, to the point where they may be scarcely noticeable. This may be understandable in terms of the departure of the probes from ideal piston sources but there does not appear to be any published information on this. It is an area which might repay further study.

The pulse form of off-axis pulses is important for the accuracy of the TOFD technique, especially in cases where the lateral wave is used as a reference. It is clear that the central pulse of the lateral wave, not the outliers, should always be used for timing. The most accurate timing method would be to use the central zero crossing of both the lateral wave and the defect signal and this would give no error. If a neighbouring zero crossing is used, provided that the corresponding positions on the lateral wave and defect pulse are measured, there will be a only small error arising from the broadening of the central lateral wave pulse. There is clearly a possibility of much larger error if the measurement points chosen on the two signals do not correspond. It is important to bear in mind that the degree of distortion of off-axis pulses can be reduced by reducing the probe diameter. Provided there is enough energy for an adequate signal, the smallest probe will give the least distorted signals and hence the highest accuracy.

# A.6 Signal averaging

In Section 4.4, we mentioned that signal averaging could be used to enhance signal strength over noise. The basis of this is developed in this section. Noise can arise from two distinct sources. We show below how the averaging process works for signals which depend on a parameter $x$, which may represent simply successive firings of stationary transducers, or may also include some change in transducer position from one firing to the next.

Suppose the signal received $R_i$ is obtained on $M$ different occasions and that the signal is a function of the parameter $x$. Suppose also that, of the observed signal $R_i(x)$, only the part $S(x)$ is the signal from the defect and the remainder $N_i(x)$ is due to noise. Each observed signal $R_i$ is taken to be degraded by a different, random, noise $N_i$. Then

$$R_i(x) = S(x) + N_i(x) \tag{A.39}$$

where the same signal $S(x)$ is assumed to occur each time. For random, uncorrelated noise we have the properties that

$$\langle N_i(x) \rangle = 0 \tag{A.40}$$

$$\left\langle N_i(x) + N_j(x) \right\rangle = \langle N_i(x) \rangle + \left\langle N_j(x) \right\rangle \quad \text{where} \quad i \neq j \tag{A.41}$$

and

$$\left\langle N_i(x) N_j(x) \right\rangle = \langle N_i(x) \rangle \left\langle N_j(x) \right\rangle \qquad \text{where} \quad i \neq j \tag{A.42}$$

where the notation $\langle Q \rangle$ means the expectation value of $Q$. The signal-to-noise power $P(x)$ is defined as

$$P(x) = \frac{S^2(x)}{\langle N^2(x) \rangle} \tag{A.43}$$

If we add $M$ signals and average them we find

$$\bar{R} = \frac{1}{M} \sum_{i=1}^{M} [S(x) + N_i(x)] \tag{A.44}$$

and the signal-to-noise power becomes

$$\bar{P}(x) = \frac{S^2(x)}{\left\langle \frac{1}{M} \sum_{i=1}^{M} [N_i(x)]^2 \right\rangle} \tag{A.45}$$

Manipulating this expression, using the results in Equations A.40 to A.42, yields

$$\bar{P}(x) = \frac{M^2 S^2(x)}{\left\langle \sum_{i=1}^{M} [N_i(x)]^2 \right\rangle} \tag{A.46}$$

$$= \frac{M^2 S^2(x)}{\left\langle \sum_{i=1}^{M} [N_i(x)] \sum_{j=1}^{M} \left[N_j(x)\right] \right\rangle}$$

$$= \frac{M^2 S^2(x)}{\left\langle \sum_{i=1}^{M} \left[N_i^2(x)\right] \right\rangle + \left\langle \sum_{i=1}^{M} \sum_{j=1}^{M} \left[N_i N_j(x)\right]_{i \neq j} \right\rangle}$$

$$= \frac{M^2 S^2(x)}{\left\langle \sum_{i=1}^{M} \left[N_i^2(x)\right] \right\rangle + \sum_{i=1}^{M} \sum_{j=1}^{M} \langle N_i \rangle \left\langle N_j(x) \right\rangle_{i \neq j}}$$

The $M$ noise samples will all have the same average square value and the second term in the denominator is zero so that, finally

$$\bar{P}(x) = \frac{M^2 S^2(x)}{M \langle N_i^2(x) \rangle} = MP(x) \tag{A.47}$$

The signal-to-noise power ratio is thus enhanced by a factor $M$, if $M$ signals are added together and the noise is random and uncorrelated. The signal-to-noise amplitude ratio is the square root of the power so that

$$SNR_{\text{average}} = \sqrt{M}\, SNR_{\text{single}} \tag{A.48}$$

Thus, averaging 64 signals that are degraded by uncorrelated random noise would improve the signal-to-noise ratio by about 18 dB, while averaging 256 such signals would give about 24 dB improvement in signal to noise.

We have seen that the advantage to be gained from signal averaging depends on two critical assumptions: that the wanted signal component remains essentially the same (i.e. is strongly correlated) from one firing of the transmitter to the next; and the noise component is uncorrelated from firing to firing.

The first of these conditions is automatically fulfilled if the transducers remain stationary between firings; if they are moved, it sets a limit, related to the ultrasonic wavelength, on how far they may be moved without upsetting the averaging process.

The second condition is fulfilled for electronic noise generated in the amplifier input stages. It is fulfilled also for electromagnetic pick-up, provided the source of the pick-up is not related to, nor synchronous with, the firing of the transducers. The remaining likely source of noise is the reception of ultrasound scattered from such features as inclusions or grain boundaries in the workpiece. For stationary transducers, noise from this source will be identical from firing to firing and so will not be attenuated by signal averaging. It may be rendered uncorrelated, if the transducers can be moved far enough between firings, the required distance being related to the characteristic length describing the distribution of scatterers. For grain scattering, this length would be the grain size. Note, however, that the requirement for a large movement to decorrelate the scattering noise is in conflict with the requirement for the wanted signal to remain correlated. In these circumstances, the actual movement may need to be a compromise between these two requirements and the advantage to be gained from averaging with probe movement (spatial averaging) may be much less than the theoretical maximum.

## A.7 Defect characterisation

In Section 5.9, we stated that the backscattered pulses originate from those parts of the defect with a change in the projected cross-sectional area. Expressing this mathematically, Lam and Tsang [1985] give for the received backscattered signal

$$S_{\text{received}} = \sum_{1}^{N} i\frac{S_{\text{transmitted}}}{\lambda} R^2 \exp\left(i2k\left(r_i - r_1\right)\right) \sum_{p=0}^{\infty} \frac{D(a,i,p)}{(i2k)^p} \tag{A.49}$$

where $A$ is the total area projection towards the transducers of that part of the defect within range $r$. The nearest part of the defect is at range $r_1$, while the various $r_i$ are the ranges at which the projected area and its derivatives have discontinuities, and $p$ is the order of such derivatives. $D(a,i,p)$ is the strength of the discontinuity while $R$ is the mean range of the defect. The ultrasonic wavevector is $k$. Typical values of the discontinuity strengths $D$ are given by Lam and Tsang as

$$D(a,i,1) = \pm\frac{L}{\sin\varepsilon} \tag{A.50}$$

for an edge of length $L$ at an incident angle of $\varepsilon$ where the $+$sign applies to a near edge and the $-$sign to a far edge. For a corner lying between directions $\theta_1$ and $\theta_2$, this gives a strength

$$D(a,i,2) = \frac{\left(\tan\theta_1 - \tan\theta_2\right)}{\sin^2\varepsilon} \tag{A.51}$$

Making use of this type of information on arrival times only, Lam and Tsang demonstrated that a microcomputer system could be used to reconstruct the shape of unknown planar, straight-edged flaws from diffraction echoes of short ultrasonic pulses.

## A.8 Transversely isotropic media

In Section 7.1.2 we discussed the effect that anisotropic media have on the speed of propagation of elastic waves, and hence on timing measurements of signal arrival times. The particular problem encountered is of a layer of austenitic cladding which crystallises with long columnar grains having a well defined $z$-axis direction but with random orientations of $x$- and $y$-axes in the plane perpendicular to $z$. This leads to a transversely isotropic material, similar to a hexagonal material but with elastic constants derived from the underlying cubic symmetry as discussed below. The elastic constants $C_{ijkl}$ are rotated about the $z$-axis and averaged. Thus, for the fourth order elastic tensor

$$C'_{ijkl} = a_{ip}a_{jq}a_{kr}a_{ls}C_{pqrs} \tag{A.52}$$

where the transformation matrices $\mathbf{a}$ are given by

$$\mathbf{a} = \begin{pmatrix} \cos\phi & \sin\phi & 0 \\ -\sin\phi & \cos\phi & 0 \\ 0 & 0 & 1 \end{pmatrix} \tag{A.53}$$

with $C_{pqrs}$ being the elastic constants of the columnar grain with its (100) direction lying along the $x'$-axis. The elastic constants $C'_{ijkl}$ then represent a columnar grain with its (100) direction lying at some angle $\phi$ relative to the $x'$-axis. Averaging these elastic constants according to

$$C^T_{ijkl} = \frac{1}{2\pi}\int_0^{2\pi} C'_{ijkl}(\phi)\,d\phi \tag{A.54}$$

yields the values [Gillan, 1980]

$$C^T_{11} = \frac{3}{4}C_{11} + \frac{1}{4}C_{12} + \frac{1}{2}C_{44} \tag{A.55}$$

$$C^T_{12} = \frac{3}{4}C_{12} + \frac{1}{4}C_{11} - \frac{1}{2}C_{44} \tag{A.56}$$

$$C^T_{13} = C_{12} \tag{A.57}$$

$$C^T_{33} = C_{11} \tag{A.58}$$

$$C^T_{44} = C_{44} \tag{A.59}$$

$$C^T_{66} = \frac{1}{2}\left(C^T_{11} - C^T_{12}\right) \tag{A.60}$$

where the superscript $T$ refers to the constants for the transversely isotropic material. The tensor has been expressed in the Voigt notation so that pairs of indices are represented by a single index according to the following scheme: $11 \rightarrow 1$; $22 \rightarrow 2$; $33 \rightarrow 3$; $23 \rightarrow 4$; $31 \rightarrow 5$; and $12 \rightarrow 6$. The values produced by Equations A.55 to A.60 are tabulated in Table A.1.

The wave equation for the displacement $U$ in a homogeneous anisotropic solid is

$$\sum_{j,k,l=1}^{3} C_{ijkl}\frac{\partial^2 U_k}{\partial x_j \partial x_l} = \rho\frac{\partial^2 U_i}{\partial t^2} \tag{A.61}$$

Plane wave solutions of this equation are given by

$$U_i = A\alpha_i \exp i\left[\omega t - k e_m x_m\right] \tag{A.62}$$

where $A$ is the amplitude, $\alpha$ the polarisation of the wave, $\omega$ the angular frequency, $t$ the time, $k$ the wavevector ($= 2\pi/\lambda$, where $\lambda$ is the wavelength). The quantities

**Table A.1** Constants defining elastic behaviour of transversely anisotropic austenitic cladding.

| | |
|---|---|
| $C_{11}$ | $263 \times 10^9 \mathrm{N\,m^{-2}}$ |
| $C_{12}$ | $98 \times 10^9 \mathrm{N\,m^{-2}}$ |
| $C_{13}$ | $145 \times 10^9 \mathrm{N\,m^{-2}}$ |
| $C_{33}$ | $216 \times 10^9 \mathrm{N\,m^{-2}}$ |
| $C_{44}$ | $129 \times 10^9 \mathrm{N\,m^{-2}}$ |
| $C_{66}$ | $82 \times 10^9 \mathrm{N\,m^{-2}}$ |
| $\rho$ | $7.9 \times 10^3 \mathrm{kgm^{-3}}$ |

$e_m$ are the direction cosines of the normal to the plane wave. On substituting this expression we obtain

$$\left[C_{ijkl}e_l e_j - \rho V^2 \delta_{ik}\right] \alpha_k = 0 \tag{A.63}$$

where $V$ is the phase velocity of the wave. Since $\alpha_k$ is arbitrary we must satisfy

$$\left|C_{ijkl}e_l e_j - \rho V^2 \delta_{ik}\right| \alpha_k = 0 \tag{A.64}$$

Setting $\Gamma_{ik} = C_{ijkl}e_l e_j$, this can be rewritten as

$$\begin{vmatrix} \Gamma_{11} - \rho V^2 & \Gamma_{12} & \Gamma_{13} \\ \Gamma_{12} & \Gamma_{22} - \rho V^2 & \Gamma_{23} \\ \Gamma_{13} & \Gamma_{23} & \Gamma_{33} - \rho V^2 \end{vmatrix} = 0 \tag{A.65}$$

The eigenvalues then give the phase velocities and the corresponding eigenvectors give the polarisation of the waves. The phase velocities define a slowness surface (reciprocal of the phase velocity $k/\omega$) and the group velocity $V_g = \partial\omega/\partial k$, corresponding to a particular wavevector **k**, is normal to the slowness surface at **k**. A section through the slowness surface for Type 308 stainless steel is shown in Figure 7.2.

## A.9 Component curvature

To extract the speed of waves which creep around curved surfaces we follow Viktorov [1958] and Peck and Miklowitz [1969] and write the Helmholtz potentials as

$$\phi = Ae^{\pm i\nu\theta}e^{-i\omega t}H_\nu^{(1)}(k_p r) \tag{A.66}$$

$$\psi = Be^{\pm i\nu\theta}e^{-i\omega t}H_\nu^{(1)}(k_s r) \tag{A.67}$$

Here $A$ and $B$ are constants to be determined by the boundary conditions and $H_\nu^{(1)}(z)$ is the Hankel function of the first kind of order $\nu$ and argument $z$. As Hankel functions of the second kind, $H_\nu^{(2)}(z)$, do not occur in this work we drop the superscript.

The arguments depend on the wavevectors of compression waves $k_p$ and of shear waves $k_s$. The boundary condition is that the stress on the surface of the cavity should vanish. The equations for the stresses, in cylindrical coordinates, are

$$\sigma_{rr} = (\lambda + 2\mu)\left[\frac{\partial^2 \phi}{\partial r^2} + \frac{1}{r}\frac{\partial^2 \psi}{\partial r \partial \theta} - \frac{1}{r^2}\frac{\partial \psi}{\partial \theta}\right] + \lambda\left[\frac{1}{r}\frac{\partial \phi}{\partial r} + \frac{1}{r^2}\frac{\partial \psi}{\partial \theta} + \frac{1}{r^2}\frac{\partial^2 \phi}{\partial \theta^2}\right] \tag{A.68}$$

$$\sigma_{r\theta} = \mu\left[\frac{2}{r}\frac{\partial^2 \phi}{\partial r \partial \theta} - \frac{2}{r^2}\frac{\partial \phi}{\partial \theta} - \frac{\partial^2 \psi}{\partial r^2} + \frac{1}{r}\frac{\partial \psi}{\partial r} + \frac{1}{r^2}\frac{\partial^2 \psi}{\partial \theta^2}\right] \tag{A.69}$$

The equation obtained from setting $\sigma_{rr} = 0$ gives a relationship between the amplitudes $A$ and $B$, provided we know $\nu$. The equation obtained from setting $\sigma_{r\theta} = 0$ gives [Viktorov, 1958]

$$\left\{\Omega_p^2 \Omega_s^2 e^{i\nu\pi} H_{\nu+2}(\Omega_p) H_{\nu-2}(\Omega_s) + H_{\nu-2}(\Omega_p) H_{\nu+2}(\Omega_s) \right. \tag{A.70}$$

$$\left. - \left[\frac{C_p^2}{C_s^2} - 1\right] H_\nu(\Omega_p)\left[H_{\nu+2}(\Omega_s) + H_{\nu-2}(\Omega_s)\right]\right\} = 0$$

with $\Omega_p = \omega/C_p$ and $\Omega_s = \omega a/C_s$, where $a$ is the radius of the cavity. The solutions of this equation give the allowed values of $\nu$ for given $\Omega_p$ and $\Omega_s$. There is a doubly infinite number of solutions to this equation [Peck and Miklowitz, 1969], with an infinite number of solutions which condense into the lateral wave travelling at the bulk compression wave speed as the radius of the cavity increases. The other infinity of solutions corresponds to the bulk shear wave velocity as the radius of the cavity increases. As well as these two infinite sets of solutions there is also one root which is a true surface wave, with amplitude dying away exponentially with distance from the cavity surface. Once the above equation has been solved, the phase velocity $V$ can be found from

$$V = \frac{\omega a}{\Re(\nu)} \tag{A.71}$$

where $\Re$ denotes the real part a complex quantity. The wave decays with an attenuation according to $e^{-\delta\theta}$, with

$$\delta = \Im(\nu) \tag{A.72}$$

and $\Im$ denotes the imaginary part. For large values of cavity radius, asymptotic solutions can be used which yield [Peck and Miklowitz, 1969]

$$\nu \sim \Omega_p + a_n (\Omega_p/2)^{\frac{1}{3}} e^{-2\pi i/3} \tag{A.73}$$

This is for the compression wave modes. The values for shear waves are obtained by substituting $\Omega_s$ in place of $\Omega_p$. The coefficients $a_n$ are the $n$th zeros of the Airy function: the first three values are -2.338, -4.088, -5.5206 [Olver, 1960]. Hurst and Temple [1982] solved Equation A.70 numerically and demonstrated that the asymptotic solutions were, in fact, good down to about $k_p a \sim 0.5$ or $k_s a \sim 0.5$ respectively. These results are shown in Figure 7.9(b).

## A.10 Confidence levels in test-block exercises

For defect detection exercises, the aim should be to determine the reliability of detection of defects in a specified class. The class might be chosen on the grounds of through-wall size or position; length; thickness; orientation; type such as lack of fusion in a weld; or in a host of other ways. The binomial distribution is important in assessment of inspection reliability, since it gives the probability of exactly $k$ successes in $n$ trials. Let us denote this probability by $P(k|p,n)$, where $p$ is the probability of success in any one trial. Then

$$P(k|p,n) = \binom{n}{k} p^k (1-p)^{n-k} \tag{A.74}$$

where $\binom{n}{k}$ denotes $n! \div \{k!(n-k)!\}$. If we want the probability of $k$ or fewer successes in $n$ independent trials we must use the cumulative binomial distribution

$$Q(k|p,n) = \sum_{r=0}^{k} \binom{n}{r} p^r (1-p)^{n-r} \tag{A.75}$$

Since the events form a complete set, that is, out of $n$ trials we are certain to get one of the results: $0, 1, \ldots, n$ successes, then

$$Q(n|p,n) = 1 \tag{A.76}$$

The probability of more than $k$ successes is given by $1 - Q(k|p,n)$. We can also put confidence limits on the results of the probability of success $p$, given an observation of $k$ successes out of $n$ trials. The value $k/n$ is the best estimate of $p$. The question is often asked: *How many trials do we need to ensure that our estimate of the reliability of this technique is, say, 95% with a high degree of confidence?* Suppose we wish to obtain this value of 95% reliability for a given defect class and we want this to 95% confidence level. We need to solve the equations

$$\sum_{r=0}^{k} \binom{n}{r} p^r (1-p)^{n-r} = 0.025 \tag{A.77}$$

for the upper bound, $p_1$, and

$$\sum_{r=k}^{n} \binom{n}{r} p^r (1-p)^{n-r} = 0.025 \tag{A.78}$$

for the lower bound, $p_2$. We can either stipulate a value for $p$, which we desire to obtain with a given confidence limit and solve for $n$ and $k$, or we can be given the results of a trial, $k$ successes in $n$ trials, say, and estimate $p = k/n$, with confidence limits $p_1$ and $p_2$. In either case the equations can be solved by trial and error, using a bisection technique, for small values of $n$. For large values of $n$, we can make use of the approximation of a binomial distribution by a normal distribution and obtain, for example, the 95% confidence interval on the value of $p$ from

$$P\left(\tilde{p} - 1.96\sqrt{\frac{\tilde{p}(1-\tilde{p})}{n}} < p < \tilde{p} + 1.96\sqrt{\frac{\tilde{p}(1-\tilde{p})}{n}}\right) \sim 0.95 \tag{A.79}$$

where $\tilde{p}$ is the best estimate of probability, that is, number of successes divided by total number of attempts. For large values of $n$, Packman, Malpani and Wells [1976] made use of the Poisson distribution, which is satisfactory provided $p$ is either very small, $\leqslant 0.1$, or very large, $\geqslant 0.9$, say. The difference in accuracy between the two distributions is illustrated by Packman et al.: if $n = 45$ and $k = 43$ then, for 95% confidence level, we obtain $p = 0.895$, whereas the true value from the binomial distribution would be $p = 0.863$. Equations A.77 and A.78 and the results quoted above are for two-sided confidence limits. Often it is appropriate to use one-sided confidence limits, which would correspond to setting $Q$ in Equation A.75 to the required confidence level and solving the equation for the lower bound value of $p$, given values of $n$ and $k$.

## A.11 Distribution of sizing errors

In Section 8.4.6, we discussed the errors made in sizing defects. A first approach to quantifying the errors in the sizing measurement is to calculate their mean and standard deviation. However, these are useful quantities only if the errors are normally distributed, or higher moments are also known. To test whether the errors are normally distributed, we apply a conventional statistical test. The statistical test we use is the Shapiro-Wilk W-statistic [Hahn and Shapiro, 1967] which can be used for 50 or fewer observations. Given $n$ observations $z_i$, we calculate the W-statistic as follows: the $n$ size errors $z_i$ are ordered such that

$$z_1 \leqslant z_2 \leqslant \ldots \leqslant z_n \tag{A.80}$$

and then the mean value $\bar{z}$ is calculated. The quantity $S^2$ is then calculated given by

$$S^2 = \sum_{i=1}^{n} (z_i - \bar{z})^2 \tag{A.81}$$

and, if $n$ is even, we set $k = n/2$ or, if $n$ is odd, $k = (n+1)/2$ and calculate

$$b = a_n(z_n - z_1) + a_{n-1}(z_{n-1} - z_2) + \cdots + a_{n-k+1}(z_{n-k+1} - z_k) \tag{A.82}$$

The coefficients $a_i$ can be found in tables [e.g. Hahn and Shapiro, 1967]. Finally,

$$W = \frac{b^2}{S^2} \tag{A.83}$$

Low values of $W$ indicate that the distribution is not very likely to be normal but the likelihood depends on the sample size $n$. For example, for a sample size of 10, a $W$ value of 0.781 would indicate a 1% chance that the data came from a normal distribution, whereas $W = 0.938$ would indicate a 50% chance. For a sample size of 20 these two values would be $W = 0.868$ and $W = 0.959$ respectively. The Shapiro-Wilk test is not a positive identification for a normal distribution but rather screens against non-normal distributions. Thus a result which gives only a 10% chance of being a random sample from a normal distribution may be well represented by a normal distribution but one which gives only a 1% chance or less is deemed unlikely to have come from a normal distribution.

## A.12 Implications for structural integrity

In Section 8.9 some of the results of probabilistic fracture mechanics analyses of pressure vessel failure rates were introduced and this section reviews some of the points in a little more detail.

The hazard presented by the failure of a component should determine the reliability required of that component. If the component is required to survive various possible excess transient stresses, for example, then non-destructive testing may well be used to identify flawed components before any catastrophic failure occurs.

Based on probabilistic fracture mechanics analyses of the failure rate expected for PWR pressure vessels, a target was suggested [Marshall, 1982] for the reliability of detecting and sizing defects according to their through-wall extent. This is usually expressed as a function of the form

$$B(a) = \varepsilon + (1 - \varepsilon)e^{-\mu a} \tag{A.84}$$

$B(a)$represents the chance of incorrectly allowing an unacceptable defect, of characteristic size (through-wall extent or length) $a$, to remain in the vessel. As such, it includes the possibility that a defect might not be detected; that, if detected, it might be incorrectly sized; and, even if correctly sized, might not be repaired satisfactorily. It is usually assumed that repair can be as good as new, so $B(a)$ is taken to represent the possibility that an unacceptable defect will go undetected, or be detected and incorrectly judged to be acceptable. The size could represent length or through-wall extent, and ought really to take into account both these factors and others, but is usually taken to be simply the through-wall extent, as this is the most critical parameter for a crack based on fracture mechanics criteria. A schematic diagram of the various regions of the $B(a)$ function is given in Figure A.6. Initially, for small acceptable defects, $B(a)$ is unity; then there comes a region of decreasing likelihood that defects will remain in the vessel, due in part to the decreasing likelihood that

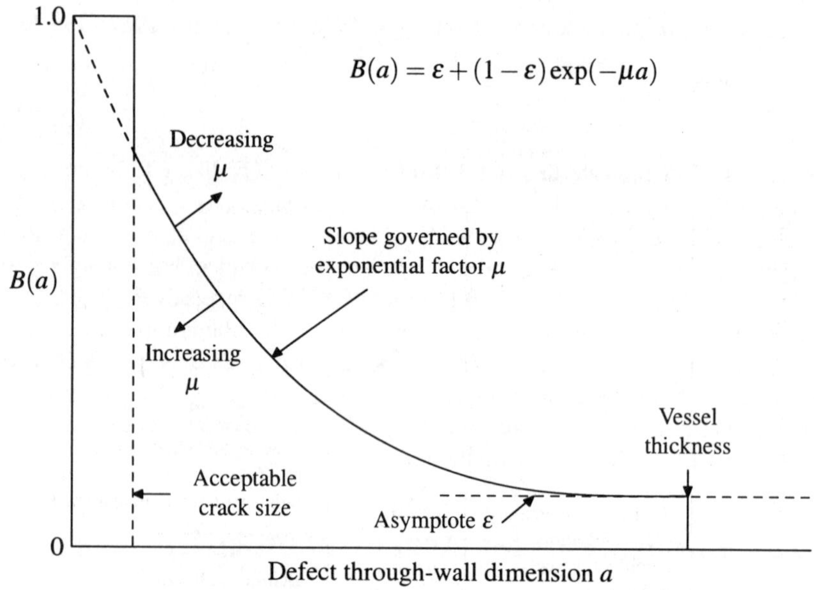


**Fig. A.6** Schematic diagram of the various regions of the probability that unacceptable defects will remain in a pressure vessel.

big defects would be created in the first place and in part to the increased likelihood of successful detection and repair; finally, there is an asymptote to which $B(a)$ tends for large defects. The asymptote represents factors beyond the capability of the non-destructive testing technique to detect and size defects accurately. An example of such a factor would be gross human error such as omitting an inspection altogether. It is expected that this asymptote will represent a low likelihood of occurrence, probably between $10^{-3}$ and $10^{-4}$ per inspection. Defects so large that that the vessel leaks or fractures into two or more parts will not go unnoticed, so $B(a)$ becomes zero at the vessel through-wall thickness.

In general, probabilistic fracture mechanics work has assumed that a single parameter of the defect, through-wall size, governs the likelihood of vessel failure. However, this parameter is not what is measured readily by most ultrasonic inspections, except by Time-of-Flight Diffraction. Classification of a defect depends on whether it represents a threat to the integrity of the structure. If it does then it is unacceptable; otherwise it is acceptable.

Marshall [1982] proposed the values $\varepsilon = 0.005$ and $\mu = 113.4$, giving

$$B(a) = 0.005 + 0.995e^{-113.4a} \tag{A.85}$$

where $a$ is in metres. This corresponds to the targets set by Marshall of a *high* degree of confidence ($B(0.025) \approx 0.06$, that is, about 95%) that defects of through-wall extent of 25 mm are detected and correctly classified while giving a *fair* chance (about

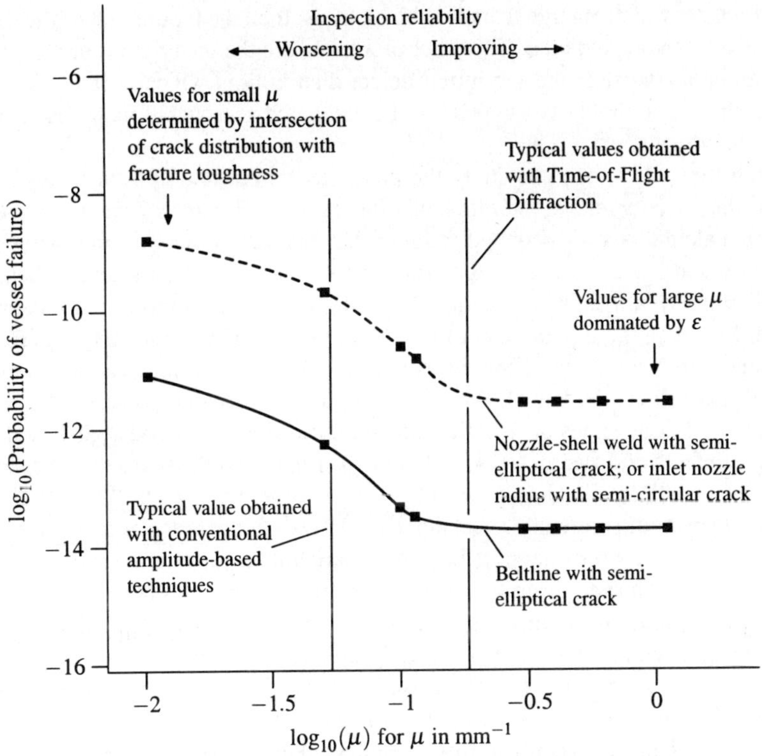


**Fig. A.7** Predicted failure rate per vessel year for a pressure vessel of a pressurised water reactor as a function of inspection unreliability.

50%) that a defect of through-wall extent 6 mm would be detected and correctly classified. This same function can be used to express the requirement for detection and correct classification of defects of other through-wall sizes. As an example, consider a defect of through-wall extent of 15 mm, for which $B(0.015) \approx 0.2$, representing about an 80% chance of correctly detecting and sizing it. This is now believed to be a conservative estimate of the reliability of ultrasonic techniques. Nevertheless, with this function, the probabilistic analyses yield a failure rate of the pressure vessel of $10^{-7}$ per vessel year. If the chance of failing to detect, or to correctly classify, a defect is only $10^{-4}$, independent of defect through-wall extent, then the failure rate of the pressure vessel decreases to below $10^{-8}$ per vessel year.

There are many assumptions in these analyses and, for more detail, the reader is referred to Marshall [1982] and Cameron [1984]. The important point which we wish to emphasise is that these are the estimated failure rates even if the chance of correctly detecting and sizing a defect of 15 mm through-wall extent is as low as 80%. This sets a scale on how reliable inspection needs to be. Once functions of this form have been deduced and are taken to be realistic and representative of the sort of results which emerge from test-block trials, then the failure rate of the vessels themselves can be predicted. The other input data are the material properties, which are well characterised, and the initial defect distribution, which is rather less well known than is desirable but which can be estimated reasonably well based on the available information.

With these data, one can study the predicted failure rate of vessels, as a function of the success rate of the ultrasonic inspections. Figure A.7 shows the results of some calculations of predicted failure rates, per vessel year, of pressure vessels in pressurised water reactors, following a large loss of coolant accident, based on the reliability of ultrasonic inspection. The reliability of the ultrasonic inspections is included through the $\mu$ parameter of the $B(a)$ function. This parameter $\mu$ represents, in essence, the capability of the ultrasonic inspection to distinguish between critical and non-critical defects. It is thus related to the resolving power at the critical defect size. Large values of $\mu$ indicate techniques which are good at distinguishing between defects of different sizes, and the $B(a)$ function quickly reaches the asymptote. Conversely, small values of $\mu$ indicate techniques having a large uncertainty in whether they would correctly reject defects relatively close to the accept-reject decision line. In other words, large $\mu$ indicates a small mean error and small associated standard deviation away from the mean for the measurement of defect through-wall size, whereas small $\mu$ implies large mean errors and associated standard deviations. In Figure A.7, taken from Cameron and Temple [1986], the variations of predicted failure rates, as a function of $\mu$, for a fixed asymptotic value of $B(a)$ of $10^{-3}$, show that there is a limit to worthwhile improvements to the accuracy of sizing techniques unless parallel improvements are made to the likelihood of gross errors (such as human error).

Theoretical modelling work on very long defects of aspect ratio 0.1 or greater and of at least 6 mm through-wall extent has shown that the chance of incorrectly accepting unacceptable defects should be as low as any externally applied asymptote, that is, certainly less than $10^{-3}$ [Cameron and Temple, 1984]. This asymptote arises in the same way as the constant in the Marshall $B(a)$ function — through external influences and mishaps (see Section 8.9). Following the arguments in Cameron and Temple [1984] leads us back to the most significant defect parameter being its through-wall extent.

# Bibliography

**Note on Back References** — numbers enclosed in brackets, thus [157], at the end of a bibliography entry, indicate the pages on which that entry is cited. They should not be confused with page numbers in journals etc., which sometimes come at the end of an entry but are never enclosed in brackets.


Achenbach, J. D. [1973]. *Wave Propagation in Elastic Solids*. North Holland, Amsterdam. [200]

Achenbach, J. D., A. K. Gautesen and H. McMaken [1982]. *Ray Methods for Waves in Elastic Solids: with Applications to Scattering by Cracks*. Pitman, Boston, London, Melbourne. [19], [69], [70], [206]

Aldridge, E. E. [1987]. U.K.A.E.A. Harwell Laboratory, unpublished work. [138]

Ammirato, F. and T. Willetts [1989]. Accuracy of ultrasonic flaw sizing techniques for reactor pressure vessels. In: J. Boogaard and G. van Dijk, editors, *Proceedings of the 12th World Conference on Non-Destructive Testing,* Amsterdam (Netherlands), 23 – 28 Apr. 1989, volume 2, pages 1077 – 1079. Elsevier, 1989. [176], [177]

Anliker, D. M. and S. A. Cilauro [1988]. Computer-assisted ultrasonic detection and measurement of cracks in pressure vessels. *Tappi Journal*, pages 41 – 45. [183]

Anon. [1983]. Offshore inspection, maintenance and repair. *Noroil*, **11**(2), 33. [110]

Anon. [1984]. Offshore inspection, maintenance and repair. *Noroil*, **12**(2), 31. [110]

Anon. [1987]. Rolls-Royce and Associates' 28 years of PWR experience. *Nuclear Europe*, (8 – 9/1987), 38. [181]

Anon. [1992]. Magnox vessels inspection: another success for TOFD. *Nucl. Eng. Int.*, **38**(462), 25 – 26. [182]

Anon. [1996]. Condition assessment services extended through joint venture. *Offshore*, **56**(9), 170, 179. [185]

Anon. [1998a]. *Offshore Oil International*. September 1998. [194]

Anon. [1998b]. Bridge inspection in Korea. *Inspection Solutions*, (63), 6. [188]

Anon. [1999]. Celebrating TOFD's 25th anniversary. *Inspection Solutions*, (65), 4 – 5. (March 1999). [192]

Anon. [2000]. Four killed as GNER express derails at 115 mph. *Railway Magazine*, **146**(1196), 6 – 7. [189]

Anon. [2001a]. Hatfield: Broken rail shattered into 300 pieces. *Railway Magazine*, **147**(1199), 6. [189]

Anon. [2001b]. A new dawn for Britain's railway? *Railway Magazine*, **147**(1199), 6. [190]

Anon. [2001c]. Total number of suspected crack sites: 3732! *Railway Magazine*, **147**(1198), 11. [189]

Arakawa, T. [1983]. A study on the transmission and reflection of an ultrasonic beam at machined surfaces pressed against each other. *Mater. Eval.*, **41**(6), 714 – 719. [140]

Ashwin, P. [1989]. Time of flight diffraction technique and applications for retaining rings and turbine discs. In: *Proceedings: Steam Turbine/Generation NDE Workshop,* Charlotte North Carolina (United States), 12 – 15 Sep. 1989, pages 29–1 – 29–23. Electric Power Research Institute. EPRI NP-6993 (1990). [184]

ASME [1974,1977,1983]. *Boiler and Pressure Vessel Code, Section XI, Rules for Inservice Inspection of Nuclear Power Plant*. American Society of Mechanical Engineers. 1974, 1977, 1983 and semi-annual addenda. [55], [177], [178]

ASME [1989]. *Boiler and Pressure Vessel Code, Section XI, Rules for Inservice Inspection of Nuclear Power Plant*. American Society of Mechanical Engineers. Mandatory appendices concerning performance demonstration and evaluation added. [197]

Atkinson, I., P. D. Birchall and A. J. Plevin [1989]. Improved characterisation of planar defects by skewed time-of-flight diffraction scanning. U.K.A.E.A. Report NRL-R-1019(R), Risley Laboratory. [102], [104]

Bainton, K. F., M. G. Silk, N. R. Williams, D. M. Davies, I. R. Lyon and V. Peters [1975]. The underwater inspection of fixed offshore platforms — a review and assessment of techniques. U.K.A.E.A. Report AERE-R8067, HMSO, London. [110], [185]

Bann, T. and A. Rogerson [1984]. An investigation into the sizing of small underclad flaws by a signal amplitude response technique and by a single probe time-of-flight diffraction technique. U.K.A.E.A. Report ND-R-1048, Risley Laboratory. [45], [46], [47]

Barbian, O. A., G. Engl, B. Grohs, W. Rathgeb and H. Wüstenberg [1984a]. A second view of the German results in the Defect Detection Trials. *Br. J. Non-Destr. Test.*, **26**(2), 92 – 96. [49]

Barbian, O. A., B. Grohs and W. Kappes [1984b]. Evaluation of time-of-flight data with the ALOK method. *Br. J. Non-Destr. Test.*, **26**(4), 214 – 217. [49], [155], [156]

Bergmann, U. and F. Bergner [1994]. Ultrasonic time-of-flight diffraction method for monitoring stable crack growth. In: F. P. Weiss and U. Rindelhardt, editors, *Institute for Safety Research, Annual Report 1994*, pages 28 – 30. Rossendorf Research Centre. [187]

Bloodworth, T. [1999]. High-accuracy defect sizing for nozzle attachment welds using asymmetric TOFD. In: *BINDT Mini-Conference on TOFD Techniques,* Wadham College, Oxford, (United Kingdom), 2 – 3 July 1999. (Proceedings not published). [125], [182]

Bowker, K. J., J. M. Coffey, D. J. Hanstock, R. C. Owen and J. M. Wrigley [1983]. CEGB inspection of Plates 1 and 2 in U.K.A.E.A. Defect Detection Trials. *Br. J. Non-Destr. Test.*, **25**(5), 249 – 255. [155], [156]

Bowker, K. J., R. K. Chapman and J. M. Wrigley [1985]. Some principles for the design of high performance automated ultrasonic defect detection systems. Report NWR/SSD/84/0158/R, Central Electricity Generating Board, London. [60], [204]

British Standards Institution [1993]. Guide to calibration and setting-up of the ultrasonic time-of-flight diffraction TOFD technique for the detection, location and sizing of flaws. British Standard BS 7706 : 1993. [195]

Broere, C., J. R. Hagedoorn and M. Lodder [1991]. Progress in ultrasonic signal imaging. In: D. Steininger, editor, *NDE Techniques for Nuclear Heat Exchangers,* San Diego, California (United States), 6 – 10 Oct. 1991, volume NE-Vol. 6, pages 49 – 53. American Society of Mechanical Engineers (1991). [183]

Browne, W. [1988]. Automated ultrasonic examination of primary circuit welds. In: N. Geary, editor, *Nuclear Technology International 1988*, pages 171 – 174. Sterling Publications Limited. [182], [183]

Browne, W. [1990a]. Advances in sub-sea ultrasonic imaging. In: *Proceedings of the International Conference on Advances in Underwater Inspection and Maintenance,* Aberdeen (United Kingdom), 24 – 25 May 1989, pages 155 – 172. Graham and Trotman (1990). [185]

Browne, W. [1990b]. Reliable and cost-effective in-service weld inspection using time-of-flight diffraction. *Welding & Metal Fabrications*, **58**(3), 153. [186]

Browne, W. [1997a]. The stunted growth of TOFD — and its cost to industry. *Insight*, **39**(9), 658. [192]

Browne, W. [1997b]. TOFD 2 — a case of a little learning. *Insight*, **39**(12), 908. [192]

Browne, W. and J. Verkooijen [1991]. Improved automated ultrasonic techniques for pipe-weld inspection. *Pipes & Pipelines International*, **36**(4), 11 – 16. [185]

Burch, S. F. [1987]. A comparison between SAFT and two-dimensional deconvolution methods for the improvement of resolution in ultrasonic B-scan images. *Ultrasonics*, **25**(5), 259 – 266. [103]

Burch, S. F. and N. K. Bealing [1986]. A physical approach to the automated ultrasonic characterization of buried weld defects in ferritic steel. *NDT Int.*, **19**(3), 145 – 153. [104]

Burch, S. F. and N. K. Bealing [1987]. Automated ultrasonic characterisation of welding defects in steel. In: J. M. Farley and P. D. Hanstead, editors, *NDT-86:* Proceedings of the 21st Annual British Conference on Nondestructive Testing, Newcastle-upon-Tyne, UK, 16 – 18 September 1986, pages 157–166. Engineering Materials Advisory Services, Ltd., Warley, West Midlands, UK. [104]

Burch, S. F. and A. T. Ramsey [1986]. Digital techniques to derive and display the phases of ultrasonic pulses. U.K.A.E.A. Report AERE-R 13026, HMSO, London. [35], [104]

Cameron, A. G. B., T. J. Jessop, P. J. Mudge, J. P. Charlesworth, M. G. Silk, K. J. Bowker, J. M. Wrigley and D. Denby [1983]. Size measurement and characterisation of weld defects by ultrasonic testing, Part 4. Report 3527/ /83, The Welding Institute, Cambridge. [108]

Cameron, R. F. [1984]. Theoretical calculations of pressure vessel failure frequencies for Sizewell B transients. U.K.A.E.A. Report AERE-R 11196, HMSO, London. [154], [178], [179], [221]

Cameron, R. F. and J. A. G. Temple [1984]. Ultrasonic inspection for long defects in thick steel components. *Int. J. Press. Vessels Piping*, **18**(4), 255 – 276. [154], [222]

Cameron, R. F. and J. A. G. Temple [1986]. Quantification of the reliability required of non-destructive inspection of PWR pressure vessels. *Nucl. Eng. Des.*, **91**(1), 57 – 68. [222]

Capineri, L., H. G. Tattersall, J. A. G. Temple and M. G. Silk [1992]. Time-of-flight diffraction tomography for NDT applications. *Ultrasonics*, **30**(5), 275 – 288. [104]

Capineri, L., G. Tattersall, M. G. Silk and J. A. G. Temple [1993]. Small size ultrasonic sources for time-of-flight diffraction tomography. In: *Ultrasonics International 93,* Conference Proceedings, Vienna (Austria), 6-8 Jul. 1993, pages 539 – 542. Butterworth-Heinemann Ltd (1993). [104]

Capineri, L., P. Grande, L. Masotti, J. A. G. Temple and C. G. Windsor [1997]. Advanced image processing techniques for automatic interpretation of time-of-flight diffraction images. In: S. Lees and L. A. Ferrari, editors, *Acoustical Imaging*, volume 23, pages 412 – 416. Plenum Press, New York, 1997. [104]

Capineri, L., P. Grande and J. A. G. Temple [1998]. Advanced image-processing techniques for real-time interpretation of ground penetrating radar images. *International Journal of Imaging Systems and Technology*, **9**(1), 51 – 59. [104]

Cecco, V. S. and G. H. Broomfield [1984]. B-scan displays of ultrasonic time-of-flight diffraction tests of compact tension specimens. U.K.A.E.A. Report AERE-R 11010, Harwell Laboratory. [186]

Cecco, V. S. and P. Carter [1983]. Ultrasonic time-of-flight diffraction for external inspection of pipe to cylindrical component welds. U.K.A.E.A. Report AERE-R 11008, Harwell Laboratory. [109]

Chapman, R. K. and J. M. Coffey [1982]. Ultrasonic scattering from smooth flat cracks: edge wave signals from finite cracks with curved edges. Report NWR/SSD/82/0034/R, Central Electricity Generating Board, London. [201], [202], [203]

Charlesworth, J. P. and B. M. Hawker [1984]. Inspection of the near-surface defect plate (DDT3) by the ultrasonic time-of-flight technique. *Br. J. Non-Destr. Test.*, **26**(2), 106 – 112. [53], [71], [164]

Charlesworth, J. P. and B. H. Lidington [1985]. The use of ultrasonic techniques for the detection of intergranular attack. In: P. J. Emerson and G. Oates, editors, *NDT-85: Proceedings of the 20th Annual British Conference on NDT, Strathclyde, 17 – 19 September 1985*, pages 509 – 522. Engineering Materials Advisory Services, Ltd., Warley, West Midlands, UK. [33]

Charlesworth, J. P. and J. A. G. Temple [1981]. Creeping waves in ultrasonic NDT. In: *Ultrasonics International '81*, pages 390 – 395. IPC Science and Technology Press, Guildford, Surrey. [145]

Charlesworth, J. P. and J. A. G. Temple [1982]. Ultrasonic inspection through anisotropic cladding. In: *Periodic Inspection of Pressurized Components*. Conference Publication 1982-9, pages 117 – 124. Intitution of Mechanical Engineers, London. [129], [132]

Coffey, J. M. and R. K. Chapman [1983]. Application of elastic scattering theory for smooth flat cracks to the quantitative prediction of ultrasonic detection and sizing. *Nucl. Energy*, **22**(5), 319 – 333. [19], [41], [72], [204]

Collingwood, J. C. [1987]. Nuclear NDT development at Harwell. *NDT Int.*, **20**(1), 33 – 41. [154]

Collingwood, J. C. and K. Newton [1987]. Effects of stress on the capability of NDT methods to detect and size fatigue cracks. In: J. M. Farley and R. W. Nichols, editors, *Non-Destructive Testing:* Proceedings of the 4th European Conference, London, 13 – 17 September 1987, pages 853 – 862. Pergamon Press, Oxford, New York. [235]

Cook, D. [1972]. Crack depth measurement with surface waves. *British Acoustical Society Proceedings,* Spring Meeting, University of Loughborough, 5 – 7 April 1972, **1**(3), Paper No. 72U19. [3]

Coster, P. [2000]. How rails fracture. *Railway Magazine*, **146**(1196), 10. [189]

Crutzen, S. [1988]. Third Programme for the Inspection of Steel Components (PISC III): An introduction. In: R. W. Nichols and S. Crutzen, editors, *Ultrasonic Inspection of Heavy Section Steel Components, The PISC II Final Report*, chapter 24, pages 643–666. Elsevier Applied Science, 1988. [165]

Crutzen, S. [1994]. PISC II status report on non-destructive examination practice and results, state of the art and PISC III results. European Commission Report EUR 15906 EN, NEA/CSNI/R(94)23,1994. [168]

Crutzen, S. J. [1985a]. PISC exercises: Looking for effective and reliable inspection procedures. *Nucl. Eng. Des.*, **86**, 197 – 218. [148]

Crutzen, S. J. [1985b]. Results of post-test NDE and destructive examinations. In: R. W. Nichols, G. Dau and S. J. Crutzen, editors, *Effective NDE for Structural Integrity*. Elsevier Applied Science Publishers, London, New York, 1988. [148]

Crutzen, S. J., W. Bürgers, F. Violin, L. Di Piazza, K. J. Cowburn and T. Sargent [1983]. Destructive examination of test plates 1 and 2 of the Defect Detection Trials (DDT Paper No 3.). *Br. J. Non-Destr. Test.*, **25**(4), 193 – 194. [164]

Crutzen, S. J., P. Jehenson, R. Nichols and M. Stephens [1985]. The PISC II project: initial conclusions regarding the procedures used in the round-robin tests. *NDT Int.*, **18**(5), 243 – 249. [148]

Curtis, G. J. and B. M. Hawker [1983]. Automated time-of-flight studies of the Defect Detection Trials plates 1 and 2. *Br. J. Non-Destr. Test.*, **25**(5), 240 – 248. [42], [53], [71], [73], [135], [161]

Curtis, G. J. and M. W. Stringfellow [1986]. Automated inspection of PISC-II plate 2 and the PWR inlet nozzle at Harwell. In: R. W. Nichols and S. J. Crutzen, editors, *Ultrasonic Inspection of Heavy Section Steel Components:* The PISC II Final Report, pages 503 – 524. Elsevier Applied Science Publishers, London, New York, 1988. [120], [122]

Daniels, W. L., B. M. Hawker and D. F. Loy [1996]. SG nozzle inspection. *Nuclear Engineering International*, **41**(498), 23 – 25. [124], [182], [198]

Dawson, D. G., P. Clough and M. G. Silk [1989]. Ultrasonic detection and sizing of thermal fatigue cracks in stainless steel cylinders. In: C. Brook and P. Hanstead, editors, *Reliability in Non-Destructive Testing,* Proceedings of the 27th Annual British Conference on Non-Destructive Testing, Portsmouth (United Kingdom), 12 – 15 Sep. 1988, pages 385 – 395. Pergamon Press, 1989. [187]

Day, P. [1992]. Experience in the routine application of Zipscan time-of-flight diffraction techniques to the in-service examination of generator end rings. *Brit. J. Non-Destr. Test.*, **34**(1), 9 – 14. [184]

Denby, D. and A. C. Duncumb [1985]. The effects of stress on the ultrasonic detectability of defects. In: *Non-Destructive Testing in the Fitness for Purpose Assessment of Welded Constructions:* Proceedings of an international conference, London 20 – 22 November 1984, pages 73 – 81. The Welding Institute, Cambridge. [140]

Dijkstra, F. H., J. A. de Raad and T. Bourna [1997]. TOFD and acceptance criteria: a perfect team. *Insight*, **39**(4), 268 – 270. [192], [194]

Dombret, P. H. [1994]. PISC III results on Action 3: Nozzles and dissimilar metal welds. In: E. Borloo and P. Lemaître, editors, *Non-Destructive Examination Practice and Results, State of the art and PISC III results,* Proceedings of the joint CEC, OECD IAEA Specialist Meeting held at Petten on 8 – 10 March 1994, pages 11 – 31. [169], [171]

Doyle, P. A. and C. M. Scala [1978]. Crack depth measurement by ultrasonics: a review. *Ultrasonics*, **16**(4), 164 – 170. [3]

Dube, N. and H. Helleringer [1989]. Time of flight diffraction technique used for low pressure steam turbine rotor inspections using the Tomoscan. In: *Proceedings: Steam Turbine/Generation NDE Workshop,* Charlotte North Carolina (United States), 12 – 15 Sep. 1989, pages 27–1 – 27–12. Electric Power Research Institute. EPRI NP-6993 (1990). [184]

European Committee for Standardisation [1996]. Time-of-flight diffraction technique as a method for defect detection and sizing. In: *Nondestructive Testing - Ultrasonic Examination*. CEN/TC 138/WG 2 N 173, 1996. [195], [196]

European Network for Inspection Qualification [1997]. European methodology for qualification of non-destructive tests. Report EUR 17299 EN, European Commission. [197]

Flach, W. T., W. T. Clayton and G. L. Lagleder [1985]. In-service inspection of reactor pressure vessels in the United States. In: *Non-Destructive Testing in the Fitness for Purpose Assessment of Welded Constructions:* Proceedings of an international conference, London 20 – 22 November 1984, pages 107 – 109. The Welding Institute, Cambridge. [47]

Freedman, A. [1962]. A mechanism of acoustic echo formation. *Acustica*, **12**, 10 – 21. [105]

Friedlander, F. G. [1958]. *Sound Pulses*. Cambridge University Press, Cambridge. [105]

Fuller, M. D., J. B. Nestleroth and J. L. Rose [1983]. A proposed ultrasonic inspection technique for offshore structures. *Mater. Eval.*, **41**(5), 571. [110]

Gardner, W. E. and H. Bosselaar [1984]. The inspection of offshore structures: defect sizing by the time-of-flight diffraction technique. In: *Offshore Steel Structure Conference,* 23 – 24 October 1984. Netherlands Industrial Council for Oceanography. [110], [111], [112], [113], [185]

Gardner, W. E. and J. A. Hudson [1982]. Ultrasonic inspection of thick section pressure vessel steel by the time of flight diffraction method. In: R. B. Clough, editor, *Quantitative NDE in the Nuclear Industry:* Proceedings of the Fifth International Conference on Nondestructive Evaluation in the Nuclear Industry, San Diego, USA, 10 – 13 May 1982, pages 250 – 257. American Society for Metals, Metals Park, Ohio, USA. [154]

Gartside, C. and J. Hurst [1994]. Application of TOFD inspection technique to fasteners in power generating plant. *Insight*, **36**(4), 215 – 217. [183]

Gillan, M. T. [1980]. Ultrasonic wave propagation in austenitic stainless steel weld metal. U.K.A.E.A. Report TP-839, Harwell Laboratory. [214]

Golan, S. [1981]. Optimization of the crack-tip ultrasonic diffraction technique for sizing of cracks. *Mater. Eval.*, **39**(2), 166 – 169. [53]

Golan, S., L. Adler, K. V. Cook, R. K. Nanstad and T. K. Bolland [1980]. Ultrasonic diffraction technique for characterization of fatigue cracks. *J. Nondestr. Eval.*, **1**(1), 11 – 19. [53]

Gordon, J. E. [1976]. *The New Science of Strong Materials or Why You Don't Fall Through the Floor*. Penguin Books, Harmondsworth, second edition. [2]

Graff, K. F. [1975]. *Wave Motion in Elastic Solids*. Oxford University Press, Oxford. [199], [203], [204]

Grohs, B., O. A. Barbian and W. Kappes [1983]. ALOK - principles and results obtained in DDT. In: *Defect Detection and Sizing:* Proceedings of a meeting sponsored jointly by The OECD Nuclear Energy Agency and The International Atomic Energy Agency, Ispra Joint Research Centre, 3 – 6 May 1983, pages 689 – 719. [49], [156]

Gruber, G. J. and G. J. Hendrix [1984]. Sizing of near-surface fatigue cracks in cladded reactor pressure vessels using satellite pulses. In: H. N. Wadley, editor, *NDE in the Nuclear Industry:* Proceedings of the 6th International Conference,

Zurich, Switzerland, 28 November – 2 December 1983, pages 83–95. American Society for Metals, Metals Park, Ohio, USA. [47]

Gruber, G. J., D. R. Hamlin, H. L. Grothues and J. L. Jackson [1986]. Imaging of fatigue cracks in cladded pressure vessels with the SLIC-50. *NDT Int.*, **19**(3), 155 – 161. [48]

Hahn, G. J. and S. S. Shapiro [1967]. *Statistical Methods in Engineering*. John Wiley, New York. [218], [219]

Haines, N. F. [1980]. The theory of sound transmission and reflection at contacting surfaces. Report RD/B/N4744, Central Electricity Generating Board, London. [140], [142]

Haines, N. F., D. B. Langston, A. J. Green and R. Wilson [1982]. An assessment of the reliability of ultrasonic inspection methods. In: *Periodic Inspection of Pressurized Components:* Conference Publication 1982-9, pages 239 – 255. Institution of Mechanical Engineers, London. [4]

Harker, A. H. [1984]. Numerical modelling of the scattering of elastic waves in plates. *J. Nondestr. Eval.*, **4**(2), 89 – 106. [6]

Harker, A. H., J. A. Ogilvy and J. A. G. Temple [1991]. Modelling ultrasonic inspection of austenitic welds. *J.Nondestr. Eval.*, **9**, 155 – 165. [139], [170]

Hawker, B. M. [1983]. The automation of inspection of thick steel sections using the ultrasonic time-of-flight technique. *Nucl. Energy*, **22**(5), 309 – 318. [38], [42], [98], [135]

Hawker, B. M. and S. F. Burch [1999]. TOFD inspection design and data interpretation. In: *BINDT Mini-Conference on TOFD Techniques,* Wadham College, Oxford, (United Kingdom), 2 – 3 July 1999. (Proceedings not published). [72], [73], [74], [98], [106]

Hawker, B. M., K. Newton and A. P. Wein [1985]. Sizing defects in complex geometries underwater by ultrasonic TOFD. In: P. J. Emerson and G. Oates, editors, *NDT-85:* Proceedings of the 20th Annual British Conference on NDT, Strathclyde, 17 – 19 September 1985, pages 171 – 185. Engineering Materials Advisory Services, Ltd., Warley, West Midlands, UK. [113], [185]

Helleringer, H. and J. Salin [1990]. Inspection of low-pressure steam turbine rotors with a Tomoscan. determination of crack height by ultrasonic time of flight diffraction. *Revue Generale Nucleaire*, (2 (Mar. – Apr. 1990)), 145 – 149. (In French). [184]

Highmore, P. and A. Rogerson [1988]. Advances in ultrasonic flaw characterisation. In: *Proceedings of the 4th European Conference on Non-Destructive Testing,* London (United Kingdom), 13 – 17 Sep. 1987, volume 3, pages 1553 – 1563. Pergamon Press. [102], [104]

Hunt, C. A. [1975]. Nondestructive measurement of cracks in gun barrels. Technical Report 20/75, R.A.R.D.E. [45]

Hurst, D. P. and J. A. G. Temple [1982]. Calculation of the velocity of creeping waves and their application to nondestructive testing. *Int. J. Press. Vessels Piping*, **10**, 451 – 464. [217]

Jessop, T. J. [1979]. Size measurement and characterisation of weld defects by ultrasonic testing, Part 1: Non-planar defects in ferritic steels. Report No. 3527/4/77, The Welding Institute, Cambridge. [151], [152], [243]

Jessop, T. J., P. J. Mudge, J. D. Harrison, J. P. Charlesworth, E. E. Aldridge, M. G. Silk, J. M. Coffey, K. J. Bowker, J. M. Wrigley and D. Denby [1982]. Size measurement and characterisation of weld defects by ultrasonic testing, Part 2: Planar defects in ferritic steels. Report No. 3527/11/81, The Welding Institute, Cambridge. [152], [153], [243]

Karal, F. C. and J. B. Keller [1959]. Elastic wave propagation in homogeneous and inhomogeneous media. *J. Acoust. Soc. Am*, **31**(6), 694 – 705. [52], [200]

Keller, J. B. [1957]. Diffraction by an aperture. *J. Appl. Phys.*, **28**(4), 426 – 444. [52], [200], [201]

Keller, J. B. [1962]. Geometrical theory of diffraction. *J. Opt. Soc. Am.*, **52**(2), 116 – 130. [52]

Kendall, K. and D. Tabor [1971]. An ultrasonic study of the area of contact between stationary and sliding surfaces. *Proc. R. Soc. London*, **Ser. A, 323**, 321 – 340. [142]

Kittel, C. [1963]. *Introduction to Solid State Physics*. John Wiley, New York, second edition. [129]

Lam, F. K. and W. M. Tsang [1985]. Flaw characterisation based on diffraction of ultrasonic waves. *Ultrasonics*, **23**(1), 14 – 20. [105], [213]

Lemaître, P. and T. D. Kobl [1995a]. PISC III Report No. 33, report on the evaluation of the inspection results of the wrought-to-wrought PISC III assemblies no. 31, 32, 33, 34, 35 and 36. European Commission Report EUR 15663 EN, European Commission Joint Research Centre, Organisation for Economic Cooperation and Development, Nuclear Energy Agency/CSNI. [172], [173]

Lemaître, P. and T. D. Kobl [1995b]. PISC III Report No. 35, report on the evaluation of the inspection results of the wrought-to-cast PISC III assembly 51 and weld a of assembly 43. European Commission Report EUR 15665 EN, European Commission Joint Research Centre, Organisation for Economic Cooperation and Development, Nuclear Energy Agency/CSNI. [173]

Lewis, P. A., J. A. G. Temple and G. R. Wickham [1996a]. Elastic wave diffraction at cracks in anisotropic materials. In: D. Thompson and D. Chimenti, editors, *Review of Progress in Quantitative Nondestructive Evaluation*, volume 15, pages 41 – 48. Plenum Press, New York. [138]

Lewis, P. A., J. A. G. Temple and G. R. Wickham [1996b]. Optimisation of ultrasonic inspection of welds in nuclear power plant. *Insight*, **38**(7). [138]

Lewis, P. A., J. A. G. Temple, E. J. Walker and G. R. Wickham [1998]. Calculation of diffraction coefficients for a semi-infinite crack embedded in an infinite anisotropic linearly elastic body. *Proc. Roy. Soc. Lond.*, **A 454**, 1781 – 1803. [73], [138]

Lidington, B. H. and M. G. Silk [1975]. Crack depth measurement using a single surface wave probe. *Br. J. Non-Destr. Test.*, **17**(6), 165 – 167. [8], [45]

Lidington, B. H., M. G. Silk, P. Montgomery and G. F. Hammond [1976]. Ultrasonic measurements of the depth of fatigue cracks. *Br. J. Non-Destr. Test.*, **18**(6), 165 – 170. [25], [26]

Lilley, J. and P. Osborne [1991]. In-line inspection using time-of-flight diffraction. *Welding & Metal Fabrication*, **59**(8), 457 – 460. [185]

Lilley, J. R. [1989]. Time-of-flight-diffraction (TOFD) techniques for crack detection and sizing in turbine rotor shafts, discs and generator retaining rings. In: J. Boogaard and G. van Dijk, editors, *Proceedings of the 12th World Conference on Non-Destructive Testing,* Amsterdam (Netherlands), 23 – 28 Apr. 1989, volume 2, pages 1104 – 1106. Elsevier, 1989. [182]

Lilley, J. R. and J. Pitcher [1989]. Underclad crack detection, sizing and monitoring with the time-of-flight-diffraction technique using zipscan. In: J. Boogaard and G. van Dijk, editors, *Proceedings of the 12th World Conference on Non-Destructive Testing,* Amsterdam (Netherlands), 23 – 28 Apr. 1989, volume 2, pages 1041–1043. Elsevier, 1989. [183]

Lock, D. L., K. J. Cowburn and B. Watkins [1983]. The results obtained in the UKAEA Defect Detection Trials on test pieces 3 and 4. *Nucl. Energy*, **22**(5), 357 – 363. [153], [164]

Lucia, A. and G. Volta [1983]. Requirements for NDI reliability as a function of the size and position of defects in RPVs. In: *Defect Detection and Sizing:* Proceedings of a meeting sponsored jointly by the OECD Nuclear Energy Agency and the International Atomic Energy Agency, Ispra Joint Research Centre, 3 – 6 May 1983, pages 793 – 822. [178]

MacDonald, D. E. [1990]. Images of flaws in generator retaining rings using SAFT reconstruction of TOFD data. In: D. Thompson and D. Chimenti, editors, *Review of Progress in Quantitative Nondestructive Evaluation*, volume 9, pages 766 – 772. Plenum Press, New York. [184]

Mak, D. K. [1985]. Ultrasonic measurement of crack depth. *Canad. Soc. Non-Destr. Test. J.*, **6**(6), 36 – 40. [42], [44]

Mak, D. K. [1986]. Correction of beam entry points for the pitch-catch technique in ultrasonic testing. *Canad. Soc. Non-Destr. Test. J.*, **7**(4), 22 – 36. [44]

Marshall, W. [1982]. *An Assessment of the Integrity of PWR Pressure Vessels:* Report by a study group under the Chairmanship of Dr W. Marshall CBE, FRS. U.K.A.E.A., London. [154], [178], [179], [219], [220], [221]

Maue, A. W. [1953]. Z. *Angew. Math. Mech.*, **33**(1/2), 1 – 10. [19], [204]

Miller, J. J. [1970]. Ultrasonic measurement of crack depth in thick-walled cylinders. Report No. AD707760 (WVT-7017)., U.S. Government. [6]

Miller, J. J., R. R. Fujczak and D. C. Winters [1973]. Measurement and analysis of fatigue crack growth in cylindrical shapes. In: *Fracture and Flaws:* Proceedings of the 13th Annual Symposium, Alburquerque, New Mexico, USA, 1 – 2 March 1973, pages 55 – 56. [45]

Mudge, P. J. [1980]. Ultrasonic time of flight measurement of fatigue pre-crack depth in fracture toughness specimens. In: C. J. Beevers, editor, *Measurement of Crack Length and Shape during Fracture and Fatigue:* Proceedings of a symposium, Birmingham (UK), May 1979, pages 393 – 399. Engineering Materials Advisory Services Ltd., Warley, West Midlands, UK. [186]

Mudge, P. J. [1982]. Size measurement and characterisation of weld defects by ultrasonic testing, Part 3: The effects of metallurgical features in ferritic steels. Report No. 3527/11/81, The Welding Institute, Cambridge. [243]

Mudge, P. J. and A. C. Duncumb [1985]. NDT of steel bridges. In: P. J. Emerson and G. Oates, editors, *NDT-85:* Proceedings of the 20th Annual British Conference on NDT, Strathclyde, 17 – 19 September 1985, pages 321 – 333. Engineering Materials Advisory Services Ltd., Warley, West Midlands, UK. [187], [188]

Murgatroyd, R. A. and D. Firth [1985]. A review and further analysis of the results of the Defect Detection Trials. *Int. J. Press. Vessel Piping*, **28**(1-5), 275 – 293 (1987). [156]

Murgatroyd, R. A., H. Seed, A. J. Willetts and H. Tickle [1983]. Inspection of Defect Detection Trials plates 1 and 2 by the Materials Physics Department, RNL. *Br. J. Non-Destr. Test.*, **25**(6), 313 – 319. [137], [156]

Murgatroyd, R. A., P. J. Highmore, S. F. Burch, T. Bann and A. T. Ramsey [1988]. PISC II parametric study on flaw characterisation using the tandem and TOFD techniques. *Int. J. Press. Vess. Piping*, **35**, 137 – 169. [105]

Newton, K. [1987]. The transparency of fatigue cracks to NDT methods used for the inspection of offshore structures. In: *Proceedings of Offshore Europe 87:* Proceedings of a conference held at Aberdeen, Scotland, September 1987. Society of Petroleum Engineers of AIME. [See Collingwood and Newton, 1987]. [115], [144], [185]

Newton, K. [1990]. The development of new techniques for underwater inspection of offshore structures. In: *Proceedings of the 9th International Conference on Offshore Mechanics and Arctic Engineering,* Houston, Texas (United States), 18 – 28 Feb. 1990, volume 3B, pages 547 – 553. The American Society of Mechanical Engineers. [185]

Newton, K., A. P. Wein and B. M. Hawker [1986]. Research into new methods for detection and sizing of defects in subsea steel constructions. In: T. Melligen, editor, *Underwater Technology Conference-86*, page 89. Norwegian Underwater Technology Centre, Bergen, Norway. [113], [114], [185]

Nichols, R. W. [1985]. Summary and conclusions. In: R. W. Nichols, G. Dau and S. J. Crutzen, editors, *Effective NDE for Structural Integrity*. Elsevier Applied Science Publishers, London, New York 1988. [156]

Nichols, R. W. and S. Crutzen [1988a]. In: R. W. Nichols and S. Crutzen, editors, *Ultrasonic Inspection of Heavy Section Steel Components, The PISC II Final Report*, page 10. Elsevier Applied Science, 1988. [166]

Nichols, R. W. and S. Crutzen [1988b]. In: R. W. Nichols and S. Crutzen, editors, *Ultrasonic Inspection of Heavy Section Steel Components, The PISC II Final Report*, page 44. Elsevier Applied Science, 1988. [166]

Norris, A. N. and J. D. Achenbach [1984]. Elastic wave diffraction by a semi-infinite crack in a transversely isotropic material. *Q. J. Mech. Appl. Math.*, **37**, 565 – 580. [138]

Nottingham, L. D. and D. E. MacDonald [1988]. Enhanced ultrasonic target identification in generator rotor retaining rings. In: J. E. Doherty and X. Edelmann, editors, *9th International Conference on Nondestructive Evaluation in the Nuclear Industry,* Tokyo (Japan), 25 – 28 Apr. 1988, pages 477 – 482. ASM International 1988. [184]

Nottingham, L. D. and D. E. MacDonald [1989]. Ultrasonic target identification in generator rotor retaining rings. In: J. Boogaard and G. van Dijk, editors, *Proceedings of the 12th World Conference on Non-Destructive Testing,* Amsterdam (Netherlands), 23 – 28 Apr. 1989, volume 2, pages 1128 – 1130. Elsevier, 1989. [184]

Nottingham, L. D. and D. E. MacDonald [1990]. Time-of-flight diffraction ultrasonic measurement of igscc in generator retaining rings. In: M. J. Whittle, J. E. Doherty and K. Iida, editors, *Proceedings of the 10th International Conference on*

*NDE in the Nuclear and Pressure Vessel Industries,* Glasgow (Scotland), 11 – 14 Jun. 1990, pages 597 – 601. ASM International, (1990). [184]

Ogilvy, J. A. [1985a]. Computerized ultrasonic ray tracing in austenitic steel. *NDT Int.*, **18**(2), 67 – 78. [137], [139]

Ogilvy, J. A. [1985b]. A model for elastic wave propagation in anisotropic media with applications to ultrasonic inspection through austenitic steel. *Br. J. Non-Destr. Test*, **27**(1), 13 – 21. [130], [137], [139]

Ogilvy, J. A. [1987]. On the theory of ultrasonic wave scattering from rough surfaces. U.K.A.E.A. Report AERE-R 12853, HMSO, London. [61]

Ogilvy, J. A. and J. A. G. Temple [1983]. Diffraction of elastic waves by cracks: application to time-of-flight inspection. *Ultrasonics*, **21**(6), 259 – 269. [19], [53], [204], [206]

Oliver, P. [1984]. The reliability of non-destructive test methods: the PISC programmes. In: *NEA Newsletter,* No. 2 (June 1984), page 15. OECD Nuclear Energy Agency, Paris. [61], [204]

Olver, F. W. J., editor [1960]. *Royal Society Mathematical Tables Bessel Functions 3.* Cambridge University Press, Cambridge. [217]

Osborne, P. [1989]. Time-of-flight diffraction for ultrasonic inspection. *Underwater Systems Design*, **11**(1), 22 – 23. [185]

Packman, P. F., J. K. Malpani and F. M. Wells [1976]. Probability of flaw detection for use in fracture control plans. In: H. Miyamoto and T. Kunio, editors, *Proceedings of a Joint Japan-USA Seminar,* Syracuse University, New York, 7 – 11 October 1974, pages 129 – 143. Northhoff International Publishing, Leyden, Netherlands. [218]

Peck, J. C. and J. Miklowitz [1969]. Shadow-zone response in the diffraction of a plane compressional wave pulse by a circular cavity. *Int. J. Solids Struct.*, **5**, 437 – 454. [215], [216]

Pennick, A. M. [1993]. Ultrasonic inspection of the Calder Hall and Chaplecross reactor pressure vessels. In: *Remote Techniques for Nuclear Plant,* Stratford-upon-Avon (United Kingdom), 10 – 13 May 1993, pages 145 – 151. British Nuclear Energy Society (1993). [183]

Pers-Anderson, E.-B. [1991]. Detection and repair of a crack in a BWR feed water nozzle safe-end weld. In: *Management of In-service Inspection of Pressure Systems,* London (United Kingdom), 12 – 13 Mar. 1991, pages 129 – 130. Institution of Mechanical Engineers (1991). [182]

PISC [1979]. A description of the PISC project; evaluation of the PISC trials results; analysis scheme of the PISC trials results; destructive examination of the PVRC plates nos 50/52, 51/53 and 204; ultrasonic examination of the PVRC plates nos 50/52, 51/53 and 204; being Volumes I to V respectively of Report No. EUR 6371 en. Commission of The European Communities, Brussels. [5], [148], [153]

PISC [1986a]. Destructive examination of the PISC-II RRT plates. In: R. W. Nichols and S. J. Crutzen, editors, *Ultrasonic Inspection of Heavy Steel Components:* The PISC II Final Report, pages 113 – 180. Elsevier Applied Science Publishers, London, New York, 1988. [165]

PISC [1986b]. Evaluation of the PISC-II trials results. In: R. W. Nichols and S. J. Crutzen, editors, *Ultrasonic Inspection of Heavy Steel Components:* The PISC II Final Report, pages 205 – 408. Elsevier Applied Science Publishers, London, New York, 1988. [165]

PISC [1986c]. The round-robin test of the PISC-II programme: plates and ultrasonic procedures used. In: R. W. Nichols and S. J. Crutzen, editors, *Ultrasonic Inspection of Heavy Steel Components:* The PISC II Final Report, pages 59 – 112. Elsevier Applied Science Publishers, London, New York, 1988. [121]

PISC [1986d]. A summary of the PISC-II project. In: R. W. Nichols and S. J. Crutzen, editors, *Ultrasonic Inspection of Heavy Steel Components:* The PISC II Final Report, pages 3 – 58. Elsevier Applied Science Publishers, London, New York, 1988. [164]

Pitcher, J. M. [1989]. Rapid detection and accurate sizing of primary circuit weld defects. In: J. Boogaård and G. van Dijk, editors, *Proceedings of the 12th World Conference on Non-Destructive Testing,* Amsterdam Netherlands), 23 – 28 Apr. 1989, volume 2, pages 1101–1103. Elsevier, 1989. [182]

Poulter, L. N. J. [1986]. Signal processing methods applied in the ultrasonic inspection of PWR inlet nozzles. *NDT Int.*, **19**(3), 141 – 144. [122], [123]

Poulter, L. N. J., A. Rogerson, A. J. Willetts and A. V. Dyke [1982]. Inspection of the Defect Detection Trials plate 4 by the Materials Physics Department, RNL. *Br. J. Non-Destr. Test.*, **26**(2), 77 – 83. [156]

Ramsdale, S. A. [1983]. *Diffraction of elastic waves by rough semi-infinite cracks.* Ph.D. thesis, University of Manchester. [69]

Ramsey, A. T. [1987]. U.K.A.E.A. Harwell Laboratory, private communication. [94], [96]

Rao, B. P. C. and B. Raj [1998]. Time-of-flight measurements with shear horizontal waves. In: *7th European Conference on Non-Destructive Testing,* Copenhagen, 26 – 29 May,1998, pages 2979 – 2986. [137]

Ravenscroft, F. A., K. Newton and C. B. Scruby [1991]. Diffraction of ultrasound by cracks: comparison of experiment with theory. *Ultrasonics*, **29**, 29 – 37. [35], [59], [206]

Reynolds, W. N. and R. L. Smith [1984]. Ultrasonic attenuation in metals. *J.Phys. D: Appl. Phys.*, **17**, 109 – 116. [128]

Rogerson, A. and R. A. Murgatroyd [1980]. Defect characterisation using ultrasonic techniques. In: R. S. Sharpe, editor, *Research Techniques in Nondestructive Testing*, volume 4, chapter 12, pages 452 – 507. Academic Press, London. [104]

Rogerson, A., L. N. J. Poulter, P. Clough and A. G. Cooper [1988]. RNL automated inspection of the PISC-II PWR inlet nozzle (Plate 3). *Br. J. Non-Destr. Test.*, **30**(2), 86 – 93. [122], [165]

Rose, J. L., M. C. Fuller, J. B. Nestleroth and Y. H. Jeong [1983]. An ultrasonic global inspection technique for an offshore K-joint. *Soc. Pet. Eng. J.*, **23**(2), 358. [110]

Rusbridge, K. L. and G. C. Roberts [1982]. The ultrasonic examination of artificial defects in diffusion bonded steel samples using time-of-flight diffraction. U.K.A.E.A. Report AERE-R 10649, Harwell Laboratory. [188]

Sawley, K. and R. Rieff [2000]. Rail failure assessment for the Office of the Rail Regulator. Report P-00-070, Transportation Technology Center, Inc. [189]

Scruby, C. B. and K. Newton [1986]. UKAEA. Harwell Laboratory, private communication. [59]

Scruby, C. B., R. J. Dewhurst, D. A. Hutchins and S. B. Palmer [1981]. Quantitative measurements of laser generated acoustic waveforms. U.K.A.E.A. Report AERE-R 10307, Harwell Laboratory. [186]

Scruby, C. B., R. J. Dewhurst, D. A. Hutchins and S. B. Palmer [1982]. Laser generation of ultrasound in metals. In: R. S. Sharpe, editor, *Research Techniques in Nondestructive Testing*, volume 5, pages 281 – 327. Academic Press, London. [186]

Sigmond, R. S. and E. Lien [1980]. Ultrasonic diffraction measurements of fatigue crack growth. *Br. J. Non-Destr. Test.*, **22**(6), 281 – 283. [186]

Silk, M. G. [1976]. Accurate crack depth measurements in welded assemblies. In: *Eighth World Conference on Nondestructive Testing,* Cannes, France, 6 – 11 September 1976. Paper 2B16. [7]

Silk, M. G. [1977]. The transfer of ultrasonic energy in the geometry of the diffraction technique for crack sizing. U.K.A.E.A. Report AERE-R 8665, Harwell Laboratory. [See Silk, 1979f]. [59]

Silk, M. G. [1978]. The fundamental sources of error in ultrasonic defect sizing. In: *Recent Developments and Special Methods of NDT:* Proceedings of the First European Conference on NDT, Mainz, 24 – 26 April 1978, volume 1, pages 43 – 54. Deutsche Gesellschaft für Zerstörungsfreie Prüfung, Berlin. [32]

Silk, M. G. [1979a]. Accurate techniques for defect sizing in pressurized components. In: *Periodic Inspection of Pressurized Components*, pages 155 – 162. Institution of Mechanical Engineers, London. [3], [25]

Silk, M. G. [1979b]. Defect sizing using ultrasonic diffraction. *Br. J. Non-Destr. Test.*, **21**(1), 12 – 15. [45], [59]

Silk, M. G. [1979c]. The propagation of polarized shear waves in steel. U.K.A.E.A. Report AERE-R 9423, Harwell Laboratory. [128]

Silk, M. G. [1979d]. The propagation of ultrasound in austenitic weldments. U.K.A.E.A. Report AERE-R 9391, Harwell Laboratory. [128]

Silk, M. G. [1979e]. A separable probe technique for accurate crack sizing using ultrasonic diffraction. In: *Ultrasonics International 79:* Proceedings of a conference held at Graz, Austria, 15 – 17 May 1979, pages 415 – 426. IPC Science and Technology Press, Guildford, Surrey. [3]

Silk, M. G. [1979f]. The transfer of ultrasonic energy in the geometry of the diffraction technique for crack sizing. *Ultrasonics*, **17**(3), 113–121. [58], [238]

Silk, M. G. [1980a]. A computer model for complex orthotropic structures. U.K.A.E.A. Report AERE-R 9666, Harwell Laboratory. [See Silk, 1981a]. [137]

Silk, M. G. [1980b]. Ultrasonic techniques for inspecting austenitic welds. In: R. S. Sharpe, editor, *Research Techniques in Nondestructive Testing*, volume 4, chapter 11, pages 393–449. Academic Press, London. [128]

Silk, M. G. [1981a]. A computer model for ultrasonic propagation in complex orthotropic structures. *Ultrasonics*, **19**(5), 208–212. [239]

Silk, M. G. [1981b]. The propagation of ultrasound in anisotropic weldments. *Mater. Eval.*, **39**(5), 462 – 466. [128]

Silk, M. G. [1981c]. Relationships between metallurgical texture and ultrasonic propagation. *Met. Sci.*, **15**(11 – 12), 559 – 565. [128]

Silk, M. G. [1982a]. Defect detection and sizing in metals using ultrasound. *Int. Metall. Rev.*, **27**(1), 28 – 50. [3]

Silk, M. G. [1982b]. The fundamental accuracy of ultrasonic time-of-flight testing techniques. In: *Periodic Inspection of Pressurized Components.* Conference Publication 1982-9, pages 125 – 133. Institution of Mechanical Engineers, London. [3]

Silk, M. G. [1982c]. Ultrasonic developments in the UK for RPV weldments. In: R. W. Nichols, editor, *Advances in Non-Destructive Examination for Structural Integrity*, pages 101 – 116. Applied Science Publishers, Essex. [3]

Silk, M. G. [1984]. The use of diffraction-based time-of-flight measurements to locate and size defects. *Br. J. Non-Destr. Test.*, **26**(4), 208 – 213. [3]

Silk, M. G. [1987]. Changes in ultrasonic defect location and sizing. *NDT Int.*, **20**(1), 9 – 14. [186]

Silk, M. G. [1987b]. The interpretation of TOFD data in the light of ASME-XI and similar rules. U.K.A.E.A. Report AERE-R 12158, Harwell Laboratory. [See Silk, 1989b]. [178]

Silk, M. G. [1989a]. Flaw growth monitoring for safer plant. *Atom*, (394), 6 – 9. [187]

Silk, M. G. [1989b]. The interpretation of TOFD data in the light of ASME XI and similar rules. *Brit. J. Non-Destr. Test.*, **31**(5), 242 – 251. [193], [240]

Silk, M. G. [1994]. Benefits of signal processing in ultrasonic inspection. *Insight*, **36**(10), 776 – 781. [104]

Silk, M. G. [1996a]. Estimation of the probability of detection of flaws in TOFD data with varying levels of noise. *Insight*, **38**(1), 31 – 36. [105]

Silk, M. G. [1996b]. An evaluation of the performance of the TOFD technique as a means of sizing flaws, with particular reference to flaws with curved profiles. *Insight*, **38**(4), 31 – 36. [106]

Silk, M. G. and C. P. Hobbs [1990]. Practical derivation of flaw behaviour: an aid to condition monitoring. *Condition Monitoring and Diagnostic Technology*, **1**(1), 18. [187]

Silk, M. G. and B. H. Lidington [1974a]. Corrections of ultrasonic time delay measurements of crack depth. U.K.A.E.A. Report AERE-M 2654, Harwell Laboratory. [8]

Silk, M. G. and B. H. Lidington [1974b]. Defect sizing using an ultrasonic time delay approach. U.K.A.E.A. Report AERE-R 7774, Harwell Laboratory. [see Silk and Lidington, 1975]. [3]

Silk, M. G. and B. H. Lidington [1975]. Defect sizing usuing an ultrasonic time delay approach. *Br. J. Non-Destr. Test*, **17**, 33 – 36. [3], [240]

Silk, M. G., B. H. Lidington, P. Montgomery and G. F. Hammond [1976]. Ultrasonic time domain measurements of the depth of crack-like defects in ferritic and austenitic steels. In: *Ultrasonic Inspection of Reactor Components,*

OECD/NEA Committee on the Safety of Nuclear Installations, Specialists' Meeting, Risley, UK 27 – 29 September 1976. Publication SNI 9/16. OECD Nuclear Energy Agency, Paris. [7]

Silk, M. G., B. H. Lidington and G. F. Hammond [1980]. A time domain approach to crack location and sizing in austenitic welds. *Br. J. Non-Destr. Test.*, **22**(2), 55 – 61. [3]

Silk, M. G., K. F. Bainton, M. J. Hillier and N. Robertson [1986a]. Investigation of the use of horizontally polarized shear waves for TOFD studies on austenitic steel. U.K.A.E.A. Report AERE-R 12145, Harwell Laboratory. [137]

Silk, M. G., M. J. Hillier, G. F. Hammond and P. C. Jones [1986b]. TOFD work at Grangemouth refinery. In: J. M. Farley and P. D. Hanstead, editors, *NDT-86:* Proceedings of the 21st Annual British Conference on Non-Destructive Testing, Newcastle upon Tyne, 16 – 18 September 1986, pages 207 – 224. Engineering Materials Advisory Services Ltd., Warley, West Midlands, UK. [186]

Silk, M. G., A. D. Whapham and C. P. Hobbs [1989]. Flaw growth monitoring as an aid to lifetime prediction. *Int. J. Materials & Product Technology*, **4**(3), 215 – 231. [187]

Slesenger, T. A., G. B. Hesketh and M. G. Silk [1985]. An introduction to the concepts and hardware used for ultrasonic time-of-flight data collection and analysis. U.K.A.E.A. Report AERE-M 3388, Harwell Laboratory. [94], [95]

Stelwagen, U. [1995]. NIL project non-destructive testing of thin plate. Final Report NDP 93-40, Dutch Welding Society, NIL. [175], [176]

Stringfellow, M. W. and J. K. Perring [1984]. Detection and sizing of inner radius defects in DDT plate 4 (simulated PWR nozzle) by the ultrasonic time-of-flight diffraction technique. *Br. J. Non-Destr. Test.*, **26**(2), 84 – 91. [53], [119], [120], [164]

Stringfellow, M. W. and J. A. G. Temple [1987]. U.K.A.E.A. Harwell Laboratory, unpublished work. [70]

Takeuchi, I., K. Morimoto, M. Hamana, M. Taniguchi and S. Hiraga [1996]. Development of evaluation system of ultrasonic testing data. *Mitsubishi Heavy Industries Technical Review*, **33**(6), 420 – 423. In Japanese. [186]

Temple, J. A. G. [1980]. Calculations of the reflection and transmission of ultrasound by cracks in steel, filled with liquid sodium. *Ultrasonics*, **18**(4), 165 – 169. [145]

Temple, J. A. G. [1981a]. Calculations of the reflection and transmission of ultrasound by cracks in steel, filled with solid sodium. *Ultrasonics*, **19**(2), 57 – 62. [145]

Temple, J. A. G. [1981b]. Calculations of the reflection and transmission of ultrasound by rough, planar defects containing water, manganese sulphide or alumina in a steel host. U.K.A.E.A. Report AERE-R 10110, HMSO, London. [145]

Temple, J. A. G. [1982]. Ultrasound reflection from, and transmission through, stratified media with rough interfaces: its relevance to ultrasonic defect detection. In: *Quantitative NDE in the Nuclear Industry*, pages 357 – 361. American Society for Metals, Metals Park, Ohio, USA. [145]

Temple, J. A. G. [1983a]. Theoretical work in relation to reliability: time-of-flight diffraction. In: R. W. Nichols and G. Dau, editors, *Non Destructive Examination for Pressurised Components*, pages 279 – 304. Elsevier Applied Science Publishers, London, New York, 1984. [59]

Temple, J. A. G. [1983b]. Time-of-flight inspection: theory. *Nucl. Energy*, **22**(5), 335 – 348. [59]

Temple, J. A. G. [1984a]. The amplitude of ultrasonic time-of-flight diffraction signals compared with those from a reference reflector. *Int. J. Press. Vessels Piping*, **16**, 145 – 159. [57], [58], [60], [203]

Temple, J. A. G. [1984b]. The effects of stress and crack morphology on time-of-flight diffraction. *Int. J. Press. Vessels Piping*, **19**(3), 185 – 211. [115], [142]

Temple, J. A. G. [1984c]. Reliable ultrasonic inspection in theory and practice: Sizing capability of time-of-flight diffraction. In: *3rd European Conference on NDT*. Florence, Italy, 15 – 18 October 1984. [164]

Temple, J. A. G. [1985]. Sizing capability of automated ultrasonic time-of-flight diffraction in thick section steel and aspects of reliable inspection in practice. U.K.A.E.A. Report AERE-R 11548, HMSO, London. [164]

Temple, J. A. G. [1987]. Calculated signal amplitudes for ultrasonic time-of-flight diffraction signals for tilted or skewed defects. *Int. J. Press. Vessels Piping*, **27**(3), 191 – 208. [61], [204]

Temple, J. A. G. [1993]. Diffraction coefficients for flat-bottomed holes from 3-Dfinite difference calculations. *Ultrasonics*, **31**(1), 3 – 12. [138]

Temple, J. A. G. and L. White [1993]. Numerical calculation of diffraction coefficients in anisotropic media. In: D. O. Thompson and D. E. Chimenti, editors, *Review of Progress in Quantitative Nondestructive Evaluation*, volume 12, pages 49–54. Plenum Press, New York. [138], [139]

Terpstra, S., J. P. Pasma and G. P. C. van Woerkom [1989]. Monitoring heights of defects in welds using the ultrasonic time-of-flight diffraction technique. In: J. Boogaard and G. van Dijk, editors, *Proceedings of the 12th World Conference on Non-Destructive Testing*, Amsterdam (Netherlands) 23 – 28 Apr. 1989, volume 1, pages 176–182. Elsevier, 1989. [187]

Toft, M. W. [1987]. Experimental studies of ultrasonic reflection from various types of misoriented defect. Report OED/STN/87/20060/R, Central Electricity Generating Board, London. [53], [55]

UKAEA [1988]. Ultrasonic scanning apparatus. British Patent No. 2,195,022. [185]

de Vadder, D. and M. Dosso [1984]. Caractérisation ultrasonore des bords de fissure par traitement numérique du signal. In: *Third European Conference on NDT*, volume 5, pages 362 – 374. Italian Society for Non-Destructive Testing, Florence, Italy. [188]

Verkooijen, J. [1995]. TOFD used to replace radiography. *Insight*, **37**, 433 – 435. [186], [194]

Viktorov, I. A. [1958]. Rayleigh-type waves on a circular cylindrical surface. *Sov. Phys. Acoust.*, **4**, 131 – 136. [215], [216]

Vopilkin, A. K. [1985]. Diffracted waves and their application in ultrasonic nondestructive testing: Ii. practical applications of diffracted waves. *Sov. J. Non-Destr. Test.*, **21**(2), 143 – 154. [188]

Waites, C. and M. J. Whittle [1998]. The status of performance demonstration and evaluation developments. *Insight*, **40**(12), 810 – 813. [196], [197]

Wall, M., B. Haywood, T. Slesenger, R. H. Gunderson and T. S. Chilton [1990]. ROV deployed ultrasonic inspection system for TLP tendons and risers. In: *IRM 90,* Aberdeen, Scotland (United Kingdom), 6 – 9 Nov. 1990. The Spearhead Group (1990). [185]

Watkins, B., K. J. Cowburn, R. W. Ervine and F. G. Latham [1983a]. Results obtained from the inspection of test plates 1 and 2 of the Defect Detection Trials (DDT paper No 2). *Br. J. Non-Destr. Test.*, **25**(4), 186 – 192. [153], [156], [164]

Watkins, B., R. W. Ervine and K. J. Cowburn [1983b]. The U.K.A.E.A. Defect Detection Trials (DDT paper No 1). *Br. J. Non-Destr. Test.*, **25**(4), 179 – 185. [118], [153], [154], [156]

Watkins, B., D. Lock, K. J. Cowburn and R. W. Ervine [1984]. The U.K.A.E.A. Defect Detection Trials on test-pieces 3 and 4. *Br. J. Non-Destr. Test.*, **26**(2), 97 – 105. [153], [156], [164]

Wedgwood, F. A. [1995]. TOFD comes of age. *Nucl. Eng. Int.*, **40**(486), 35 – 37. [181]

Welding Institute [1979]. [See Jessop, 1979]. [151]

Welding Institute [1982a]. [See Jessop et al., 1982]. [151]

Welding Institute [1982b]. [See Mudge, 1982]. [151]

Whapham, A. D., S. Perring and K. L. Rusbridge [1985a]. Effects of stress on the ultrasonic response of fatigue cracks. U.K.A.E.A. Report AERE-R 10854, Harwell Laboratory. [See Whapham, Perring and Rusbridge, 1985b]. [116], [140]

Whapham, A. D., S. Perring and K. L. Rusbridge [1985b]. Effects of stress on the ultrasonic response of fatigue cracks. In: *Proceedings of the 7th International Conference on NDE in the Nuclear Industry,* Grenoble 28 January – 1 February 1985, pages 389 – 392. American Society for Metals, Metals Park, Ohio USA. [243]

Whitehouse, D. J. and J. F. Archard [1970]. The properties of random surfaces of significance in their contact. *Proc. R. Soc. London, Ser A*, **316**, 97 – 121. [142]

Whitehouse, D. J. and M. J. Phillips [1978]. Discrete properties of random surfaces. *Phil. Trans. R. Soc. London, Ser A*, **290**, 267 – 298. [142]

Whittle, M. J. and J. M. Coffey [1981]. The PISC exercise: a discussion of its relevance to ultrasonic inspection of pressure vessels. *Br. J. Non-Destr. Test.*, **23**(2), 71 – 74. [148], [149]

Winchester, R. [1989]. Astable ROV design concept structural inspection device (SID) version. In: *Proceedings of the International Conference on Advances in Underwater Inspection and Maintenance,* Aberdeen (United Kingdom), 24 – 25 May 1989, pages 19 – 28. Graham and Trotman (1990). [185]

Wooldridge, A. B. [1979]. The effects of compressive stress on the ultrasonic response of steel-steel interfaces and of fatigue cracks. In: *Improving the Reliability of Ultrasonic Inspection:* Proceedings of a symposium, 1979, pages 6 – 18. British Institute of Non-Destructive Testing, Northampton, UK. [140]

Wüstenberg, H., A. Erhard, H. J. Montag and G. Schenk [1982]. Measurement of crack depth with ultrasonic methods - through-transmission and reflection modes. In: P. Höller, editor, *New Procedures in Nondestructive Testing:* Proceedings of the Germany-US Workshop, Fraunhofer Institute, Saarbrücken, Germany, 30 August – 3 September, 1982. Springer Verlag. [156]

Yokote, Y., T. Ishizuka, T. Tahara, A. J. Bagdasarian, R. J. Gougler and R. M. Stellina [1994]. Detection and sizing of defects in heavy wall pressure vessel welds. In: *Determining Material Characterization: Residual Stress and Integrity with NDE,* 1994 Pressure Vessels and Piping Conference, Minneapolis, Minnesota (United States), 19 – 23 Jun. 1994, volume PVP-Vol. 276, NDE-Vol. 12, pages 125 – 132. ASME (1994). [183], [184]

Zeelenberg, E. [1998]. Development of acceptance criteria for TOFD. In: *7th European Conference on Non-Destructive Testing,* Copenhagen, 26 – 29 May,1998, pages 1210 – 1211. [194]

# Index